Third Edition

Mosby's
HANdbook
of DISEASES

CRF	Chronic renal failure
CSF	Cerebrospinal fluid
CSF	Colony-stimulating factors
CT	Computed tomography
CVA	Cardiovascular accident, cerebrovascular accident
CVC	Central venous catheter
CVP	Central venous pressure
D&C	Dilatation and curettage
DDT	Dichlorodiphenyltrichloroethane
DI	Diabetes insipidus
DIC	Disseminated intravascular coagulation
DM	Diabetes mellitus
DMD	Duchenne's muscular dystrophy
DNA	Deoxyribonucleic acid
DST	Dexamethasone suppression test
DUB	Dysfunctional uterine bleeding
EBV	Epstein-Barr virus
ECG	Electrocardiogram
ECMO	Extracorporeal membrane oxygenation
EEG	Electroencephalogram
EF	Edema factor
ELISA	Enzyme-linked immunosorbent assay
EMG	Electromyogram
ERCP	Endoscopic retrograde cholangiopancreatography
ESWL	Extracorporeal shock wave lithotripsy
FDA	Food and Drug Administration
FRC	Functional residual capacity
FU	Fluorouracil
FVC	Forced vital capacity
G6PD	Glucose-6-phosphate dehydrogenase
GBS	Guillain-Barré syndrome
GDM	Gestational diabetes mellitus
GERD	Gastroesophageal reflux disease
GFR	Glomerular filtration rate
GI	Gastrointestinal
HAM	Hypoparathyroidism, Addison's disease, and moniliasis
HAV	Hepatitis A virus
Hb	Hemoglobin
HbsAG	Hepatitis B surface antigen
HBV	Hepatitis B virus
Hct	Hematocrit
HCV	Hepatitis C virus
HDV	Hepatitis D virus
HELLP	Hemolysis, elevated liver enzymes, low platelet count

Continued on inside back cover

Third Edition

Mosby's
Handbook
of Diseases

Ref.
RT
65
L37
2005

Rae W. Langford, EdD, RN

Private Practice
Rehabilitation Nurse Consultant
Legal Nurse Consultant
Research and Statistics Consultant
Houston, Texas

June D. Thompson, DrPh, RN

Former Director of Nursing Research,
Education, and Standards
University Hospital
University of New Mexico Health Sciences Center
Albuquerque, New Mexico

ELSEVIER
MOSBY

ELSEVIER
MOSBY

An Affiliate of Elsevier

11830 Westline Industrial Drive
St. Louis, Missouri 63146

MOSBY'S HANDBOOK OF DISEASES ISBN: 0-323-03011-4
Copyright © 2005, Mosby, Inc. All rights reserved.

NOTICE

Nursing is an ever-changing field. Standard safety precautions must be followed, but as new research and clinical experience broaden our knowledge, changes in treatment and drug therapy may become necessary or appropriate. Readers are advised to check the most current product information provided by the manufacturer of each drug to be administered to verify the recommended dose, the method and duration of administration, and contraindications. It is the responsibility of the licensed health care provider, relying on experience and knowledge of the patient, to determine dosages and the best treatment for each individual patient. Neither the publisher nor the author assumes any liability for any injury and/or damage to persons or property arising from this publication.

Previous editions copyrighted 2000, 1996.

International Standard Book Number 0-323-03011-4

Acquisitions Editor: Cindy Tryniszewski
Developmental Editor: Laura Sieh Chu
Publishing Services Manager: Pat Joiner
Project Manager: Rachel E. Dowell
Designer: Paula Ruckenbrod

Printed in China

Last digit is the print number: 9 8 7 6 5 4 3 2 1

Valerie O'Toole Baker, APRN, BC, MSN
Assistant Professor of Nursing
Gannon University
Erie, Pennsylvania

Margaret A. Lynch, MSN, RNCS
Family Nurse Practitioner
The Cambridge Hospital
Cambridge, Massachusetts

Cecilia Jane Maier, MS, RN, CCRN
Assistant Professor
Mount Carmel College of Nursing
Columbus, Ohio

Francess M. Warrick, MS, RN
Program Coordinator-Vocational Nursing
El Centro College
Dallas, Texas

Debra S. Wellman, RN, MSN, CNA
Clinical Assistant Professor
Indiana University School of Nursing
Bloomington, Indiana

Preface

Scholars throughout time have documented the discovery of new information. Those discoveries are exploding. The material contained in one Sunday *New York Times* is equivalent to all the information discovered in the late eighteenth century. It is no longer sufficient to memorize and retain facts. It is imperative to locate, synthesize, and use information that is relevant in our lives. If we were to simply compile all available health care knowledge, the results would be overwhelming. Instead, it is vital that we mine, cull, cut, and polish that knowledge and place the resulting *crown jewels* at the fingertips of professionals like you.

The *Handbook of Diseases,* third edition, is a *crown jewel* product. This handbook contains information highlights for more than 350 diseases and conditions relevant to children and adults. Each disease and condition is organized in a succinct and consistent format so that you can immediately find essential information: (1) a definition of the disease or condition; (2) the etiology and incidence of the problem; (3) the pathophysiology; (4) risk factors; (5) clinical manifestations; (6) frequently ordered diagnostic studies; and (7) therapeutic management, including indications for surgery, common medications, and general interventions, prevention, and education.

The *Handbook* is designed for you, the reader. The A to Z format in this book permits quick and easy access. All diseases and conditions are listed in alphabetical order starting with Abruptio Placentae and ending with Zollinger-Ellison Syndrome. A cross reference is indicated where applicable so that whether you know the disease or condition by its scientific name, *Herpes Zoster,* or by its common name, *Shingles,* you can still look it up quickly. Common abbreviations are prominently displayed on the inside front and back covers. New to the third edition are 32 additional diseases and conditions including Anthrax, SARS, and Smallpox. Also new to this edition is a special icon ⓠ that helps to pull your eye to potentially life threatening or critical situations.

So, when you need current and crucial health care knowledge at your fingertips, you will find that this succinct little handbook is a *crown jewel* in your pocket.

Rae W. Langford, EdD, RN

June M. Thompson, DrPH, RN

Contents

Z

Abruptio Placentae

A premature separation of a normally implanted placenta from the uterine wall, usually occurring in the third trimester of pregnancy

Etiology and Incidence

Etiology is unknown but has been linked to hypertension, cocaine use, smoking, and blunt force trauma to abdomen. Abruptio placentae occurs in 0.4% to 3.5% of all deliveries and accounts for 15% of all perinatal deaths. About one third of infants born to women with abruptio placentae die from either prematurity or intrauterine hypoxia. There is a 1% maternal mortality rate.

Pathophysiology

The placenta releases from the wall of the uterus, and retroplacental bleeding occurs. The degree of release may vary from a few millimeters to complete detachment. Blood can accumulate under the placenta (concealed hemorrhage) or can be passed out the cervix (external hemorrhage).

Risk Factors

Hypertension
Cocaine use
Cigarette use (15% to 25% of cases linked to smoking)
Blunt force abdominal trauma (auto accident and maternal battering)
Previous separation of placenta (risk of recurrence 4%; risk after two separations rises to 25%)
Multiple fetuses
Premature rupture of membranes for more than 24 hours

Clinical Manifestations

Signs and symptoms vary with degree of separation and hemorrhage. Severe cases involve profuse vaginal bleeding; maternal shock (hypotension, dizziness, rapid pulse, dyspnea, and pallor); sudden, severe pain; tender, tightly contracted uterus; and fetal distress or fetal death.

Complications

Complications include hypofibrinogenemia with disseminated intravascular coagulation (DIC), uteroplacental apoplexy (Couvelaire uterus), and renal failure. Preexisting preeclampsia compounds complications.

Diagnostic Tests

History and physical examination
Abdominal ultrasound to rule out placenta previa

Therapeutic Management

Surgery	Cesarean section only for obstetrical indications (e.g., fetal distress); Cesarean section contraindicated for severe and/or uncorrected bleeding.
Medications	Corticosteroids to accelerate lung development
General	If bleeding not life threatening, if fetal heart rate (FHR) normal, and if fetus not near term: bed rest until bleeding stops; monitor FHR; fluid and volume replacement by intravenous administration; blood replacement if necessary to prevent shock.
	If bleeding continues or increases: prompt vaginal delivery, with rupture of membranes (reduces possibility of DIC), is indicated.
Prevention/ Promotion	Cease use of cocaine and/or tobacco
Education	Education about fetal monitoring; medication effects and side effects

Abuse, Child

Maltreatment of any child under the age of 18 by a caregiver that results in serious harm, risk of serious harm, or death. It is generally categorized as (1) abuse (physical, emotional, and/or sexual) or (2) neglect (physical, emotional, and/or educational). Each state provides specific legal definitions of child abuse and neglect.

Etiology and Incidence

Precise causal mechanisms are unknown, but history of abuse to the abuser is strongly linked—as are poverty, stress, lack of parenting skills, and emotional instability. More than 2 million reports on child maltreatment are filed with the Child Protection Service (CPS) annually. Nearly 1 million of these cases are substantiated. More than 5% of children under age 18 are victims of abuse in the United States. Somewhere between 2000 and 4000 deaths are attributable to abuse annually and 80% of these occur in children less than 5 years of age. Females and handicapped children are at greater risk. Incidence increases with age, and adolescents are twice as likely as infants to be abused. The perpetrators are most likely to be parents (77%), relatives of the child (11%), and other caretakers (2%).

Pathophysiology

Physical abuse is the infliction of physical injury as a result of punching, beating, kicking, biting, burning, shaking, or otherwise harming the child. The parent or caretaker may rationalize the injury as discipline or punishment.

Sexual abuse includes fondling a child's genitals, intercourse, incest, rape, sodomy, exhibitionism, and commercial exploitation through prostitution or the production of pornographic materials. Many experts believe that sexual abuse is the most underreported form of child maltreatment because of the secrecy or "conspiracy of silence" that so often characterizes these cases.

Emotional abuse (psychological or verbal abuse and/or mental injury) includes acts or omissions by the parents or other caregivers that have caused or can cause serious behavioral, cognitive, emotional, or mental disorders. In some cases of emotional abuse, the acts of parents or other caregivers alone, without any harm evident in the child's behavior or condition, are sufficient to warrant child protective services intervention.

Child neglect is characterized by failure to provide for the child's basic needs. Neglect can be physical, educational, and/or emotional.

Physical neglect includes refusal of or delay in seeking health care, abandonment, expulsion from the home, refusal to allow a runaway to return home, and inadequate supervision.

Educational neglect includes the allowance of frequent truancy, failure to enroll a child of mandatory school age in school, and failure to attend to a special educational need.

Emotional neglect includes such actions as noted inattention to the child's needs for affection, refusal of or failure to provide needed psychological care, spouse abuse in the child's presence, and permission of drug or alcohol use by the child. The assessment of child neglect necessitates consideration of cultural values and standards of care, and recognition that the failure to provide the necessities of life may be related to poverty.

Risk Factors

Child	Unwanted child
	Child who appears unkempt or unclean, or who has torn, dirty clothes
	Child who is different in any way from his or her siblings
	"Difficult" child or unruly child
Parent or Caregiver	Caucasian (more than 50%)
	Inappropriate or negative parental comments; indifference to the child's welfare
	Lack of parenting skills
	Parent or caregiver history of being abused as a child
	Parents who express little tolerance for the child, have poor impulse control, and/or seem angry and depressed
Society/ Environment	Stress in household (e.g., divorce, unemployment)
	Lack of basic resources (e.g., housing, food, clothing)
	Lack of financial resources

Clinical Manifestations

Physical Abuse	Physical signs include unexplained bruising on soft tissue areas such as the face, back, neck, buttocks, upper arms, thighs, ankles, and back of legs; multiple bruises at different stages of healing; burns; bites; cuts; unexplained head or abdominal injuries; multiple fractures; or x-ray evidence of multiple old fractures. Child's comments or behavior exhibit fear of being hit or hurt. Child wearing long-sleeve shirts or similar clothing to hide injuries.
Sexual Abuse	Patterns are evident, such as torn, stained, or bloody underclothing; bruising, redness, swelling, or bleeding of the genitalia, vagina, or rectum; statements that it hurts to walk or sit; and complaints of pain or itching in the genital area. The child may play out their abuse with dolls or playmates.
Emotional Abuse	Child exhibits inappropriate behavior or developmental delays with speech or social interactions, facial tics, rocking motions, and odd reactions to persons in authority. Emotional abuse often seen in combination with other forms of abuse or neglect.
Neglect	Patterns are evident for a lack of care and attention. Child may have to provide care for self that is inappropriate for his or her age or developmental level. Child may be unresponsive, withdrawn, or may not respond to the caregiver's coaxing. Nonorganic failure to thrive or malnutrition should be considered when a healthy baby at birth appears to have lost weight or physical tone, especially when the infant is 25% below the expected growth curve.

Complications

Severe injury, disability, developmental delay, mental impairment, and death are all complications of chronic and/or severe physical abuse. Abuse victims have increased likelihood of becoming abusers.

Diagnostic Tests

Diagnosis is typically made by social service, health care, and legal experts after history, investigation, and physical examination.

A physical exam is conducted to reveal injuries or evidence of past injuries; general state of health and hygiene (height or weight parameters that are less than expected, malnourishment, and unkempt appearance). Information, drawing, or play behaviors from child that include evidence of abuse are also diagnostic tools as are observation of child–parent interactions (eye contact, touching, verbal interaction, and/or parental concern).

Therapeutic Management

Surgery	None
Medications	None
General	Initial interventions are geared toward stabilizing injuries and preventing further abuse.
	◑ If serious signs are obvious, report the situation to the local source for immediate investigation. If the child is perceived to be in immediate danger, seek child protection through the local child protection agency. If the signs are vague or inconsistent, document observations and report to appropriate local source for investigation.
	Long-term interventions include monitoring, therapy, and support for child and abuser(s).
Prevention/ Promotion	Mechanisms of prevention include risk factor identification, parenting classes, home visits, early intervention, support groups for parents, and counseling. Social agency referrals for financial assistance, food, clothing, and shelter needs.
Education	Education about realistic expectations for child behavior at various stages of development, appropriate forms of discipline; information on available community resources, such as Parents Anonymous or Parents United International.

Abuse, Domestic (Intimate Partner Violence)

Abuse or violence commonly describing spouse or partner abuse; includes physical and/or sexual violence (use of physical force) or threats of such violence or psychological and/or emotional abuse and/or coercive tactics

Etiology and Incidence

Intimate partner violence is a form of family violence. Intimate partner violence accounts for approximately 22% of violent crimes against women versus 3% for men. Women are significantly more likely to be physically or sexually assaulted by a current or former intimate partner than by an acquaintance, family member, or stranger. This cause of violence is the leading cause of injury and death to American women. Accurate data about the incidence of spouse or partner abuse are difficult to calculate. Lifetime prevalence estimates of intimate partner violence in the United States range from 5% to 51% with the most ranging between 25% and 35%. It is a crime committed every 15 seconds. Domestic violence is also the most common unreported crime in America. Victims of domestic violence are primarily in heterosexual relationships, but new data show that domestic violence is now also being reported in both male and female homosexual relationships.

Pathophysiology

Physical abuse is the deliberate infliction of injury to a spouse or partner. Common behaviors of the spouse or partner include kicking, biting, hitting, pushing, choking, and assaulting with weapons. Pregnant women often sustain injuries to the abdomen and potentially to the unborn child.

Sexual violence may also be referred to as *marital* or *partner rape*. This is a form of violence whereby sex is used to hurt, degrade, dominate, humiliate, and gain power over the victim. It is an act of aggression.

Emotional or *psychological abuse* is a form of violence that has the power to destroy the victim's self-esteem over time. This form of abuse is often seen as verbal intimidation and threats, ridicule and humiliation, stalking and monitoring the victim's activities, isolating the victim from friends and family, and controlling their access to money, education, and jobs.

Risk Factors

Victim	Feels worthless, degraded, isolated
	Cut off from family and friends
	Leaving spouse or partner not seen as an alternative
	Perceives family must be kept together at any cost
	Lacks positive self-esteem, which prevents telling about abuse
	Often economically dependent on the abuser
Batterer	Denies any violent behavior
	Exhibits extreme possessiveness and jealousy
	History of violence in the family
	Refuses to accept responsibility for abuse, blames behavior on stress, alcohol, drugs, or the victim
	Uses alcohol and/or drugs
Society/ Environment	Lack of understanding that violence is learned and used as tension release
	Women viewed as property
	Continued exposure to violence in entertainment, sports, and media
	Lack of public awareness about severity of the problem
	Reinforcement of sexual roles that condone aggressive male behavior

Clinical Manifestations

General	Victim may not have obvious physical injury, but vague signs or symptoms, such as sleep and appetite disturbances, fatigue, dizziness, weight change, and other physical symptoms associated with depression, anxiety, or posttraumatic stress. Other illnesses, such as gastrointestinal and autoimmune disorders, have also been associated with abuse.

Women also seek help for problems that are seemingly unrelated to abuse (e.g., a blood pressure check, a routine physical, treatment of allergies, or an upper respiratory infection).

Physical Abuse	Physical signs include bruising (face, neck, arms, legs, abdomen, or back), cuts, broken bones, black eyes, burns, marks of strangulation, wounds or bruises at different stages of healing, and swelling or puffiness in the face or around the eyes. Other signs include a history that does not match the presenting injuries and reports of being hit or injured.
Sexual Violence	Physical signs include bruising around the breasts or genitalia; genital, vaginal, or rectal swelling or lacerations; torn, stained, or bloody underclothing; and reports of being assaulted or raped.
Emotional and/or Psychological Abuse	Reports of being intimidated are evident, as are given looks or gestures, being yelled at, or being in an environment where things are being thrown or smashed. Threats to harm a child or children or to keep them from the victim are made. Victim is isolated from family and friends, and there is economic domination.

Complications

Severe injury, disfigurement, and death are all complications of chronic and/or severe physical abuse.

Diagnostic Tests

The Abuse Assessment Screen includes a standard list of questions that should routinely be asked when assessing all individuals at risk.

1. When you and your partner argue, are you ever afraid of him or her?
2. When you and your partner verbally argue, do you think he or she tries to emotionally hurt and/or abuse you?

3. Does your partner try to control you? Where you go? Who you see? How much money you can have?
4. Has your partner (or anyone) ever slapped you, pushed you, hit you, kicked you, or otherwise physically hurt you?
5. Since you have been pregnant or when you were pregnant, has your partner ever bit you, slapped you, pushed you, hit you, kicked you, or otherwise physically hurt you?
6. Has your partner ever forced you into sex when you did not want to participate?

With any yes, say, "Thank you for sharing. Can you tell me more about the last time?"

Further definitive diagnosis is typically made by social service, health care, and legal experts after a more detailed history, investigation, and physical examination.

Therapeutic Management

Surgery	None
Medications	None
General	◑ If serious signs are obvious, report the situation to the local authorities for immediate investigation and victim protection. If the individual is perceived to be in an immediately dangerous situation, seek protection through the local Adult Protective Services or the county Department of Social Services. If the signs are vague or inconsistent, document observations and report to the appropriate local authorities for investigation.
	Victim: Establish trust, use nonjudgmental approach; establish a "safety plan" for escape; referral for counseling, placement for safe haven, for needed financial and/or basic services
	Abuser: Counseling programs

Prevention/ Promotion	Awareness through education and empowerment training
	Screening of all women ages 14 and older as required of all health care settings by The Family Violence Prevention Fund and the Joint Commission on Healthcare Organizations
Education	Raise awareness by conducting education about the incidence and causes of domestic violence. Provide empowerment, assertiveness training, and awareness education to teens and young adults.

Abuse, Elder

An act or failure to act that results in risk of harm, harm, neglect, or exploitation of the elderly. Elder abuse may occur in many forms (e.g., physical, emotional, psychological, or sexual abuse; neglect; abandonment; and financial or material exploitation). Abuse may be classified as *domestic* (e.g., perpetuated by spouse, sibling, child, friend, or caregiver), *institutional* (e.g., perpetuated by personnel in nursing, foster, group homes, or board and care facilities) or *self* (perpetuated by the elder).

Etiology and Incidence

Precise causal mechanisms of elder abuse and neglect are unknown but mental and/or physical illness, substance abuse, and excessive dependence play a key role as does a history of family violence. It is estimated that 1 in 10 individuals over the age of 65 suffers from some form of abuse in the United States. The incidence of abuse is greatly underreported and as many as 85% of cases may be unrecorded. The most common abuse is by one spouse on another (60%) or by an adult child living in the home (25%).

Pathophysiology

Physical abuse is the deliberate infliction of injury on an elder that results in injury to the body, physical pain, or impairment. Physical abuse may include, but is not limited to, such acts of violence as striking, hitting, beating, pushing, shoving, shaking, slapping, kicking, pinching, and burning. In addition, the inappropriate use of drugs and physical restraints, force-feeding, and physical punishment of any kind are also examples of physical abuse.

Sexual abuse is nonconsensual sexual contact of any kind with an elderly person. Sexual contact with any person incapable of giving consent is also sexual abuse. This includes, but is not limited to, unwanted touching, sexual assault or battery—such as rape, sodomy, coerced nudity, and sexually explicit photographing.

Emotional or psychological abuse is the infliction of anguish, pain, or distress through verbal or nonverbal acts such as insults, threats, intimidation, humiliation, and harassment.

Neglect is the refusal or failure to fulfill any part of a person's obligations or duties to an elder. Refusal or failure to provide life necessities such as food, water, clothing, shelter, personal hygiene, medicine, comfort, and personal safety may be evidence of this.

Abandonment is the desertion of an elderly person by an individual who has assumed responsibility for providing care. Financial or material exploitation occurs when conducting illegal or improper use of an elder's funds, property, or assets. Examples include cashing an elder's personal check without authority, forging the person's signature, misusing or stealing the individual's possessions or money, and coercing or deceiving the elder into signing documents.

Self-neglect is characterized if the elderly person acts to threaten his or her own health or safety. The individual's refusal or failure to provide self with adequate food, water, clothing, shelter, personal hygiene, medication, and personal safety may be evidence of this.

Risk Factors

Elders	*General:* Increasing levels of debility (abuse rate increases as functional abilities decline)
	Female: Poor physical or mental health (e.g., depression, confusion, fragility, chronic disease or disability, and reduced functional abilities)
Family/ Caregiver	Mental or emotional disorders, alcoholism, or drug addiction
	Poor personal health, incapable of providing adequate care
	Caregiver strain, burnout
	Limited resources or support
Society/ Environment	History of family violence
	Poverty or limited financial resources

Clinical Manifestations

Physical Abuse	Signs include cuts, lacerations, or other wounds; bruises; welts; black eyes; broken bones, sprains, or dislocations; any injury

that is incompatible with the history; broken eyeglasses and/or frames; physical signs of being subjected to punishment or being restrained; laboratory findings of medication overdose or underuse of prescription drugs; elder report of being hit, slapped, kicked, or maltreated; caregiver's refusal to allow visitors to see elder alone.

Sexual Abuse	Bruises around the breasts or genitalia; unexplained venereal disease or genital infections; unexplained vaginal or rectal bleeding; torn, stained, or bloody underclothing; elder report of being assaulted or raped
Psychological/ Emotional Abuse	Appearance of being emotionally upset or agitated; hesitation to talk openly; extremely withdrawn and noncommunicative; unusual behavior usually attributed to dementia, implausible stories, and/or report of being verbally or emotionally abused
Neglect	Dirt, feces and/or urine, or other health and safety hazards in the elder's living environment; dehydration; malnutrition; untreated bed sores; poor personal hygiene; untreated health care problems; elder report of being mistreated
Abandonment	Desertion of an elder at a hospital, nursing facility, or similar institution; desertion at a shopping center or other public location; elder's own report of being abandoned
Financial or Material Exploitation	Unusual, sudden, or inappropriate activity in bank accounts; signatures on checks that do not resemble the older person's signature; unusual concern by caregiver that an excessive amount of money is being spent on care of the older person; numerous unpaid bills; overdue rent; abrupt changes in a will or other financial

	documents; unexplained disappearance of funds or valuable possessions; unexplained or sudden transfer of assets to a family member or someone outside the family
Self-neglect	Dehydration; malnutrition; untreated or improperly attended medical conditions; poor personal hygiene; hazardous or unsafe living conditions; inappropriate or inadequate clothing; overall lack of self-care

Complications

Severe injury, disfigurement, and death are all complications of chronic and/or severe physical abuse.

Diagnostic Tests

Diagnosis is typically made by social service, health care, and legal experts after history, investigation, and physical examination. Laboratory tests and drug screening may be done to determine the extent of malnutrition, dehydration, and medication levels.

Therapeutic Management

Surgery	None
Medications	None
General	❶ If serious signs are obvious, report the situation to the local authorities for immediate investigation and elder protection. If the elder is perceived to be in an immediately dangerous situation, seek elder protection through the local Adult Protective Services or the county Department of Social Services. If the signs are vague or inconsistent, document observations and report to appropriate local authorities for investigation.

	Seek respite care services, counseling, support groups for abuser and victim. Also seek social agency referrals for financial assistance and functional assistance (e.g., housekeeping, cooking, and shopping).
Prevention/ Promotion	Skill-building workshops for family members, coordinated care of elderly needs, public education about the problem, and coordination among state agencies and service providers are all mechanisms for prevention.
Education	Education about alternative forms of venting frustrations; information about available community resources

Acne Vulgaris

> Inflammatory disease of the sebaceous glands and hair follicles that is characterized by comedones, papules, pustules, nodules, and pus-filled cysts on or under the skin on the face, neck, chest, or upper back

Etiology and Incidence

Etiology is unknown, although genetics, hormonal dysfunction, and oversecretion of sebum are strongly implicated. Predisposing factors include stress, certain medications (steroids, phenytoin, iodides and bromides, and/or oral contraceptives), mechanical skin irritants, climate, and exposure to industrial halogenated hydrocarbons. Acne is the most common skin disease in the United States. It usually begins in puberty and affects about 80% of adolescents in some form. Males are affected more often, but females have more severe and prolonged cases.

Pathophysiology

Androgens stimulate sebaceous glands and increase oil production. Hyperkeratosis occurs, and the hair follicles in the sebaceous glands are blocked, causing comedones (blackheads and whiteheads) to form and enlarge. Proliferation of anaerobic bacteria causes rupture of the hair follicle and the contents are released into the dermis, resulting in sterile inflammatory pustules, cysts, and abscesses. Chronic and recurring lesions form distinctive acne scars.

Clinical Manifestations

Superficial acne	Comedones, pustules, oily skin
Deep acne	Inflamed nodules, pus-filled cysts, abscesses, and scarring

Complications

Permanent scarring

Diagnostic Tests

Physical examination

Therapeutic Management

Treatment varies, depending on the severity of the acne.

Surgery	Excision of large cysts and abscesses, cryosurgery to freeze cysts and nodules, dermabrasion for scarring
Medications	Topical antimicrobial and antiinfective drugs; comedolytics and or oral antiinfective drugs for pustules; isotretinoin (baseline liver and lipid panels and pregnancy test required before use) if antibiotics are unsuccessful; oral estrogen-progesterone in females
General	Extraction of blackheads
	Emotional support to boost self-esteem
Education	Avoid picking or squeezing comedones or pustules; avoid exposure to coal tar products, cocoa butter, greasy cosmetics or hair gels. Diet has little or no influence on acne; excessive cleansing is counterproductive. Over-the-counter preparations have no proven efficacy and may aggravate acne outbreaks.

Acquired Immunodeficiency Syndrome (AIDS)

(See HIV Infection)

Acute Respiratory Distress Syndrome (ARDS)

Acute respiratory failure associated with pulmonary injury and characterized by noncardiogenic pulmonary edema, hypoxemia, and severe respiratory distress

Etiology and Incidence

ARDS is precipitated by a variety of acute processes that injure the lung. Trauma is the most common cause; other causes include anaphylaxis, aspiration of gastric reflux, pneumonia, inhalation burns from fire or chemicals, drug reactions, drug overdose, near drowning, and oxygen toxicity. The condition may also develop as the result of an underlying disease process (e.g., leukemia, tuberculosis, pancreatitis, uremia, or thrombocytopenic purpura) or as a byproduct of a medical procedure (e.g., coronary artery bypass, multiple blood transfusions, mechanical ventilation, or hemodialysis).

The incidence of ARDS in the United States is estimated at 150,000 cases per year and mortality is about 50% despite supportive therapy. Those patients with gram-negative septic shock and ARDS have a 70% to 90% mortality rate. ARDS is also called *shock lung, wet lung, stiff lung, white lung, Da Nang lung,* and *adult hyaline membrane disease.*

Pathophysiology

The exact cause of the damage to the alveolar-capillary membrane is poorly understood. However, the pathophysiologic changes are divided into three phases. The exudative phase occurs immediately after the injury or insult to the lung. Neutrophils cause increased capillary permeability, which leads to increased fluid accumulation, and surfactant-producing cells are also damaged, leading to atelectasis. This compromises gas exchange, contributing to hypoxemia. Hyaline then lines the alveolar membrane, decreasing lung compliance. A ventilation-perfusion mismatch contributes to hypoxemia, which is nonresponsive to increased concentrations of oxygen. The proliferative phase begins 1 to 2 weeks after the initial injury and is an attempt to regenerate the lung tissue. The space is flooded with lymphocytes, monocytes, and granulocytes, and creates a widespread fibrosis. The fibrotic phase is the final phase; diffuse fibrosis and scarring results in decreased lung compliance and pulmonary hypertension, and the need for long-term mechanical ventilation.

Clinical Manifestations

Early	Cough, restlessness, and dyspnea—particularly on exertion—followed by rapid, shallow respirations, inspirational chest retractions, and wheezing with bilateral fine scattered crackles
Late	Intracostal and suprasternal chest retractions; bloody, sticky sputum; racing heart rate; clammy, mottled, cyanotic skin; severe difficulty breathing; confusion; coma

Complications

Complications include secondary bacterial superinfections, tension pneumothorax, multiple-system organ failure, metabolic and respiratory acidosis, and cardiac arrest.

Diagnostic Tests

Pulmonary Function	Decreased functional residual capacity (FRC) and compliance, low and/or normal pulmonary capillary wedge pressure, increased shunt fraction
Arterial Blood Gases	Decreased PaO_2, low and/or normal $PaCO_2$, elevated pH
Lactic Acid	Elevated
Radiology	Blurred margins and alveolar infiltrates on early chest x-rays, normal cardiac silhouette

Therapeutic Management

Mechanical ventilation with positive end-expiratory pressure and continuous positive airway pressure is generally required until the underlying problem has been identified and treated.

Surgery	None
Medications	No specific drugs; morphine and pancuronium bromide (Pavulon) are used in the management of mechanical ventilation; antiinfective drugs may be used for underlying infections.
General	Correction of underlying cause of injury; hyperalimentation to prevent nutritional depletion; blood gas monitoring to prevent oxygen toxicity; careful aseptic technique and monitoring of secretions to prevent superinfection; intubation and ventilation; tracheobronchial suctioning to clear secretions; cardiac monitoring; bed rest; fluid volume replacement; regulation of activity to reduce hypoxia; prone positioning; communication tools (e.g., alphabet or picture boards, response switches).
Education	Instruction to family in communicating with intubated patient; patient teaching in anxiety reduction techniques such as guided imagery or progressive relaxation

Adenovirus

A family of viruses that causes conjunctivitis and/or upper respiratory infections
(See also Conjunctivitis and Pneumonia, Bacterial/Nonbacterial)

Etiology and Incidence

Adenoviruses are a cluster name for more than 40 specific viruses that cause common illnesses. For example, adenovirus is the causative agent for 4% to 5% of all respiratory illnesses. The most common respiratory diseases are acute febrile respiratory disease in children, acute respiratory diseases in adults, and viral pneumonia in both children and adults. Ocular diseases caused by adenovirus include acute follicular conjunctivitis and epidemic keratoconjunctivitis (mostly seen in Japan).

Pathophysiology

Acute febrile respiratory disease is the most common of the adenoviruses. Air, water, or direct contact spreads the infection. Viral pneumonia in infants causes pneumonia in a lobe of the lung, and depending on severity, it may be considered lobular pneumonia. Acute pharyngoconjunctival fever commonly has a water-borne transmission, a 5-to-8-day incubation, and lasts 1 to 2 weeks. Conjunctivitis is a common manifestation of infections with several different adenovirus serotypes. It occurs most often in young adults, typically parents of children with acute pharyngoconjunctival fever.

Clinical Manifestations

Manifestations vary depending on the type of adenovirus and the affected body system.

Acute Febrile Respiratory Disease (Seen in Children)	The most common outbreak occurs in the home or day-care center. Some children have fever only, some have fever and pharyngitis, and others have fever, pharyngitis, bronchitis, and a nonproductive cough. Regional lymph nodes may be swollen and tender.

Acute Respiratory Disease (Seen in Adults)	Symptoms include malaise or tiredness, fever (lasting 2 to 4 days), chills, and headache. Respiratory signs include nasopharyngitis, hoarseness, and dry cough. Cervical lymph nodes may be swollen and tender. A fine, red macular rash may appear on the body.
Viral Pneumonia (Seen in Infants)	It is rare, but when seen, it is sudden and affects infants from a few days to 1-month old.
Acute Pharyngoconjunctival Fever	A triad of symptoms result, including fever, pharyngitis, and conjunctivitis.
Conjunctivitis	This is the sensation of a foreign body in the eye. Watering and local redness of the palpebral and bulbar conjunctiva are symptoms. Discharge from the eye is not purulent. A mild sore throat may also develop.

Complications

Secondary bacterial infections.

Diagnostic Tests

Clinical Evaluation	Identification that an infection is caused by an adenovirus is usually presumptive and is made on clinical examination.
Virus Isolation	Although rarely done, except in military situations, it is possible to isolate the virus in 7 to 10 days using respiratory or ocular secretions.

Therapeutic Management

Surgery	None
Medications	Acetaminophen may be necessary for febrile episode. Aspirin should be avoided in children because of concerns of developing Reye's syndrome.

General	*Mild symptoms:* Supportive rest is recommended, including bed rest if needed.
	Severe symptoms: Children may become quite ill. Severe pneumonia in children may require hospitalization and supportive care.
	Careful hand washing and cleanliness are required when around or caring for infected individuals. Air, water, or direct contact may spread the virus. When possible, separate ill child or adult from others in the household or classroom.
Prevention/ Promotion	Avoid exposure; careful hand washing; avoidance of finger-face contact
Education	Instruction on hand washing technique

Adrenal Insufficiency, Primary (Addison's Disease)

A progressive, chronic disease process resulting from a decline in the production of adrenocortical steroids as the adrenal cortex is destroyed

Etiology and Incidence

Most cases (70% to 80%) are the result of atrophy of the adrenal cortex caused by autoimmune processes; the rest result from destruction of the entire gland. Clinical signs often are manifested during periods of metabolic stress. About 4 in 100,000 individuals are affected across all age groups.

Pathophysiology

A decline in cortisol and corticosterone production by the adrenal cortex results in multiple disturbances in fat, protein, and carbohydrate metabolism, which in turn give rise to diminished production of liver glycogen and increased production of insulin. This leads to hypoglycemia and muscle weakness. Electrolyte imbalances and dehydration are caused by an increase in sodium (Na) secretion and a decrease in potassium (K) secretion, leading to low serum concentrations of sodium chloride (NaCl) and high serum concentrations of K. The decrease in cortisol also leads to an increase in adrenocorticotropic hormone (ACTH) and beta-lipotropin, which stimulates melanin production and causes hyperpigmentation. Over time, resistance to infection and stress diminishes. Dehydration may lead to reduced cardiac output and ultimately circulatory collapse.

Clinical Manifestations

Early	Weakness, fatigue, orthostatic hypotension, tanning, freckles, vitiligo, darkened mucosal areas
Midcourse	Nausea, vomiting, diarrhea, abdominal pain, headaches, dizziness, fainting, intolerance to cold, hypoglycemia, amenorrhea, and decreased resistance to infection

Late   Weight loss, dehydration, hypotension, confusion, restlessness, emotional lability, and small heart size

Complications

Acute stress or trauma, in which the body's store of glucocorticoids is exhausted, may trigger an adrenal crisis, which is characterized by generalized muscular debility; severe abdominal, back, and leg cramps; peripheral vascular collapse; and acute renal failure.

Diagnostic Tests

ACTH Stimulation Test	No increase in cortisol
Blood Chemistry	Elevated K and blood urea nitrogen; decreased Na, bicarbonate, and fasting glucose; Na:K ratio less than 30:1; elevated hematocrit, eosinophils, and lymphocytes
CBC	Decreased WBCs
Radiology	Small heart, adrenal size, and calcifications; renal or pulmonary tuberculosis

Therapeutic Management

Surgery	None
Medications	IV hydrocortisone, NaCl replacement; vasopressors to elevate blood pressure; hydrocortisone and/or fludrocortisone PO maintenance for life; antibiotics with evidence of infection; antitubercular drugs with evidence of tuberculosis
General	Fluid replacement IV and PO; high-calorie diet; cardiac monitoring for peaked T waves; rest; monitoring for signs of infection; monitoring of urine output

Education   Important to recognize signs and symptoms of corticosteroid excess and/or deficiency so drugs can be adjusted accordingly; stress life-long need for maintenance medications and how drugs work; emphasize need to wear ID band so appropriate therapy can be administered in an emergency and to carry emergency kit with hydrocortisone and syringe for injection.

Aldosteronism, Primary (Conn's Syndrome)

A hypertensive disorder resulting from excess production of aldosterone by the adrenal gland

Etiology and Incidence

Most cases are caused by an adenoma of the adrenal gland. Other causes are adrenal nodular hyperplasia and adrenal carcinoma. Only 0.5% to 2% of those with hypertension are affected. The condition is three times more likely to affect women, and the typical age ranges from 30 to 50 years.

Pathophysiology

Excess production of aldosterone leads to hypernatremia, hypervolemia, and hypokalemic alkalosis. Mild to severe arterial hypertension occurs because of the increased volume and arteriolar sodium levels. Hypokalemia results from increased renal excretion of potassium, and metabolic alkalosis occurs because of an increase in hydrogen ion secretion. Over time, this leads to transient paralysis and tetany.

Clinical Manifestations

In many cases the only manifestation is a mild to moderate hypertension. Other signs and symptoms include episodic weakness, fatigue, paresthesia, polyuria, polydipsia, and nocturia. Glycosuria, hyperglycemia, and personality disturbances are occasionally manifested.

Complications

Marked alkalosis with transient paralysis, tetany, and positive Chvostek's and Trousseau's signs.

Diagnostic Tests

Plasma Renin Activity	Decreased (measured after restricted sodium and/or diuretic therapy)
Aldosterone Levels	Increased (measured after sodium loading)
Blood Chemistry	Normal or increased sodium, decreased potassium

CT Scan	To detect presence of adenoma
Blood Pressure	Elevated
Edema	Absent

Therapeutic Management

Surgery	Adrenalectomy
Medications	Spironolactone (Aldactone)
General	Low-sodium diet
Education	Instruction about medication, diet, and surgical options

Allergic Rhinitis (Hay Fever)

An acute IgE-mediated hypersensitive reaction causing watery, itchy eyes, sneezing, nasal congestion, and clear watery nasal discharge.

Etiology and Incidence

Airborne allergens; pollens from trees, weeds, or grasses; and fungal spores are causes for seasonally related symptoms. Spring reactions are mostly caused by tree pollens, summer reactions are due to grass and/or weed pollens, and fall reactions are caused by weed pollens. Dust mites and animal allergens; smoke or other nasal irritants; and perfumes, detergents, and/or soaps are also known causes of allergic rhinitis. Allergic rhinitis is the most common allergic response and an estimated 30 million to 50 million Americans are affected.

Pathophysiology

Susceptible persons exposed to a causal agent react by producing an antibody, immunoglobulin E (IgE), which is directed at fighting the antigen. The IgE binds to mast cells (found in tissues) and basophils (found in the bloodstream) in the body. Both types of cells contain granules filled with histamine or other chemicals known collectively as mediators. When the antigen enters the body, it attaches to the IgE on the mast cells. The mast cells then break apart and release histamine. The histamine interacts with the receptors and irritates areas of the nose, eyes, and throat. Histamine release results in swelling of the nasal mucosa, runny nose, and itchy eyes. Persons who have hay fever are thought to have more IgE. This may contribute to overreaction of the immune system in hypersensitive individuals.

Risk Factors

Familial tendencies
Known exposure to sensitive allergens

Clinical Manifestations

The nose, roof of the mouth, pharynx, and eyes begin to itch gradually or abruptly after exposure to allergens. Symptoms include watery, itchy eyes; sneezing; nasal congestion; and clear, watery nasal discharge. Pruritus may follow. Severe cases may manifest frontal headaches, irritability, anorexia, depression, and insomnia.

Complications

Complications include chronic year-long rhinitis, secondary infections, and asthma.

Diagnostic Tests

History and Physical Examination	Exposure to known allergens; previous seasonal history of similar signs; clinical manifestations as described above
Laboratory Tests	CBC with WBC differential; sputum, nasal, and bronchial secretions may be evaluated for presence of eosinophils
Skin Testing	Used to identify and/or confirm responsible causal agents

Therapeutic Management

Surgery	None
Medications	Corticosteroid nasal inhalers as front line treatment; antihistamines to reduce mucus; decongestants to reduce swelling
	Desensitization injections (allergy shots) for severe cases that do not respond to episodic treatment
General	Recognition and avoidance of exposure to the particular causal agents responsible for the allergic response
Prevention/ Promotion	Maintain allergen-reduced environment (e.g., allergen-proof casings for bedding, carpet removal, reduction of dust-collecting surfaces; use of air purifiers and/or dust filters; air conditioners to lower humidity and prevent mold; removal of animals from bedrooms or house if sensitive). Make use of mast cell stabilizer nasal spray, such as cromolyn sodium, for prophylaxis.

Education   Instruction on avoidance of allergen triggers; instruction on medication effects and side effects, and use of nasal aerosols and sprays

Alopecia Areata (AA)

Recurrent, nonscarring hair disorder that results in sudden circumscribed or total loss of hair in individuals with no obvious skin disorder or systemic disease

Etiology and Incidence

Precise etiology for alopecia is unknown, but the latest research indicates that it is an autoimmune disorder that results from a genetic abnormality and may be triggered by some physiologically or emotionally stressful event. Prevalence is estimated to be 1 in 1000 in the population in the United States. It occurs equally in males and females and across all age ranges. Incidence is in excess of 4 million in the United States. In addition, many mild cases and cases not involving the scalp go unreported.

Pathophysiology

The pathophysiology of AA remains unclear, but it appears to be a T-cell–mediated autoimmune disease. The body produces antibodies that attack structures of the anagen phase hair follicle. There is a lymphocytic infiltrate that forms around the follicle with T-helper and T-suppressor cells.

Risk Factors

Familial tendencies
Family history of other autoimmune diseases

Clinical Manifestations

These include localized or extensive loss of hair in singular or multiple patches from any hair-bearing area of the body. The scalp is most frequently affected. Spontaneous regrowth and relapse is common. AA usually otherwise asymptomatic, but may experience burning or itching at site of hair loss. Nail pitting and other nail abnormalities may be seen with severe AA.

Complications

AA is a physically benign disease, but it can cause tremendous emotional and psychological upheaval in many affected individuals and their families.

Diagnostic Tests

History and physical exam of patterns of hair loss

Microscopic exam of plucked hair for an anagen and/or telogen count

Light hair pull can indicate presence of active disease and/or hair loss

Scalp biopsy can be helpful if diagnosis uncertain

Therapeutic Management

No treatment has been found that prevents or halts disease progression

Surgery	None
Medications	Topical applications of steroids (fluocinolone acetonide, betamethasone dipropionate); topical immunotherapy (squaric acid dibutyl ester, diphencyprone) and minoxidil have been used with varying degrees of success
General	Phototherapy to promote hair regrowth works in some cases; dermatography to camouflage eyebrows; wigs and/or hairpieces to camouflage scalp hair loss; support groups and supportive counseling
Education	Educate about chronic relapsing nature of disease; reassure that condition is medically benign; educate that hair regrowth is unpredictable; educate about realistic expectations from treatment (e.g., no cure, current treatments for hair regrowth varyingly effective); and inform about community resources such as the National Alopecia Areata Foundation

Alzheimer's Disease

A

A chronic, progressive, neurological disorder characterized by degeneration of the neurons in the cerebral cortex and subcortical structures, resulting in irreversible impairment of intellect and memory

Etiology and Incidence

The cause is not fully known. However, four genes have been linked to the disorder and are in some way responsible for removing toxic protein fragments from the brain. Theories have also been advanced involving autoimmune disease and viruses. Alzheimer's disease has become the most common degenerative brain disorder, affecting approximately 4 million individuals in the United States, and is the eighth leading cause of death, claiming nearly 55,000 lives a year. Nearly 10% of those over age 65 and as many as 40% of those over age 85 are affected, with a higher incidence seen in women.

Pathophysiology

Selective neuronal cells—primarily those involved in the transmission and reception of acetylcholine—degenerate in the cerebral cortex and basal forebrain, resulting in cerebral atrophy of the frontal and temporal lobes, with wide sulci and dilated ventricles. Senile plaques and neurofibrillary tangles are present. The basic pathophysiological processes accompanying the brain damage are unknown.

Risk Factors

Advancing age
ApoE4 genotype
Family history of Alzheimer's

Clinical Manifestations

Early	Short-term memory loss, impaired insight and/or judgment, momentary disorientation, diminished abilities for abstract thought, emotional lability, anxiety, depression, decline in ability to perform activities of daily living (ADLs)

Midcourse	Apraxia, ataxia, alexia, astereognosis, auditory agnosia, agraphia, prolonged disorientation, progressive memory loss (long and short term), aphasia, lack of comprehension, decline in care abilities, insomnia, loss of appetite, repetitive behavior, socially unacceptable behavior, hallucinations, delusions, paranoia
Late	Total dependence in ADLs, bowel and bladder incontinence, loss of speech, loss of individuation, myoclonic jerking, seizure activity, loss of consciousness

Complications

The end stage of Alzheimer's disease invites complications commonly associated with comatose conditions (e.g., incontinence, skin breakdown, joint contractures, fractures, emaciation, aspiration pneumonia, and infections).

Diagnostic Tests

A definitive diagnosis can be made only through autopsy.

Clinical Evaluation	Any of the above manifestations after depression, delirium, and other dementia disorders (e.g., head injury, brain tumor, alcoholism, drug toxicity, and arteriosclerosis) have been ruled out; family history
Mental Status Examination	Decreased orientation, impaired memory, impaired insight and/or judgment, loss of abstraction and/or calculation abilities, altered mood
CT Scan/ MRI	Brain atrophy; symmetrical, bilateral ventricular enlargement
EEG	Slowed brain wave activity, reduced voltage
Blood	Levels of ApoE4

Therapeutic Management

Surgery	None at present but experimental trials with fetal neuronal transplants are being conducted.

A

Medications	Cholinesterase inhibitors (donepezil, rivastigmine, and galantamine) used to improve memory and other cognitive deficits in individuals with mild to moderate dementia. Memantine, used for the treatment of mid- and late-stage Alzheimer's, can be used in combination with cholinesterase inhibitors. These drugs do not alter the underlying dementia. Vitamin E has been shown to be effective in delaying functional decline. Medications are used for treating specific symptoms or behavioral manifestations (i.e., antidepressants, antianxiety agents, stimulants, antipsychotics, and sedatives); experimental drugs include cholinergic, dopamine, and serotonin precursors; neuropeptides; and transcerebral dilators. Gene therapy is on the horizon.
General	Structured, supportive, familiar environment; orientation and cueing program for daily tasks; safety program; family support and counseling; respite care; institutionalization when home care is no longer possible
Prevention/ Promotion	Vitamin E 2000 IU per day
Education	Emphasize to caregiver ways to create safe environment; use of orientation and cueing; importance of support and respite care to prevent caregiver burnout

Amyotrophic Lateral Sclerosis (ALS)
(Lou Gehrig's Disease)

A rapidly progressive, degenerative disease of the upper and lower motor neurons characterized by atrophy of the hands, arms, legs, and eventually the entire body. Seventy percent of individuals die within 5 years of diagnosis.

Etiology and Incidence

The etiology of ALS is unknown, but proposed explanations include genetics, metabolic disturbances, and external agents. Although the incidence worldwide is 60 to 70 people per 100,000, with large clusters of cases in the western Pacific, the incidence in the United States is only about 5 in 100,000. The disease usually occurs in men between 40 and 70 years of age.

Pathophysiology

Patterns of degeneration occur in the brain and spinal cord. The anterior horn cells deteriorate, resulting in denervation of muscle fibers. Atrophy of the precentral gyrus and loss of Betz's cells occur in the cortex. Motor neurons are lost in the brainstem, although neurons that control the sensory and urinary sphincters are spared. The corticospinal tract and large motor neurons in the spinal cord also atrophy.

Clinical Manifestations

Early	Weakness, cramps in the hands and forearms
Midcourse	Fatigue, dyspnea, slurred speech, dysphagia, asymmetric spread of muscle weakness to the rest of the body, spasticity, fasciculations, hyperactive deep tendon, and extensor plantar reflexes
Late	Paralysis of vocal cords; paralysis of chest muscles, necessitating ventilatory support and enteral feeding

Complications

Disuse syndrome, contractures, skin breakdown, wasting, and aspiration pneumonia can complicate the end stage of ALS.

Diagnostic Tests

A

Clinical Evaluation	Any of the above manifestations, motor involvement unaccompanied by sensory abnormalities
Electromyography (EMG)	Fibrillation, positive waves, fasciculations, giant motor units
Blood	Possible elevation in creatinine phosphokinase
Spinal Tap	Elevated total protein, normal cell and IgG concentrations
CT Scan	Normal until cerebral atrophy late in disease
Myelogram	Normal until spinal cord atrophy late in disease

Therapeutic Management

Surgery	Cricopharyngeal myotomy to alleviate dysphagia, tracheostomy, esophagostomy or gastrostomy
Medications	Riluzole (glutamate antagonist) to delay need for tracheostomy; muscle relaxants (e.g., baclofen) to control spasticity; tricyclic antidepressants to control saliva; phenytoin to reduce cramping
General	Physical therapy to maintain muscle strength; occupational therapy for ADLs support; speech therapy to aid communication; splints for neutral joint alignment; leg braces, canes, or walkers to aid ambulation; nutritional support, tube feedings; cardiac monitoring; mechanical ventilation; counseling for individual and family; respite care or placement if family is unable to provide care
Education	Assist patient and family to learn and use communication devices; teach ways to reduce aspiration and provide safe environment; provide support resources

Anal Fissure

A small ulceration, tear, or slitlike crack in the lining of the anus

Etiology and Incidence

The exact cause of anal fissures is unknown. Predisposing factors include passing large and hard stools, laxative abuse, scarring from anal surgery, and chronic diarrheal diseases such as ulcerative colitis and Crohn's disease, bacterial or viral infections, and malignancy. Anal fissures are most common in young and middle-aged adults but can occur at any age. Men are affected more frequently than women.

Pathophysiology

Fissures may be acute or chronic. The fissure rests on the internal sphincter and causes it to go into spasm, which is believed to perpetuate the fissure. An external skin tag may be present at the lower end of the fissure. Defecation stimulates spasms of the internal anal sphincter that cause the sphincter to contract and trap drainage. Any problem that causes local trauma or a loss of elasticity of the anal canal may predispose the individual to anal fissures.

Risk Factors

Chronic diarrheal diseases (Crohn's, ulcerative colitis)
Bacterial infection (tuberculosis [TB], sexually transmitted diseases [STDs])
Viral infection (herpes simplex, cytomegalovirus, human immunodeficiency virus [HIV])
Malignancy (Kaposi's sarcoma, lymphoma)
Frequent passing of large, hard stools
Laxative abuse
Frequent anal intercourse or use of other anal dilators

Clinical Manifestations

Pain	Complaints of pain, tearing, or burning sensation during bowel evacuation

| Bowel Habits | Change in bowel habits with evacuation spasms that result in prolonged gnawing discomfort |
| Rectum | Slight bleeding or rectal discharge may be present with bowel evacuation, skin tags |

Complications

Constipation secondary to painful bowel evacuation or secondary infection of fissure area

Diagnostic Tests

| Digital Rectal Examination | To assess sphincter tone, anal papillae, tenderness, and presence of blood and stool |
| Proctoscopy/ Anoscopy | To visualize the anorectal area and locate the anal fissure |

Therapeutic Management

Surgery	Lateral internal anal sphincterotomy when conservative measures fail
Medications	Bulk stool agents, analgesic and/or anesthetic ointments; topical application of silver nitrate or glyceryl trinitrate ointment; injection of botulinum toxin in side of internal sphincter for chronic fissures
General	Treatment of underlying cause; sitz baths, warm topical compresses, medicated pads (e.g., Tucks) or witch hazel pads to cleanse; high fiber diet; increased oral fluid intake
Prevention/ Promotion	Balanced diet, adequate fluid intake, and exercise to promote regular bowel habits; avoidance of anal dilating devices
Education	Education about etiologies and preventive strategies

Anaphylaxis

An immediate, acute, systemic reaction resulting from an immunoglobulin E (IgE)-mediated antigen-antibody response that can range from mild to life threatening

Etiology and Incidence

The most common causes are insect stings, drugs, blood products, and parenteral enzymes. Anaphylaxis occurs in both genders and across all age groups and races. Individuals with known allergies or previous sensitivity reactions are at greater risk.

Pathophysiology

Histamine, leukotrienes, and other mediators are released when the antigen agent reacts with the IgE (antibody) on the basophils and mast cells. This causes smooth muscle contraction and vascular dilation. Vasodilation and escape of plasma into tissues cause urticaria and angioedema, and a decrease in plasma volume, leading to shock. The escape of fluid from the alveoli causes pulmonary edema and angioedema. A prolonged reaction can produce cardiac arrhythmias and cardiogenic shock.

Clinical Manifestations

Mild	Queasiness, anxiety, hives, itching, flushing, sneezing, nasal congestion, runny nose, cough, conjunctivitis, abdominal cramps, tachycardia
Moderate	Malaise, urticaria, periorbital edema; pulmonary congestion; hoarseness; edema of the tongue, larynx, and pharynx; dysphagia; bronchospasm; dyspnea; wheezing; nausea; vomiting; diarrhea; hypotension; syncope; confusion
Severe	Cyanosis, pallor, stridor, occluded airway, hypoxia, respiratory arrest, cardiac arrhythmia, circulatory collapse, seizures, incontinence, coma, death

Complications

Lack of timely and appropriate treatment results in shock, cardiac and respiratory collapse, coma, and death.

Diagnostic Tests

Clinical Evaluation	Rapid development of above signs and symptoms after exposure to a likely offending agent
CBC	Normal or elevated Hct
Blood Chemistry	Normal until circulatory collapse
Radiology	Normal or hyperinflation, edema
ECG	Normal until hypoxemia develops

Therapeutic Management

❶ Treatment centers on immediate and aggressive management of emerging symptoms. Maintaining the airway and blood pressure is critical.

Surgery	Tracheostomy
Medications	Epinephrine and other drugs to counteract effects of mediator release and to block further mediator release, vasopressors to maintain blood pressure
General	Maintenance of airway; suctioning; monitoring of vital signs; monitoring of blood gases for acidosis; IV volume replacement; ECG monitoring for dysrhythmias
Prevention/ Promotion	Instruction in prophylaxis for those at risk (i.e., avoid known allergens, wear a medical alert identification bracelet or necklace that identifies allergies, and ensure that all medical records have allergies highlighted in a prominent place)
	If allergic reaction is severe, investigate the possibility of carrying an anaphylaxis kit with preloaded epinephrine syringes.
Education	Prophylaxis instruction

Anemia (Aplastic, Hemolytic, Iron Deficiency, Pernicious, Posthemorrhagic)

An inadequate number of circulating RBCs and an insufficient amount of Hgb to deliver oxygen to tissues, resulting in pallor, fatigue, shortness of breath, and predisposition to cardiac complications. The type and cause dictate manifestations and treatment; various types are addressed below.

Aplastic Anemia

A reduction in the number of circulating RBCs resulting from bone marrow failure and generally accompanied by agranulocytosis and/or thrombocytopenia

Etiology and Incidence

The etiology is unknown in half of diagnosed cases; the other half is induced by chemicals, drugs, viruses, or radiation. The incidence is low.

Pathophysiology

Exposure to a known or unknown toxin depresses production of erythrocytes, platelets, and granulocytes in the bone marrow. Common toxins include ionizing radiation, chemical agents (e.g., benzene, dichlorodiphenyl trichloroethane [DDT], and carbon tetrachloride), and drugs (e.g., antitumor or antimicrobial agents).

Clinical Manifestations

The onset is usually insidious, occurring weeks or months after exposure to the toxin. Fatigue, weakness, dyspnea, and waxy pallor of the skin and mucous membranes are characteristic. Thrombocytopenia causes hemorrhage into mucous membranes, skin, and optic fundi. Agranulocytosis leads to severe infection.

Complications

Chronic anemia leads to increasing hemorrhage and repeated infections, which result in death in about half of those diagnosed.

Diagnostic Tests

CBC	Decreased RBCs (normochromic, normocytic), WBCs, and Hgb
Platelet Count	Decreased
Serum Iron	Increased
Bone Marrow Biopsy	Hypocellular and/or hypoplastic; fatty, fibrous tissue
Reticulocyte Count	Markedly decreased

Therapeutic Management

Surgery	None
Medications	Corticosteroids to stimulate granulocyte production; antibiotics for infection; androgens to stimulate bone marrow; antithymocyte globulin or cyclosporine for immunosuppression
General	Removal of causative agent; bone marrow transplant from an human leukocyte antigen (HLA)-matched donor (sibling); blood transfusions; hemorrhage precautions

Hemolytic Anemia

Abnormal or premature destruction of RBCs and the inability of the bone marrow to produce sufficient RBCs to compensate

Etiology and Incidence

The etiology is typically related to an extracorpuscular factor (e.g., trauma, burns, surgery, chemical agents, drugs, infectious organisms, and systemic diseases). Less common are intracorpuscular causes such as a glucose-6-phospate dehydrogenase (G6PD) deficiency.

Pathophysiology

The precipitating factor results in a shortened life span for erythrocytes and an increase in erythrocyte destruction by the reticuloendothelial system. The bone marrow is unable to produce sufficient replacement cells to keep pace with the destruction, and anemia ensues.

Clinical Manifestations

Hemolysis can be acute or chronic. The symptoms of chronic hemolysis resemble those of other anemias: fatigue, weakness, dyspnea, and pallor. Individuals with chronic symptoms may suffer from a physiological or emotional stressor that triggers a hemolytic crisis. Acute hemolytic crisis, which is rare, is characterized by chills; fever; headache; pain in the back, abdomen, and joints; splenomegaly; hepatomegaly; lymphadenopathy; and reduced urinary output.

Complications

Chronic symptoms can lead to jaundice, arthritis, renal failure, and other organ failure. Crisis can lead to paresthesia, paralysis, chills, vomiting, shock, and/or organ failure.

Diagnostic Tests

Sickle Cell Test	To rule out sickle cell anemia
CBC	Decreased Hgb and Hct
Serum Tests	Elevated lactate dehydrogenase and bilirubin
Bone Marrow Aspiration	Hyperplasia
Reticulocyte Count	Elevated
Urine/Fecal Urobilinogen	Elevated

Therapeutic Management

Surgery	Splenectomy
Medications	Corticosteroids to depress extracorpuscular factors and diminish inflammatory response; diuretics to prevent tubular necrosis; folic acid to increase RBC production
General	Elimination of causative agent; erythrocytopheresis (RBC exchange); transfusion; oxygen therapy for hypoxemia; fluid and electrolyte management

Iron Deficiency Anemia

A chronic anemia characterized by depleted iron stores and small, pale RBCs lacking in Hgb

Etiology and Incidence

Iron deficiency anemia is usually caused by chronic blood loss or by an increased need for or decreased intake of iron. It is the most common of the anemias, with a worldwide incidence rate of approximately 30%. It occurs most often in women, children, and the elderly in underdeveloped countries.

Pathophysiology

Some factor (e.g., chronic blood loss or a decrease in iron intake) leads to iron deficiency. This occurs in orderly steps. Initially, iron loss exceeds intake, and the iron stores in the bone marrow are used and depleted. A compensatory mechanism increases absorption of dietary iron but depletion continues, and insufficient iron is available for RBC formation. This leads to a decrease in Hgb production, microcytosis, and a decrease in oxygenation of the tissue.

Risk Factors

Acute and/or chronic blood loss
Iron-deficient diet
Pregnancy
Alcoholism

Clinical Manifestations

Usual signs and symptoms associated with anemia (pallor, fatigue, and weakness) plus symptoms specific to the iron deficiency, such as glossitis, cheilosis, koilonychia (spoon-shaped fingernails), and pica.

Complications

Exhaustion, infection, and respiratory and cardiac complications are possible if the condition goes untreated.

Diagnostic Tests

CBC	Decreased RBCs, Hgb, and Hct
Peripheral Blood Smear	Decreased mean corpuscular volume and mean corpuscular Hgb concentration, microcytosis, hypochromia
Iron Capacities	Decreased serum iron, serum ferritin, and iron ferritin; increased iron-binding capacity
Bone Marrow Aspiration	Erythrocyte: granulocyte ratio of 1:1 (normal, 1:3 to 1:5); lack of marrow iron; ringed sideroblasts

Therapeutic Management

Surgery	None
Medications	Iron replacement PO or parenterally
General	Correction of underlying cause (e.g., treatment of bleeding, transfusion, increased dietary intake of iron)
Prevention/ Promotion	Iron supplements during pregnancy
	Recognition of groups at risk (pregnant women, alcoholics, individuals experiencing blood loss, malnourished individuals)
Education	Nutritional education about foods rich in iron

Pernicious Anemia

A chronic, progressive anemia characterized by the production of megaloblasts, which are enlarged RBCs with immature nuclei

Etiology and Incidence

A deficiency in or underuse of vitamin B_{12} usually causes pernicious anemia. It is a fairly common anemia in adults over age 50 who are of Scandinavian origin.

Pathophysiology

Most commonly, the gastric mucosa develops a defect caused by an unknown factor and atrophies. This inhibits the secretion of intrinsic factor (IF), which binds and transports dietary vitamin B_{12} to the ileum for absorption. The lack of IF prevents vitamin B_{12} from entering the body, and existing stores of the vitamin are depleted, leading to the production of enlarged, immature RBCs.

Clinical Manifestations

Usual signs and symptoms associated with anemia (pallor, fatigue, weakness, and dyspnea) plus symptoms that stem from the physiological changes in the gastrointestinal tract (e.g., glossitis, gingivitis, indigestion, epigastric pain, loss of appetite, diarrhea, constipation, and weight loss); peripheral neurological changes occur, with paresthesia in the hands and feet.

Complications

If the condition goes untreated, the neurological changes become more profound, with involvement of the spinal cord and loss of vibratory sense, ataxia, spasticity, and disturbances in bowel and bladder function. Depression, paranoia, and delirium may follow. Splenomegaly and hepatomegaly occur along with organ failure, neurological degeneration, or infection, eventually causing death.

Diagnostic Tests

Peripheral Blood Smear	Oval macrocytes, hypersegmented neutrophils, enlarged platelets
Schilling Test	Radioactive-tagged vitamin B_{12} is not excreted in urine
CBC	Decreased Hgb, leukocytes, erythrocytes, and thrombocytes
Bone Marrow Aspiration	Hyperplasia; increased large-cell megaloblasts
Gastric Analysis	Lack of free hydrochloric acid

Therapeutic Management

Surgery	None
Medications	Lifelong parenteral vitamin B_{12} replacement (dietary vitamin B_{12} replacement is not effective); oral iron if Hgb does not rise

| **General** | Treatment of underlying cause of gastric atrophy, if possible; oxygen to increase arterial levels; oral hygiene; orientation if confused; safety precautions for neurological effects |
| **Education** | Instruction about vitamin B_{12} replacement as a life change |

Posthemorrhagic Anemia

An anemia characterized by a decrease in Hgb in the blood and related to rapid, massive hemorrhage

Etiology and Incidence

Rapid blood loss may be caused by traumatic rupture, incision, or erosion of a large blood vessel (ulcer or tumor). The prognosis depends on the rate and site of the bleeding and the total blood loss.

Pathophysiology

With blood loss, blood volume diminishes, hemodilution occurs, and oxygenation of the tissue declines.

Clinical Manifestations

The rate of blood loss determines the signs and symptoms, which may include dizziness; faintness; weakness; pallor; thirst; sweating; rapid, weak pulse; rapid respiration; and orthostatic hypotension.

Complications

Lack of prompt treatment or failure to control the bleeding results in shock, coma, and death.

Diagnostic Tests

CBC	RBCs, Hgb, and Hct are deceptively high during initial period of hemorrhage because of vasoconstriction; values begin to decline within hours of the onset of bleeding if hemorrhage is not controlled
Peripheral Smear	Normocytic cells, agranulocytosis
Coagulation Time	Reduced

Therapeutic Management

Surgery	If indicated to control hemorrhage
Medications	Iron replacement
General	Control of bleeding; blood transfusions; IV fluids, oral fluids as tolerated; oxygen; absolute bed rest; diet high in protein and iron

Angina Pectoris

Transient chest pain resulting from myocardial ischemia
(See also Coronary Artery Disease and Myocardial
Infarction)

Etiology and Incidence

Angina is caused by an imbalance in the demand for oxygen and
the myocardial oxygen supply. Coronary atherosclerosis is often
an underlying factor. Aortic stenosis, hypertension, anemia,
hypovolemia, coronary thrombosis, coronary artery spasm, cardiomyopathy, and cocaine ingestion can also play a role. It is
estimated that more than 6.5 million people in the United
States suffer from angina.

Pathophysiology

In the usual pathogenic process, atherosclerosis eventually
causes an obstruction that leads to decreased coronary blood
flow, which in turn reduces the myocardial oxygen supply and
delivery. An increase in oxygen demand through exertion, exercise, coronary artery spasm, or an underlying pathological
condition causes oxygen demand to outstrip supply, and pain
results.

Risk Factors

(See Coronary Artery Disease)

Clinical Manifestations

The chief symptom of stable angina is a highly variable, transient, substernal pain that typically arises with exertion (e.g.,
exercise, heavy meal, emotional excitement, and sexual intercourse) and subsides with rest. It may be a vague ache or an
intense crushing sensation that may or may not radiate to the
left shoulder, arm, or jaw or through to the back. Attacks are
exacerbated by cold. Because characteristics tend to be constant
for a given individual, a change in symptom patterns (e.g., an
increase in the frequency or intensity of attacks) should be
viewed as serious. When these changes occur, the condition is
called *unstable angina*. Unstable angina is associated with the
deterioration of atherosclerotic plaque and may not be relieved

by rest. Variant angina is usually in response to coronary artery spasm and may occur at rest.

Complications

🔔 Unstable angina is often a precursor to myocardial infarction (MI).

Diagnostic Tests

Tests include clinical evaluation of the nature of the pain; treadmill test to induce attack and detect ECG changes; and test dose of nitroglycerin to see if pain is relieved. Serum lipids and cardiac enzymes are used to screen for risk factors. Nuclear imaging, angiography, and PET are used to check myocardial perfusion and underlying CAD.

Therapeutic Management

Surgery	Coronary artery bypass for selected cases with severe angina, localized coronary artery disease (CAD), no history of MI, and good ventricular function; percutaneous coronary intervention to compress plaque and stent placement to keep coronary artery open; angioplasty to remove obstructive atherosclerotic lesion
Medications	Antiplatelet aggregation therapy is first line of drug treatment. Nitrates, beta-blockers, and calcium channel blockers are used to prevent myocardial insufficiency and relieve pain. Prophylactic aspirin is given for individuals with known CAD, and aspirin and heparin to treat intracoronary clotting in unstable angina and prevent progression to MI.
General	Rest and cessation of activity until pain subsides Unstable angina necessitates immediate hospitalization, bed rest, and ECG monitoring for possible MI
Prevention/ Promotion	Reduction of risk behaviors (e.g., smoking); diet to reduce cholesterol levels and/or weight if necessary; consistent exercise program to condition myocardium

| **Education** | Identify precipitating factors and instruction to prevent or control those factors; teach to recognize and report unstable angina symptoms |

Ankylosing Spondylitis

A systemic inflammatory disorder affecting primarily the spinal column and the large peripheral joints and eventually resulting in hardening and deformity of the affected skeleton

Etiology and Incidence

Studies support a genetic basis with environmental links, but the exact cause is unknown. A higher than expected level of human leukocyte antigen (HLA)-B27 tissue antigen is seen in 90% of Caucasians and 50% of African Americans with the disease. It is three to four times more common in men than in women, and onset typically occurs between the ages of 20 and 40.

Pathophysiology

The disease most commonly begins in the sacroiliac area of the spine. The intervertebral disks become inflamed and cartilage and bone deteriorate, leading to the formation of fibrous tissue, which infiltrates the disk space and then ossifies. This inflammation and ossification process gradually progresses up the lumbar, thoracic, and cervical spine, leaving behind bamboolike vertebral calcifications.

Clinical Manifestations

Early	Recurrent pain in the lower back or large peripheral joints; morning stiffness that is relieved by activity; stooped posture; limited motion of lumbar spine or limited range of motion (ROM) in affected joints; fatigue; fever; anorexia; weight loss; diminished chest expansion; red, painful eyes
Late	Kyphosis, fixed flexion of hips, vertebral fractures, impotence, incontinence, diminished bladder and rectal sensation, angina, pericarditis, pulmonary fibrosis (rare)

Complications

Occasionally the disease is severe and rapidly progressive, resulting in severe, pronounced skeletal deformities that greatly inhibit performance of activities of daily living (ADLs). In rare cases, atlantoaxial subluxation occurs, resulting in compression of the spinal cord. Development of secondary amyloidosis, a rare event, can cause death.

Diagnostic Tests

Clinical Evaluation	Spine and/or joint pain or limitation, any manifestations described above, family history
Radiology	Narrowing in sacroiliac joints, vertebral squaring, calcification, demineralization
HLA-B27 Antigen	Positive in 90% of cases
Erythrocyte Sedimentation Rate	Mildly elevated
Immunoglobulin M Rheumatoid Factor	Negative

Therapeutic Management

Surgery	Rare, spinal osteotomy to correct kyphosis, cervical fusion to keep neck upright, and total joint replacements for severe joint deformities
Medications	Analgesics; nonsteroidal antiinflammatory drugs (NSAIDs) to reduce pain, spasm, and swelling and to facilitate exercise; methotrexate may be used for intractable pain
General	Physical therapy, regular stretching, ROM, and strength-building exercises, straight posture, proper alignment of joints, use of firm mattress in prone position with no pillows, avoidance of prolonged time in any one position, traction and/or back brace in special cases
Education	Centers on postural training (avoiding spinal flexion, heavy lifting, prolonged walking, standing or sitting) and natural stretching exercises (swimming, badminton, and tennis)

Anorectal Abscess

A local abscess (cavity containing pus surrounded by inflamed tissue) in the area of the rectum and anus

Etiology and Incidence

An anorectal abscess is an infection that can occur anytime there is trauma and a break in the anal and/or rectal wall tissue. Causes include traumatic anal intercourse, chronic diarrheal conditions, such Crohn's disease, and hematological and immune-deficient conditions. Common infective organisms include *Escherichia coli*, staphylococci, and streptococci. Anorectal abscesses are more common in men.

Pathophysiology

The abscess commonly develops from an infection beginning in an anal crypt and moving along anal ducts through the internal sphincter. The infection may also develop in an anal fissure, prolapsed internal hemorrhoid, traumatic injury, and superficial skin lesions. If not treated, the abscess may progress to an anorectal fistula.

Risk Factors

Chronic diarrheal or inflammatory bowel diseases
Traumatic anal intercourse or use of anal dilators
Passing large and/or hard stools

Clinical Manifestations

Early signs include a change in bowel habits with purulent discharge and increased odor. As the abscess becomes worse, increased throbbing, constant pain exacerbated by sitting or walking, anorectal swelling, and redness are present. Fever and malaise may also be present.

Complications

Secondary and/or systemic infection and sepsis are possible.
❶ Abscesses in human immunodeficiency virus (HIV)-positive and diabetic patients constitute an emergency requiring immediate surgical intervention.

Diagnostic Tests

Proctoscopy	To visualize the lesion and determine the extent of the abscess

Therapeutic Management

Surgery	Prompt surgical drainage of the abscess is required.
Medications	Stool softeners or antiinfectives depending on the causative organism and the extent of infection
General	Perianal area should be kept clean by packing and irrigating abscess after surgery if required; Sitz bath, rubber ring, or pillow for sitting; low residue diet
Prevention/ Promotion	Avoidance of traumatic anal intercourse or use of anal dilators
	Balanced diet, adequate fluid intake, and exercise to promote regular bowel habits
Education	Instruction on wound care, cleaning after bowel movements; importance of follow-up care

Anorectal Fistula

A tubelike tract with one opening in the anal canal or rectum and the other in a secondary, or external, opening—such as the perianal skin

Etiology and Incidence
Anorectal fistulas usually arise spontaneously and occur secondary to drainage of a perirectal abscess. Predisposing causes include traumatic injury, Crohn's disease, chlamydial infections, tuberculosis, cancer, and radiation therapy. Anorectal fistulas are common in all age groups and occur equally in males and females.

Pathophysiology
The primary, or internal, opening is usually at a crypt near the pectinate line. The exit of the fistula may be to the outside via the skin, vagina, buttocks, or bladder. Feces may enter the fistula and cause an infection.

Risk Factors
Nonspecific cryptoglandular infection (skin or intestinal flora)
Chronic diarrheal diseases (Crohn's, ulcerative colitis)
Diseases such as tuberculosis (TB), lymphogranuloma venereum, and actinomycosis
Malignancy (leukemia and lymphoma)
Chemotherapy and radiation therapy
Trauma, such as surgery (episiotomy and prostatectomy), anal intercourse, and foreign body insertion into anus

Clinical Manifestations
Perianal pain, swelling, and fever are common as is intermittent or constant discharge. If the fistula drains to the outside, persistent, bloodstained, and purulent and/or stool drainage may occur.

Complications
Secondary and/or systemic infections are seen along with septicemia. ◑ Fistulas in human immunodeficiency virus (HIV)-positive and diabetic patients constitute an emergency requiring immediate surgical intervention.

Diagnostic Tests

Rectal	Inspection of the skin may reveal one or more secondary openings. A cordlike track may be palpated. A probe may be inserted into the tract to determine depth and direction.
Anoscopy	To assess and further evaluate fistula tract
Proctosigmoidoscopy	Required to determine internal point of origin and to rule out other fistula formation sources
Rectal Biopsy/ Colonoscopy	Done if malignancy or inflammatory bowel disease suspected

Therapeutic Management

Surgery	Fistulotomy or fistulectomy treatment of choice; colostomy, rectal advancement flaps
Medications	Analgesics for pain; antiinfectives for presence of infection, immunocompromise, cellulitis, or valvular heart disease; stool softeners and/or laxatives
General	Treat underlying cause
	Sitz baths and wound irrigation; packing and wound care as required; pillow or rubber ring for sitting comfort
Prevention/ Promotion	Avoidance of traumatic anal intercourse or use of anal dilators
Education	Instruction on wound care, cleansing after bowel movements; importance of follow-up care

Anorexia Nervosa

An eating disorder characterized by drastically reduced food intake and intense exercise, leading to marked weight loss and eventual emaciation. Anorectic individuals have a disturbed sense of body image and attempt to achieve control, autonomy, and competence in their lives by manipulating their food intake and body weight.

Etiology and Incidence

Etiology is unknown, but social factors appear to play a role. Various theories suggest societal influences, dysfunctional family systems, disturbed mother-child relationships, and metabolic or genetic vulnerabilities. Onset usually occurs in adolescence in young white women of middle or upper socioeconomic status. Men account for only 5% of cases, and the disorder is not seen in areas where food is in short supply. Estimates of the incidence of anorexia in the United States range from 1 in 800 to 1 in 100 among adolescent girls. Reports of anorexia in young black women with professionally educated and employed parents are increasing. The incidence among men and adults is also rising. The mortality rate averages 15% of reported cases.

Pathophysiology

The pathological processes are those seen in malnutrition and starvation. Eventually all body systems become involved as they are deprived of vital nutrients.

Risk Factors

Adolescence
Characteristics such as perfectionism, overachievement, compulsiveness, and meticulousness
Female gender
Preoccupation with weight, food, or diets

Clinical Manifestations

Early signs and symptoms include meticulousness; perfectionism; preoccupation with weight; increase in physical activity; restriction of intake; preoccupation with food, recipes, and meal planning; hoarding and hiding food; and meal preparation for others. This is followed by marked weight loss, amenorrhea, social isolation, increasingly secretive behavior, and denial. Other common manifestations include bradycardia, low blood pressure, hypothermia, lanugo, hirsutism, edema, and depression.

Complications

As malnourishment continues, all body systems are affected. Cachexia ensues, and endocrine disorders, electrolyte imbalances, metabolic acidosis, and cardiac dysfunction appear. Sudden death from ventricular dysrhythmia is possible, as is eventual death from total system failure.

Diagnostic Tests

Diagnosis is made through a constellation of symptoms and patterns described above, in concert with loss of at least 15% of body weight, particularly in individuals in high-risk groups. A key to diagnosis is the eliciting of a central fear of fatness undiminished by weight loss.

Therapeutic Management

Surgery	None
Medications	Doxepin to reduce anxiety and depression; fluoxetine to prevent relapse
General	*Short term:* Hospitalization to stabilize fluid and electrolytes and stop weight loss
	Long term: Psychotherapy, family therapy, and dietary supplements to induce weight gain

Anthrax

An acute infectious bacterial disease found predominantly in hooved animals and occurring in humans in three forms: cutaneous, inhalation, and gastrointestinal. Recent bioterrorist attacks and threats have increased the need to recognize and treat this disease.

Etiology and Incidence

Anthrax is caused by the spore-forming, rod-shaped bacterium *Bacillus anthracis.* Cutaneous anthrax occurs when the bacteria enter a break in the skin; inhalation anthrax occurs when the bacterial spores are inhaled; and gastrointestinal anthrax occurs after the consumption of contaminated meat. Incidence is rare, with about five cases per year reported in the United States. There were 22 cases of anthrax caused by terrorist activity in 2001.

Pathophysiology

Bacillus anthracis produces a toxin with three protein components: edema factor (EF), protective antigen factor (PA), and lethal factor (LF). PA binds to cell surface receptors and forms a channel so that EF and LF can enter the cell and form toxins. These toxins inhibit bacterial phagocytosis and macromolecular synthesis and cause cellular necrosis. The toxins also increase host susceptibility to infection by suppressing or blocking various cell functions and inducing cytotoxic effects. Toxins are then disseminated by the vascular and lymphatic systems, causing systemic toxicity, bacteremia, lymphangitis, and lymphadenopathy.

Clinical Manifestations

Cutaneous	Begins as an itchy, raised, red-brown skin bump that develops into a vesicle and then a painless ulcer with a depressed, black necrotic center. Lymph nodes in the adjacent area may be swollen and there may be fever, fatigue, and headache.

	Eschar from the ulcer dries and drops off with little or no scarring after 1 to 2 weeks.
Gastrointestinal	Severe abdominal pain, fever, fatigue, anorexia, hematemesis, bloody diarrhea; in some cases there may be lesions in nose, mouth, and throat
Inhalation	Starts with brief prodrome that resembles a viral respiratory illness followed by hypoxia, dyspnea, fever, muscle aches, headaches, and fatigue

Complications

Cutaneous forms respond readily to treatment, but 20% of untreated cases result in death. Gastrointestinal anthrax can spread systemically and is fatal in 30% to 60% of cases if not treated immediately. Once the spores travel to the lymphatic system in inhaled anthrax, respiratory failure and shock occur and death usually ensues regardless of treatment.

Diagnostic Tests

Diagnosis made by history of possible exposure; physical exam for presenting symptomatology and by isolation of *B. anthracis* in blood, skin lesions, or respiratory secretions. Serologic testing with enzyme linked immunosorbent assay can confirm diagnosis. An anthracis test (available in specialized labs) can be used to detect anthrax cell-mediated immunity. Chest x-rays may detect mediastinal widening, pleural effusion, and infiltrates in inhalation anthrax.

Therapeutic Management

Surgery	Tracheostomy for ventilator support in inhalation anthrax
Medications	Antiinfectives (penicillin, doxycycline, Cipro, and/or Floxin) are primary treatment
General	IV hydration, ventilator support in inhalation form; notify local state authorities in all suspected cases
Prevention/ Promotion	Anthrax vaccine recommended in limited use for those at risk (e.g., military, veterinarians,

and livestock handlers.) Risk of side effects is high and schedule is six doses over 18-month period. Treatment for exposure is usually a 60-day course of antibiotics or a combination treatment with anthrax vaccine and antibiotics.

Education   Instruction on medication effects, side effects, and need to take full course of medications

Anxiety Disorders

A group of disturbances in which anxiety is the predominant experienced symptom

Etiology and Incidence

Anxiety is a subjective experience that is a normal part of everyday living. Normal anxiety is proportionate to a given threat or situation and is used constructively to alter a situation or object. Approximately 4% to 6% of the general population experience pathological anxiety, which is disproportionate to a threat and can actually paralyze a person's problem solving, daily functioning, and overall productivity. Anxiety disorders include generalized anxiety disorder (the incidence for men and women is equal); panic disorder with agoraphobia (the incidence for women is three times that of men); and obsessive-compulsive disorder (equally common in men and women).

Pathophysiology

Anxiety ranges from a healthy state of alertness and attention to a pathological state. The biology of anxiety disorders is obscure, although it appears that some biochemical and hereditary traits are apparent. Psychological and interpersonal factors may predispose a person to anxiety disorders. These include early psychic trauma, pathogenic parent-child relationships, pathogenic family patterns, and loss of social supports. Generalized chronic anxiety is a continuous hyperalert and hyperanxiety state that produces apprehension and dread that are disproportionate to the situation. Panic states are acute, sudden anxiety attacks that may last for a few minutes to 1 hour or more. The frequency of these attacks may range from several times a day to less than one per month. During the attack, the person has fears of imminent death or physical catastrophe. Other fears include humiliation or appearing foolish or stupid. Obsessive-compulsive behavior is not necessarily pathological. It becomes pathological when the individual feels compelled to carry out an activity again and again. Obsessions are persistent, intrusive, and inappropriate ideas, thoughts, and/or actions.

Risk Factors
Familial tendency
Chronic stressful situations
Isolation
Feelings of being overwhelmed
Low self-esteem or threats to self-esteem

Clinical Manifestations

Behavioral	Expressed feelings of apprehension disproportionate to the external risk; dread; irritability; anger; frustration; terror; blocking; panic; incapacitation and immobilization; impaired memory, attention, and concentration; irrational fear with avoidance of a dreaded activity, event, or object; scattered thoughts or lack of focus on details; lack of confidence; low self-esteem; sense of worthlessness and rejection; stuttering; rapid, pressured speech; repetitive questioning about same thing
Physical	Heart palpitations; tachycardia; dizziness; light-headedness; dyspnea; gasping for air; heartburn; tremors; generalized weakness; nausea; vomiting; change in appetite; insomnia; difficulty falling asleep; restlessness; elevated blood pressure and pulse; urinary frequency; diarrhea or occasional constipation

Complications
Individuals with undiagnosed and/or untreated anxiety disorders may have difficulty coping with every day activities of daily living (ADLs). Over time, they may exhibit signs of other psychological or physiological conditions.

Diagnostic Tests

Laboratory	Exclusion of other medical disorders or conditions such as thyroid dysfunction
ECG	Screen for cardiopathology

Therapeutic Management

Surgery	None
Medications	Benzodiazepines, selective serotonin reuptake inhibitors, tricyclic antidepressants, monoamine oxidase inhibitors
General	Provide quiet, nonstressful, nondemanding environment; reduce physiological stressors; encourage individual to evaluate own actions and causes of actions; help to expand coping strategies, problem solving, and assertiveness skills
	Electroconvulsive therapy, behavior and/or cognitive therapy, and anxiety reduction strategies (e.g., progressive relaxation, deep breathing, visual imagery, and soothing music)
	Limit CNS stimulants (e.g., caffeine, nicotine)
Education	Education to distinguish normal from abnormal anxiety; instruction in anxiety reduction strategies; identification of available resources and support systems; instruction in effects and side effects of medications and importance of taking medications as instructed

Aortic Aneurysm

A

> A localized dilation or ballooning of the aorta

Etiology and Incidence

Most cases are caused by arteriosclerosis. Smoking and hypertension contribute to the formation of aneurysms. Trauma, syphilis, infection, connective tissue disorders, and arteritis are also causes. Aneurysms can develop anywhere along the aorta, but 75% occur in the abdominal aorta. About 25% develop in the thoracic aorta, and the remainder occur in peripheral aortic branches. White males over age 40 have the highest incidence of aortic aneurysms in the United States.

Pathophysiology

With arteriosclerosis, fibrosis and intimal thickening develop as a result of long-term hypertrophy and atrophy of the smooth muscle coat, generally as a result of aging. The vessel becomes less elastic, and the vessel wall thins in spots. Pressure on these spots causes ballooning, which increases over time. Aneurysms caused by infection occur when the infection infiltrates and damages the aortic wall. Aneurysms caused by blunt chest trauma arise from damage to the aorta and subsequent leakage and hematoma formation.

Clinical Manifestations

Many people are asymptomatic, even with huge aneurysms. Signs and symptoms, when present, are dictated by location and compression or erosion of adjacent tissues.

Abdominal	Deep, boring, steady visceral pain in lumbosacral area, often relieved by positioning; feeling of abdominal pulsation or pain; tenderness on palpation; wide aortic pulsation on palpation
Thoracic	Deep, diffuse chest pain; pain in spine; cough; wheezing; hemoptysis; dysphagia; hoarseness; tracheal deviation; and abnormal chest wall pulsations

Complications

🔴 The most serious threat posed by an aneurysm is rupture. Depending on the severity of bleeding, hypovolemic shock and death usually follow quickly. The success rate for surgery for a ruptured abdominal aortic aneurysm is only 50%.

Diagnostic Tests

Abdominal/ Chest X-ray	Calcification of aneurysm wall
Ultrasound/CT Scan/MRI	To determine extent and size of aneurysm
Contrast Aortography	To determine origin of major vessels arising from aortic site; useful for resection

Therapeutic Management

Surgery	Resection and replacement with a synthetic conduit recommended for all aneurysms >6 cm and for most 4 to 6 cm
Medications	Intensive antibiotic therapy for mycotic aneurysms before resection, antihypertensives to decrease blood pressure and myocardial contractility
General	Monitoring if surgery is not done

Appendicitis

An acute inflammation of the appendix

Etiology and Incidence

The etiology is not clear but appears to be related to obstruction of the appendiceal lumen by a fecal mass, stricture, or infection. Acute appendicitis is one of the most common reasons for abdominal surgery. The incidence is about 1 in 1000 persons in the United States, and the condition is most common in adolescents and young adults and is slightly more prevalent in men.

Pathophysiology

The lumen is obstructed, blood flow is diminished, hypoxia develops, the mucosa ulcerates, and bacteria invade the wall, causing an infection and producing edema. This further impedes blood flow, causing tissue necrosis, gangrene, and perforation.

Clinical Manifestations

The typical symptom is progressively severe abdominal pain, which begins in the midabdomen and shifts to the lower right quadrant after 6 to 10 hours. The pain may be accompanied by a low-grade fever, malaise, nausea, and vomiting.

Complications

Perforation causes peritonitis.

Diagnostic Tests

Clinical Evaluation	Localized rebound tenderness at McBurney's point
WBCs	Moderately elevated with left shift
Laparoscopy	For visualization when diagnosis is in doubt

Therapeutic Management

Surgery	Appendectomy, which may be done by laparoscope, decreasing recovery time
Medications	Antibiotics for prophylaxis after surgery
General	None

Arthritis (Osteoarthritis, Rheumatoid)

Osteoarthritis (Degenerative Joint Disease)

A chronic, degenerative disease process occurring primarily in the hips and knees and characterized by deterioration of the joint cartilage, formation of new bone in subchondral areas and joint margins, and joint hypertrophy

Etiology and Incidence

The etiology of primary osteoarthritis is unknown and may have genetic ties, but it is not related to the normal aging process. However, almost all individuals over 40 have degenerative changes in weight-bearing joints with signs and symptoms increasing with age. Secondary osteoarthritis usually follows a predisposing event such as trauma, disease, developmental processes, or obesity. Osteoarthritis is the most common of all articular disorders, affecting approximately 35 million Americans. Men and women are equally affected until the age of 50 when the incidence becomes higher for women.

Pathophysiology

The water content of the hyaline cartilage increases, and the protein-carbohydrate molecules decrease. The cartilage becomes softer and sheds flakes into the joint. The shedding rubs away the cartilage and increases the friction coefficient in the joint, setting up an erosive cycle. As the cartilage erodes, underlying bone is exposed. Fibrous tissue forms in the joint capsule, causing inelasticity and limiting joint movement. New bone, formed in the subchondral area and at joint margins, is stiff and subject to microfractures and callus formation. Deterioration of the weight-bearing surface combined with the bony overgrowth leads to joint hypertrophy and deformity.

Risk Factors

Family history
Obesity
Sedentary lifestyle
Joint trauma and/or infection

Clinical Manifestations

Early	Deep, aching joint pain that is aggravated by exercise and that worsens as the day progresses; stiffness after inactivity
Midcourse	Reduced joint motion, tenderness, crepitus, grating sensation, flexion contractures, joint enlargement
Late	Tenderness on palpation, pain with passive range of motion (PROM), increase in degree and duration of pain, joint deformity, and subluxation

Complications

Osteoarthritis of the spine can cause compression of the spinal cord, leading to weakness in the extremities, incontinence of bowel and bladder, and impotence.

Diagnostic Tests

Clinical Evaluation	Any of above manifestations, Heberden's or Bouchard's nodules of finger joints
Gait Analysis	Altered motion patterns
Radiology	Narrowed joint space, increased density of subchondral bone, pseudocysts in subchondral marrow, osteophytes at joint periphery
Erythrocyte Sedimentation Rate	Normal and/or moderate increase
Synovial Analysis	High viscosity; yellow, transparent color; negative culture; WBC 200 to 2000/μl; <25 polymorphonuclear leukocytes

Therapeutic Management

Surgery	Arthroscopy, osteotomy, laminectomy, fusion, total joint replacement if conservative therapy fails

Medications	Nonsteroidal antiinflammatory drugs (NSAIDs), Cox2 inhibitors (celecoxib, rofecoxib), muscle relaxants, and intraarticular steroid injections provide some transient relief. Topical agents (capsaicin) may provide temporary pain relief. Dietary supplements glucosamine and chondroitin sulfate are used for pain relief and improving joint mobility.
General	Isometric, isotonic, isokinetic, strengthening, stretching, ROM, and balance exercises; rest; massage and moist heat for pain; elastic bandages for support; canes and walkers to aid mobility; weight reduction to reduce joint load
Prevention/ Promotion	Maintain normal weight; eat balanced diet; follow regular program of moderate exercise; avoid high-heeled shoes.
Education	Enhance joint stability (avoid soft chairs, recliners, and pillows under knees; wear sturdy, low-heeled shoes; remove environmental hazards; and use mobility aids and joint support devices); follow planned exercise program; lose weight if overweight; and follow individualized pain relief regimen

Rheumatoid Arthritis

A chronic, systemic, degenerative disease characterized by inflammation of the connective tissue and manifested primarily in and around peripheral joints

Etiology and Incidence

The etiology is unknown, although the disease often is characterized as an autoimmune disorder, and a familial link is suspected. The latest research links an abnormal immune reaction to carbohydrates as an underlying cause. Smoking has also been linked to the disease. Approximately 2.1 million people in the United States are affected, with women three times more likely to be affected than men. Onset usually occurs between ages 35 and 50, although the disease has been diagnosed in children between ages 8 and 15.

Pathophysiology

Joint inflammation begins with congestion and edema of the synovial membrane and joint capsule, which develops into synovitis. Thickened layers of granulation tissue invade and destroy the cartilage and joint capsule. The fibrous granulation tissue deforms, ossifies, occludes, and immobilizes the joint. Eventually the disease spreads to major organ systems, including the heart, lungs, kidneys, and eyes.

Clinical Manifestations

Early	Nonspecific symptoms of fatigue, malaise, low-grade fever, anorexia, and weight loss
Midcourse	Tenderness, pain, and stiffness in affected joints (most often the fingers) that occur in a bilateral, symmetric pattern and spread to the wrists, elbows, knees, and ankles; diminished joint function; paresthesia; joint contractures and deformities
Late	Subcutaneous rheumatoid nodules, leg ulcers, lymphadenopathy, inflammation and dryness of mucous membranes, episcleritis, pericarditis, valvular lesions, splenomegaly, pneumonitis

Complications

Acute rheumatoid arthritis is characterized by abrupt onset and progressive, relentless deterioration of joints and then other major body systems without remission and with poor or no response to medical treatment. The prognosis in these cases is poor.

Diagnostic Tests

Clinical Evaluation	The American Rheumatoid Association (ARA) looks for a presence of four or more of the following: (1) morning stiffness

lasting more than an hour; (2) inflammation in at least three joints with swelling observed in fingers, wrist, elbow, knee, ankle, and/or toe joints; (3) the swelling in at least one joint should be the wrist, fingers, or toes; (4) symmetric joint swelling; (5) subcutaneous nodules; (6) positive rheumatoid factor; (7) bone erosion; or (8) decalcification seen on x-ray.

Rheumatoid Factor	Positive in 80% of cases
Synovial Analysis	Opaque color; increased volume and turbidity; decreased viscosity and complement; 3000 to 50,000 WBCs/µl; polymorphonuclear cells predominant
Erythrocyte Sedimentation Rate	Elevated in 90% of cases
CBC	Hypochromic anemia, elevated WBCs
Radiology	Soft tissue swelling, narrowed joint space, marginal erosions, destruction of auricular cartilage

Therapeutic Management

Surgery	Synovectomy for pain relief, repair of ruptured tendon sheaths to prevent deformity and subluxation, osteotomy to change weight-bearing surfaces, total joint replacement to increase mobility
Medications	Aspirin, NSAIDs, Cox2 inhibitors, and disease-modifying antirheumatic drugs such as gold compounds, penicillamine, methotrexate, cyclosporine, and hydroxychloroquine to reduce pain and inflammation; oral or intraarticular injections of corticosteroids to reduce inflammation; biological therapy (etanercept, infliximab) to slow disease progression

General   Whirlpool, moist compresses, paraffin gloves to reduce pain and edema; therapy and exercise to increase ROM, strength, and endurance; balance of activity and rest; splints, canes, or walkers to aid mobility; emotional support to adapt to disability; use of occupational and physical therapies; weight control and balanced diet

Education   Stress importance of regular individualized exercise program, ROM, and planned activity schedule to maintain joint mobility; identify ways to modify activities of daily living (ADLs) to protect joints from stress; training with assistive devices to enhance ADLs; identify effects and side effects of long-term medication use and need for regular medical and laboratory monitoring

Asbestosis

A diffuse, interstitial pulmonary fibrosis resulting from inhalation of asbestos

Etiology and Incidence

The cause is prolonged exposure to airborne asbestos particles. Susceptibility increases with increasing length and intensity of exposure. The incidence is greatly increased by chronic occupational exposure. Families of workers are also at risk from fibers carried home on clothing. The general public may engender some risk from long-term exposure to asbestos dust in old buildings in which asbestos was used as insulation or from asbestos in shingling or building material. There are 5 to 10 new cases per 100,000 persons in the United States annually.

Pathophysiology

Asbestos particles are deposited on bronchiole or alveolar walls and are ingested by cells, leading to an edematous process in the wall that results in nonnodular alveolar and interstitial fibrosis, reduced lung volume and compliance, and impaired gas transfer.

Risk Factors

Exposure to asbestos fibers in an occupational setting that involves the mining, milling, or use of asbestos, where the suppression of asbestos dust is poorly controlled and exposure is not adequately limited

Smoking

Clinical Manifestations

Symptoms begin with exertional dyspnea and decreased exercise tolerance. As the disease progresses, dyspnea is chronic even at rest and a dry cough may develop.

Complications

Asbestos is a cocarcinogen with tobacco, and asbestos workers who smoke are 90 times more likely to develop lung cancer than smokers who are not exposed to asbestos.

Diagnostic Tests

Clinical Evaluation	History of long-term exposure to asbestos
Radiology	Interstitial markings in lower lung, thickening, plaques, calcification
Pulmonary Function	Early: Normal Later: Reduced lung capacity and compliance
Arterial Blood Gases	Early: Normal Later: Decreased PO_2, increased PCO_2

Therapeutic Management

Surgery	Lung transplant in select population
Medications	None
General	No effective treatment is available. Chest physiotherapy, increased fluids, steam inhalation to loosen secretions, and oxygen therapy help with symptom management. Exercise to maximize lung function and to prevent respiratory infection (flu and pneumonia vaccines). Avoid further exposure to asbestos.
Prevention/ Promotion	Enforce industrial safety regulations to control exposure (e.g., adequate dust suppression measures and wearing respirators) Remove asbestos from public buildings when it poses a health threat Cease smoking
Education	Reinforce teaching about safety measures for workers who work around asbestos (dust suppression and respirator use); smoking cessation programs for asbestos workers

Asthma

A chronic inflammatory disorder of the airways, which leads to airway obstruction; characterized by airway hypersensitivity to a variety of stimuli, resulting in transient bronchospasm and constriction of the airways, which manifest as wheezing, chest tightness, shortness of breath, and cough

Etiology and Incidence

Asthma is triggered by either extrinsic or intrinsic agents. Extrinsic agents include allergens such as dust, smoke, pet dander, mold spores, chemicals, and foods. Intrinsic agents include underlying respiratory infections, emotional stress, exercise, acid reflux, and fatigue. Many attacks are triggered by a combination of agents. Asthma affects more than 14.5 million people in the United States, and 5500 people a year die as a result of the disease. It is the most common chronic disease of children and adults, beginning in childhood about half the time and in adolescence or adulthood half the time. In childhood, boys are affected twice as often as girls, but this ratio evens out by adolescence. The prevalence and mortality rates are increasing rapidly worldwide. The last 2 decades have seen close to a 50% increase in incidence of this disease. It is theorized that this increase is related to the shift to urban living centers and the increase in pollution.

Pathophysiology

Various agents trigger a reaction in the tracheal and bronchial linings, which causes bronchospasm of the smooth muscle and constriction of the airways. The airways become inflamed and edematous and produce excess thickened secretions, which aggravate the blockage. Eosinophils infiltrate the airway walls, and injure and desquamate the epithelial lining. Expiratory capacity is reduced, causing trapping of gas in the airways, hyperinflation, and labored breathing. Because the obstruction is not uniform, blood flow continues in some areas of hypoventilation, producing a ventilation-perfusion imbalance and resulting in arterial hypoxemia.

Clinical Manifestations

Symptoms vary from mild to pronounced, depending on the acuteness and severity of the attack

Mild   Diffuse wheezing, slight dyspnea, chest
            tightness
Moderate   Marked wheezing; dyspnea at rest; hyperpnea;
            chest tightness; nostril flaring; dry cough;
            upright, forward-leaning posture; prolonged
            expiration
Severe   Decreased wheezing; severe dyspnea; chest
            retractions; nasal flaring; shallow, rapid
            respirations; anxiety; fatigue; inability to
            speak more than a few words before stopping
            for breath; upright posture; cyanosis

Complications

Atelectasis, pneumothorax, and status asthmaticus with respiratory failure are common complications.

Diagnostic Tests

The following tests are useful during acute attacks:

Clinical   Above-mentioned manifestations are seen
Evaluation   plus pulsus paradoxus; decrease in airway
                exchange, rhonchi, wheezes; increased pulse
                and respirations. During stable periods, may
                be assessed for asthma triggers and severity
                of disease based on frequency and severity of
                attacks, response to bronchodilators, degree
                of lung damage seen on x-ray, and exercise
                tolerance.
Arterial   *Mild:* pH, PaO_2, $PaCO_2$ normal; forced vital
Blood Gases   capacity (FVC) 80% of normal
                Moderate: pH increased; PaO_2, $PaCO_2$
                decreased; FVC 50% of normal
                Severe: pH, PaO_2 decreased; $PaCO_2$ increased;
                FVC 25% of normal
Sputum   Increased viscosity, plugs

CBC	Eosinophilia
Radiology	Chest x-ray normal to hyperinflation, increase in lung markings, possible atelectasis
Pulmonary Function	Total lung capacity, functional reserve capacity, and respiratory volume increased; vital capacity normal or decreased
Peak Expiratory Flow rate (PEFR)	Decreased; also used to monitor treatment effectiveness

Therapeutic Management

Surgery	None
Medications	Stepwise pharmacologic approach recommended by National Asthma Education and *Prevention Program*
	Step 1: (Mild intermittent asthma) no maintenance drugs, short-acting inhaled β_2 agonists (albuterol and terbutaline) as needed
	Step 2: (Mild persistent asthma) low dose inhaled corticosteroids and/or leukotriene receptor antagonists (montelukast and zafirlukast) for maintenance; short acting inhaled β_2 agonists for quick relief
	Step 3: (Moderate persistent asthma) low and/or medium dose inhaled corticosteroids plus long-acting, inhaled β_2 agonists (salmeterol) or long-acting oral β_2 agonists (albuterol sustained release tabs) for maintenance; short-acting inhaled β_2 agonists for quick relief
	Step 4: (Severe persistent asthma) high dose inhaled corticosteroids and systemic corticosteroids plus long-acting inhaled β_2 agonists (salmeterol) or long-acting oral β_2 agonists (albuterol sustained release tabs) for maintenance; short-acting inhaled β_2 agonists for quick relief

    🕭 Severe prolonged attacks not responding to high dose inhaled steroids and bronchodilators are treated as an emergency with intravenous steroids and repeat doses of inhaled bronchodilators in a controlled setting, such as an emergency department or hospital.

General   *Severe prolonged attack:* Hospitalization with oxygen administration, intravenous fluid and electrolyte replacement, maintenance of patent airway, and close monitoring

Maintenance: Avoid triggering agents, maintain influenza shots and pneumonia vaccines, avoid or seek early treatment for respiratory infections, regular exercise program, and attend support groups

Prevention/   Keep environment free of triggers
Promotion   Use maintenance medications consistently
Education   Education about effects of disease, effects and side effects of medications; reinforcement of asthma management plan (avoidance of personal triggers, breathing techniques, consistent adherence to maintenance therapy) to reduce or prevent attacks; proper use and maintenance of equipment (peak flow meter, metered dose inhaler, spacer, and nebulizer)

Attention Deficit Disorder (ADD)/Attention Deficit Hyperactivity Disorder (ADHD)

A persistent pattern of developmentally inappropriate inattention and easy distractibility, with or without impulsivity, hyperactivity, or severe restlessness

Etiology and Incidence

The exact etiology is unknown and is probably multifactorial. There appears to be a strong genetic and/or familial link and neurotransmitter abnormalities in the brain are thought to play a role. Maternal smoking during pregnancy has also been associated with ADD and/or ADHD. Prevalence estimates range from 10% to 15% in school children in the United States, with males 4 to 10 times more likely to be diagnosed. Males are more likely to be diagnosed with ADHD and females are more likely to be diagnosed with ADD. Increasing numbers of adults are being diagnosed and the prevalence estimates range from 2% to 6% in adults.

Pathophysiology

Two dopamine receptor genes (D2 and D4) and the DAT gene have been implicated in ADD and ADHD. There is evidence of decreased frontal cortical activity with decreased levels of dopamine transmission and abnormal glucose metabolism. There is a distinct pattern of neuropsychological deficit including difficulty in working memory and executive function.

Risk Factors

Familial pattern
Thyroid hormone abnormality in small number of familial cases
Use of cigarettes, drugs, alcohol during pregnancy

Clinical Manifestations

DSM IV criteria list the following manifestations:

Children

Inattention	Inattention to details and/or makes careless mistakes; difficulty sustaining attention; seems not to listen; loses things; fails to

	finish tasks; difficulty organizing; avoids tasks that require sustained attention; easily distracted; forgetful
Impulsivity/ Hyperactivity	Impulsivity—blurts out answer, difficulty waiting turn, interrupts and/or intrudes on others; hyperactivity—fidgets or squirms, cannot stay seated, excessive running and/or climbing, always on the go, difficulty engaging in quiet play; talks excessively
Associated Symptoms	Clumsiness, emotional lability, anxiety, aggressiveness, sleep disturbances, bossiness, dysphoria, mood swings, poor social skills, and poor peer relationships
Adults	
Inattention	Lack of attention and/or careless mistakes; difficulty sustaining attention; difficulty following verbal instructions; misplaces things; fails to finish tasks; difficulty organizing; avoids tasks that require concentration; easily distracted; forgetful
Hyperactivity/ Impulsivity	Fidgets; trouble sitting still; restless and/or jittery; trouble doing things quietly, always on the go; talkative; acts before thinking; easily frustrated and/or impatient; interrupts people's conversations
Associated Symptoms	Multiple jobs and relationships, misjudgment of time; mood lability and flash anger outbursts; many projects started but few completed

Complications

There is a high correlation between untreated ADD and ADHD and traumatic injury in adolescents. Untreated adults have lower educational and occupational attainment and lower job satisfaction. There is a high rate of substance abuse among those with untreated ADHD.

Diagnostic Tests

No specific diagnostic tests are available, although use of single-photon emission computed tomography (SPECT) and positron emission tomography (PET) scanning and EEG and MRI is being studied. Diagnosis is chiefly through social, medical, and school histories coupled with a careful clinical exam, use of ADHD rating scales, and continuous performance and neuropsychological testing.

DSM IV criteria set out the following parameters:

For children at least six clinical manifestations in either inattention or impulsivity and/or hyperactivity category must have occurred often, have persisted for at least 6 months, have onset before age 7, be more severe than is typical for the age level, and have occurred in two or more settings. For adults, at least six of the manifestations in either category must be seen often and have persisted for at least 6 months. Three symptoms are necessary for diagnosis in adults over age 50. At least some of the symptoms had to have been present in childhood. There must be evidence of significant impairment in at least two settings (e.g., at work, at home, when driving, and during social or leisure activities).

Therapeutic Management

Surgery	None
Medications	Stimulants such as methylphenidate (Ritalin), dextroamphetamine (Dexedrine) and amphetamine salts (Adderall); atomoxetine (Strattera), a selective norepinephrine reuptake inhibitor, recently approved for adults; second line drugs include imipramine, desipramine, bupropion, and venlafaxine
General	Children may function better in specialized educational settings. Environmental structure, routines, limit setting, and self-monitoring techniques can help manage symptoms; support groups may improve social skills; cognitive therapy in combination with medication has shown promise in symptom reduction.
Education	Educate the person about long-term need for drug therapy and medication side effects. Note: stimulant medications should not be taken in combination with products containing organic acids, such as citric or ascorbic acid, as they interfere with drug absorption.

Autism (Autistic Disorder)

Complex, pervasive developmental disorder of early childhood accompanied by a host of intellectual and behavioral deficits that can vary greatly in scope and severity

Etiology and Incidence

The causal mechanisms are unknown, but it is thought to be a genetically linked, autosomal-recessive nonspecific neuronal injury and has been associated with other neurological conditions, such as encephalitis, phenylketonuria, and fragile X chromosomal disorder. There are an estimated 3 to 5 per 10,000 school-aged children diagnosed with autism in the United States. Boys are affected four times more frequently than girls, although girls are more severely affected and onset is typically seen well before the age of 3.

Pathophysiology

Pathogenesis is unknown, but children with autism have abnormal electroencephalograms with cerebellar vermal hypoplasia, epileptic seizures, persistence of primitive reflexes, metabolic abnormalities, and delayed hand dominance.

Risk Factors

Genetics
Maternal rubella
Male gender

Clinical Manifestations

Cognitive	Impaired language communication (absence of speech; abnormalities of pitch, tone, rate, or rhythm; immature, stereotyped grammar; echolalia; pronominal reversal; and concrete and idiosyncratic word use); impaired understanding; mental retardation (mild to severe)
Development	Poor sucking and feeding responses; persistence of primitive reflexes; advanced gross motor skills; exceptional abilities (e.g.,

	memory); lack of developmentally appropriate play
Behavioral	Hyperactivity; short attention span; impulsivity; aggressive behavior; temper tantrums; repetitive behaviors and/or mannerisms (rocking, hand clapping, spinning, swaying); self-injurious behavior (head banging and biting); elaborate routines and/or rituals; intense concern with sameness; preoccupation with inanimate objects
Emotional	Solitary play; interpersonal isolation; lack of emotional reciprocity; unyielding to touching, hugging, holding; inappropriate responses to danger; excessive fear of harmless objects
Perceptual	Idiosyncratic reactions to stimuli (e.g., high pain threshold; sensitivity to light, sound, or touch); fascination with sensory stimulation
Social	Lack of appropriate peer relations; lack of interest in or inappropriateness of social interaction; little sense of personal space boundaries

Complications

Autism is a severely disabling condition. Prognosis is strongly tied to the level of language skills and intellectual function. Most will require life-long supervised and structured care. Some individuals may develop schizophrenia in adolescence or young adulthood.

Diagnostic Tests

Diagnostic criteria from DSM IV TR require:

A.   A total of six indicators from three categories with at least two from category 1.

Category 1: Qualitative impairment in social interaction manifested by: (a) noticeable impairment in use of multiple nonverbal behaviors; (b) failure to develop appropriate peer relations; (c) lack of spontaneous seeking to share enjoyment, interests, or achievements; (d) lack of social and/or emotional reciprocity.

Category 2: Qualitative impairments in communication manifested by: (a) delay in or lack of spoken language; (b) marked impairment in ability to initiate and/or sustain conversation; (c) stereotyped, repetitive, idiosyncratic language; (d) lack of varied spontaneous play appropriate to developmental level.

Category 3: Restrictive, repetitive, stereotyped behavior and/or activity patterns manifested by: (a) preoccupation with restricted patterns of interest; (b) inflexible adherence to specific nonfunctional routines and/or rituals; (c) repetitive motor mannerisms or complex whole body movements; (d) persistent preoccupation with parts of objects.

B. Delays or abnormal functioning in a least one of the following before age 3: (1) social interaction, (2) language, or (3) symbolic play.

C. Disturbance not better accounted for by Rett syndrome or childhood disintegrative order; psychological and intelligence testing.

Therapeutic Management

Surgery	None
Medications	Neuroleptics for aggressive and/or self-destructive behavior; antiseizure drugs for concomitant seizure disorder
General	Behavioral training, structured environment at home and school; educational focus on language and social development; speech therapy; ongoing cognitive and language testing during childhood; placement in structured care environment
Education	Instruction in behavioral training and structured environments for parents and educators; information about community resources such as Autism Society of America

Back Pain, Low (Acute and Chronic)

B

Pain in the lumbar, lumbosacral, or sacroiliac regions, or in the spine with possible radiation down one or both buttocks and legs

(See also Herniated Disk)

Etiology and Incidence

Back pain may be related to acute or chronic processes and there are multiple causes for such pain. Causes include primary mechanical derangements (e.g., strain, spasm, joint or disk degeneration, compression fracture, and stenosis); infection (e.g., abscess and osteomyelitis); neoplasia (e.g., myeloma, lymphoma, and metastases); metabolic disease (e.g., osteoporosis, osteomalacia, and hemochromatosis); rheumatologic disorders (e.g., ankylosing spondylitis, psoriatic arthropathy, and polymyalgia); referred pain (e.g., abdominal visceral, retroperitoneal vascular process, and herpes zoster); and miscellaneous processes (e.g., Paget's disease, fibromyalgia, and psychogenic pain). Low back pain is the most common musculoskeletal complaint among adults and is experienced in 70% to 80% of the general population. Symptoms tend to be recurrent and become more persistent and severe with age.

Pathophysiology

Pathophysiology is related to causation. Aging also causes intervertebral disk degeneration and small tears in the anulus fibrosus, compression of end plate cartilage, and microfracture of the subchondral bone, which can contribute to increased severity and persistence of the pain.

Risk Factors

Occupations that necessitate repetitive lifting, heavy lifting, or sudden maximal lifting efforts
Occupational exposure to heavy equipment vibrations
Prolonged sitting or standing, poor postural habits
Tobacco use
Extreme obesity
Pregnancy

Major skeletal abnormalities
Spinal stenosis

Clinical Manifestations

Acute	Self-limiting pain, spasm, and/or stiffness in lower back tied to a specified event such as overexertion, strain, trauma, or stress that remits within 1 to 8 weeks
Chronic	Pain is long term; onset, character, location, and radiation of pain symptoms vary with the cause for the back pain

Complications

Long-term incapacity from chronic pain, structural weakness, or spinal instability.

Diagnostic Tests

Testing and exam are done for differential diagnosis of low back pain.

Clinical Evaluation	Assessment of onset, character, location, and radiation of pain symptoms; assessment of sensory, motor, and reflex deficits
Radiology	X-rays of spine and sacroiliac joint to detect fractures, dislocations, inflammation, destructive lesions, and vertebral collapse
CT Scan/MRI	Detection of herniated intervertebral disks, spinal stenosis, and disk bulges
Electromyography	Detect/confirm nerve root compression
Radionuclide Bone Scan	Identify metastatic lesions, characterize spondylolysis
Erythrocyte Sedimentation Rate	Elevation in metastatic processes, infection, and/or ankylosing spondylitis
HLA-B27 Antigen	Positive in ankylosing spondylitis

Therapeutic Management

Surgery	Diskectomy, microdiskectomy, percutaneous diskectomy for herniation and sciatica with progressive deficit; laminectomy and foraminotomy for severe spinal stenosis; spinal fusion for spinal instability or severe arthritic changes
Medications	Nonsteroidal antiinflammatory drugs (NSAIDs), narcotics for pain and inflammation; muscle relaxants for spasm; tissue injections of steroids and anesthetics for tender points in myofascial or fibromyalgia; tricyclic antidepressants for chronic low back pain or fibromyalgia
General	Rest in flexed knee hip position for 1 to 2 days; local heat and massage; deep heat after acute stage; lumbosacral stretching exercises; lumbosacral corset for obese or pregnant individuals with chronic ligament strain; mattress with firm support; elevated toilet seat for chronic pain; structured pain management program for chronic nonresponsive pain
Prevention/ Promotion	Avoid prolonged standing, sitting
	Use upright posture when sitting or standing; avoid slumping and slouching
	Use good body mechanics when lifting, break down larger loads, avoid forward bent and twisted lifting positions, and avoid sudden maximal effort movements
	Include abdominal strengthening and lumbosacral flexion exercises in a regular exercise program
	Weight reduction if overweight
	Tobacco cessation for users
Education	Education about preventive actions

Bell's Palsy

> Unilateral facial paralysis with sudden loss of the ability to use the muscles that control expression on one side of the face

Etiology and Incidence

The cause is unknown but is thought to be related to a virus or immune disorder. Onset often occurs in concert with an outbreak of herpes simplex in or around the ear. Most individuals are 20 to 60 years of age, and men and women are affected equally.

Pathophysiology

Cranial nerve VII (facial nerve) is compressed at the temporal bone pathway by edema produced by an unknown cause. As a result, the muscles controlling expression on one side of the face are paralyzed.

Clinical Manifestations

Facial weakness, numbness, heaviness, and pain behind the ear followed by inability to work facial muscles on one side are apparent. The extent of the symptoms depends on the severity of compression. Symptoms can include inability to wrinkle the forehead, upward rolling of the eyeball, inability to close the eyelid, and unilateral lack of smile or frown expression. Taste, lacrimation, and salivation may also be affected.

Complications

Facial contractures, corneal ulceration, and synkinesia are possible complications. Paralysis may be transient or permanent. Any return of function usually occurs in 1 to 6 months.

Diagnostic Tests

Diagnosis is based on clinical evaluation and history of onset. An electromyogram (EMG) may be used to test percutaneous nerve excitability.

Therapeutic Management

Surgery	Hypoglossal-facial nerve anastomosis to restore partial facial function if none has returned by 6 to 12 months
Medications	Methylcellulose drops are used for affected eye, analgesics as required for pain, and steroids to reduce edema of facial nerve. Acyclovir is often used in conjunction with steroids when herpes virus infection is suspected.
General	Hot wet packs and patching of affected eye; stimulation of facial nerve, facial exercises, gentle upward massage, and physical therapy to prevent facial contracture
Education	Education that paralysis is likely to resolve within 6 weeks; teach to chew food on unaffected side to improve taste and avoid food trapping; maintain scrupulous oral hygiene to prevent parotitis, caries, or gum disease from accumulated food

Black Lung Disease (Coal Worker's Pneumoconiosis)

Chronic, progressive, nodular pulmonary disease involving diffuse deposition of coal dust in the lungs

Etiology and Incidence

The cause is inhalation and prolonged retention of bituminous or anthracite coal dust. Susceptibility increases with length and intensity of exposure, smallness of inhaled particles, and silica content of the coal. Anthracite coal miners in the eastern United States have the highest incidence.

Pathophysiology

The deposition of coal dust triggers a phagocytic reaction and increases the production of macrophages. As the dust overwhelms the pulmonary clearing mechanism, fibroblasts appear and lay down a network of reticulin fibers that enmesh the dust. The collections of macrophages and reticulin fibers around the bronchioles, known as coal macules, lead to dilation of the alveoli; this is known as the simple disease phase. If allowed to progress, the macules enlarge and coalesce, and a massive fibrosis occurs, which destroys pulmonary structures as the vascular bed, alveoli, and airways are invaded; this is the complicated phase.

Risk Factors

Prolonged exposure to coal dust.

Clinical Manifestations

Simple Phase	Asymptomatic
Complicated Phase	Exertional dyspnea, hypoxia, black sputum

Complications

Pulmonary hypertension and cor pulmonale may develop in severe cases. Smoking, bronchitis, emphysema, and other respiratory diseases aggravate the disease process.

Diagnostic Tests

Clinical Evaluation	History of exposure to coal dust, usually at least 10 years underground
Radiology	*Simple phase:* Small, rounded opacities in both lung fields
	Complicated phase: Large opacities greater than 1 cm mixed with numerous small opacities
Pulmonary Function	*Simple phase:* Normal vital capacity
	Complicated phase: Decreased
Arterial Blood Gases	*Simple phase:* Normal, decreased PO_2
	Complicated phase: Increased PCO_2

Therapeutic Management

Surgery	None
Medications	None
General	*Simple phase:* Eliminate further exposure, prevent secondary infections
	Complicated phase: Chest physiotherapy and steam inhalation to loosen and remove secretions; increased fluid intake to thin secretions; oxygen (advanced stage)
Prevention/ Promotion	Prevention is an occupational safety issue and involves suppression of the coal dust at the coalface in the coal mines.

Bladder Cancer

Transitional cell carcinomas account for 90% of all bladder cancers, and squamous cell tumors and adenocarcinomas account for the remaining 10%. It is also classified as invasive or noninvasive (superficial). Invasive tumors grow in the bladder wall, spreading quickly to the underlying musculature, whereas noninvasive tumors occur on the superficial surface of the bladder wall.

Etiology and Incidence

Known carcinogens include tobacco tars and industrial chemical agents found in rubber, dye, paint shops, chemical manufacturing, petrochemical, and printing plants. Chronic irritants (e.g., schistosomiasis and bladder calculi) are predisposing factors. Bladder cancer is the fourth most common cancer in men and the eighth most common in women. More than 57,000 new cases are diagnosed each year in the United States and 12,500 people die annually. The morbidity and mortality rates are three times higher for men than women, and the median age for disease diagnosis is 65.

Pathophysiology

Transitional cell tumors are characterized by multicentric and papillary growth into the bladder lumen, with potential invasion into the bladder muscle, pelvis, pelvic structures, and surrounding lymph nodes. The lungs, bones, and liver are common sites of metastasis.

Risk Factors

Tobacco use (increases risk twofold to fourfold)
Occupational exposure (e.g., aluminum worker, dry cleaner, worker in a plant producing preservatives or polychlorinated biphenyls, chimney sweep, miner, and exterminator)
Chemical exposure (benzidine, 2-naphthylamine, p-aminodiphenyl, 4-nitrobiphenyl)
Chronic bladder irritation (bladder calculi, schistosomiasis)
History of multiple urinary tract infections
Overuse of drugs such as acetaminophen or phenacetin
Beer (nitrosamine) consumption

Diet high in fried, fatty meats; other fats; and low vitamin A
intake

History of treatment with cyclophosphamide (Cytoxan) or
pelvic radiation

Clinical Manifestations

Frequency and burning on urination, hematuria, dysuria, and
pyuria are the most common presenting signs and symptoms.
Pain in the legs, pelvis, and lower back may develop with invasion and metastasis.

Complications

Fistulas of the ureter or small bowel (or both) and obstruction
of the small bowel are possible.

Diagnostic Tests

Filling defects on a cystogram and positive results on urine
cytological tests suggest a neoplasm. The definitive diagnosis is
made by cystoscopy and transurethral resectional biopsy. CT
scan or MRI with bimanual examination is used for staging.

Therapeutic Management

Surgery	*Noninvasive tumors:* Endoscopy, transurethral resection, and fulguration; laser therapy
	Invasive tumors: Radical cystectomy with urinary diversion, usually an ileal conduit with external pouch
Medications	Chemotherapy
	Noninvasive tumors: Intravesical instillations with bacille Calmette-Guérin (BCG); alpha interferon, thiotepa, or valrubicin are secondary treatment choices
	Invasive tumors: Systemic chemotherapy with multidrug combinations, such as methotrexate, vinblastine, Adriamycin, and cisplatin (MVAC). Other agents used include mitoxantrone, vincristine, etoposide, ifosfamide, Taxol, gemcitabine, piritrexim, and gallium nitrate

| General | Radiation as a preoperative regimen or as adjunct to chemotherapy |
| Education | Care of and instruction about ileal appliance; stress need for routine follow-up |

Blepharitis

An inflammation of the eyelid margins

Etiology and Incidence

A common chronic condition associated with seborrheic dermatitis of the scalp, eyebrows, and external ears. Severe cases may be bacterial in origin (commonly staphylococcal). Allergies may aggravate the condition. It is often impossible to isolate the exact causative agent. Other common conditions associated with chronic blepharitis are diabetes, gout, anemia, and rosacea. Infections of the nose and mouth may also be transferred to the eyes and lids by frequent eye rubbing.

Pathophysiology

Blepharitis may be seborrheic or ulcerative. Seborrheic (nonulcerative) blepharitis is commonly associated with seborrhea of the face, eyebrows, external ears, and scalp. Inflammation of the eyelid margins occurs, with redness, thickening, and often the formation of scales and crusts or shallow marginal ulcers. Ulcerative blepharitis is caused by bacterial infection (usually staphylococcal) of the lash follicles and the meibomian glands.

Risk Factors

Chronic diseases such as diabetes, gout, anemia, and rosacea
History of sties, chalazia
Infections of the mouth and/or throat
Seborrheic dermatitis or allergies

Clinical Manifestations

Seborrheic Blepharitis	*General:* Foreign-body sensation
	Eyelids and lashes: Red lid margins, flaking and scaling around lashes, itching and burning sensation, and loss of lashes
	Cornea and conjunctiva: Light sensitivity, conjunctivitis, and possible corneal inflammation
Ulcerative Blepharitis	*General:* Foreign-body sensation
	Eyelids and lashes: Crusts on the eyelids, leaving a bleeding surface when removed;

small pustules develop in lash follicles; shallow ulcers may develop; eyelids become "glued" together during sleep by dried drainage

Cornea and conjunctiva: Light sensitivity, conjunctivitis, and possible corneal inflammation

Complications

Lid margins thicken over time with misdirected growth and/or loss of eyelashes. Corneal pannus, ulcerative keratitis, and lid ectropion can occur in severe chronic cases.

Diagnostic Tests

Clinical evaluation with characteristic manifestations
Detailed history to locate possible source
Possible laboratory isolation of causative agent

Therapeutic Management

Blepharitis is stubborn to treat and is often resistant to various therapies.

Surgery	None
Medications	Topical (ointment, drops) and systemic antiinfectives for infective agents; flavanoid type of compounds (resveratrol, silymarin) being tested to reduce inflammation
General	Eyelid hygiene consists of scrubbing the lid margins and lashes daily; massaging lid margins to stimulate flow of secretions then cleansing with a cotton swab dipped in a diluted solution of baby shampoo; use of seborrheic dermatitis medicated shampoos; and hot compresses to lids loosen debris
Education	Education that this is a chronic condition with no cure that often resists treatment; instruction in scrubbing and washing techniques

Bone Cancer, Primary

B

Skeletal malignancy arising from osseous, cartilaginous, fibrous, or reticuloendothelial tissue of the bone (multiple myeloma is excluded from this category)

Etiology and Incidence

Etiology is unknown. Primary bone tumors are rare, accounting for only 0.2% of all malignancies in the United States. The tumors affect primarily children and adolescents (Ewing's sarcoma and osteosarcoma) and adults over age 65 (fibrosarcoma, chondrosarcoma, and reticulum cell sarcoma).

Pathophysiology

Osteosarcomas are the most common primary bone tumor. Cancer cells originate in the mesenchyma of the medullary cavity of the bone (usually long bones around or in the knee) and proliferate rapidly, absorbing normal bone and promoting tissue destruction. The bone becomes sclerotic or lytic, or both, and an aggressive periosteal reaction ensues, accompanied by a soft tissue mass. The lungs are the most common metastatic site and spread to regional lymph nodes is rare. Fibrous tumors are similar in character to osteosarcomas.

Risk Factors

History of Paget's disease, fibrous dysplasia, or enchondromatosis
History of prior radiation

Clinical Manifestations

An initially painless mass is the most common presenting sign. Pain or swelling, or both, at the affected site is also common.

Complications

Pathological fractures occur with progressive destruction of normal bone tissue. Survival rate is about 50% with combination therapy and early treatment.

Diagnostic Tests

X-rays and bone scans of the involved bone allow visualization of the tumor. The definitive diagnosis is made through a biopsy of the tumor. MRI is conducted to visualize tumor size and location and enhance resection abilities.

Therapeutic Management

Surgery	En bloc resection and reconstruction of affected limb; amputation of affected limb
Medications	Systemic chemotherapy with methotrexate; intraarterial perfusion with doxorubicin as an adjunct before surgery
General	Radiation used with Ewing's sarcoma, rehabilitation after amputation, gait training, fitting of prosthesis
Education	Care of and instruction for artificial limb; stress need for routine follow-up

Brain Abscess

An intracerebral infection consisting of an encapsulated collection of pus

Etiology and Incidence

Causes include extension of existing cranial infection (e.g., ear infection, sinusitis, mastoiditis, osteomyelitis, and periodontal infection); penetrating head wounds; blood-borne transmission from a distant infection (e.g., bacterial endocarditis, abdominal/pelvic infections, and bronchiectasis); IV drug abuse; or immunodeficiency. The incidence is highest in individuals with sinusitis, or with ear or pulmonary infection. The number of abscesses is increasing with the rise in immunodeficiency disorders and IV drug abuse.

Pathophysiology

The brain produces a poorly localized inflammatory response to the invading pathogen. Brain tissue subsequently liquefies and becomes necrotic, producing a cystic mass, which is encapsulated by glia and fibroblasts. As this mass enlarges, it increases intracranial pressure, causing signs and symptoms similar to those of a brain tumor.

Risk Factors

Blood-borne infections (e.g., bacterial endocarditis, peritonitis)
Immunodeficiency infections
Infections of the face and head (e.g., otitis media, sinusitis, mastoiditis, acne, or abscesses of teeth or gums)
IV drug use
Open head injury

Clinical Manifestations

Headache, nausea, vomiting, seizures, altered mental status, drowsiness, confusion, nuchal rigidity, and low-grade fever can occur. The duration of symptoms varies considerably from hours to weeks.

Complications

The illness is progressive and usually fatal if left untreated. With treatment, the mortality rate is 30%, and more than half of survivors suffer some neurological sequelae.

Diagnostic Tests

Clinical Evaluation	Above manifestations and predisposing conditions
Lumbar Puncture	**Contraindicated**
CT Scan/MRI	Visualization of abscess

Therapeutic Management

Surgery	Biopsy, drainage, and evacuation of abscess through stereotactic techniques or craniotomy
Medications	IV antibiotics as initial choice, depending on suspected organism and probable source of infection; later choices made from culture and sensitivity, along with Gram's stain results; steroids to reduce brain edema and intracranial pressure (ICP); anticonvulsants to control seizure activity
General	Serial-order CT scans to monitor progression; monitoring for hyponatremia and inappropriate antidiuretic hormone secretion; prevention of complications of extended bed rest (e.g., antiembolism stockings, range of motion (ROM) exercises, and turning); early, aggressive rehabilitation to prevent or reduce neurological sequelae
Prevention	Prevention of brain abscess through prompt treatment of infections of face and head

Brain Cancer

(See Brain Tumor, Primary)

Brain Tumor, Primary

B

An expanding, intracranial lesion, which may be either benign or malignant. However, since both types can be lethal if inaccessible or left untreated and malignant tumors rarely metastasize beyond the central nervous system, the distinction serves mainly to describe the rate of growth and invasiveness. Tumors are divided into six classes, according to their origin: (1) skull, (2) meninges, (3) cranial nerves, (4) neuroglia, (5) pituitary and/or pineal body, and (6) congenital.

Etiology and Incidence

The etiology is unknown. Brain tumors are diagnosed in about 10,000 persons per year in the United States. Undiagnosed brain tumors are found in about 2% of all routine autopsies. They can occur at any age but are most prevalent between ages 30 and 50. The overall occurrence is evenly divided between the genders. Common childhood tumors include cerebellar astrocytomas, medulloblastomas, gliomas, ependymomas, and assorted congenital tumors. Common adult tumors include meningiomas, schwannomas, and cerebral astrocytomas.

Pathophysiology

As the tumor grows, the surrounding brain tissue is compressed or infiltrated (or both), causing focal disturbances. The flow and absorption of cerebrospinal fluid (CSF) are altered and/or obstructed, causing increased intracranial pressure (ICP). Blood vessels are compressed, altering or obstructing blood flow and resulting in tissue necrosis and seizures. If tumors arise in certain locations, brain tissue can shift, leading to herniation, infarction, and hemorrhage in the pons and midbrain.

Clinical Manifestations

The signs and symptoms depend heavily on the tumor's location, size, and rate of growth. Slow-growing tumors are often asymptomatic until they have grown quite large.

General	Headache, nausea, vomiting, impulsivity, diminished judgment, memory impairment, depression, seizures, drowsiness, lethargy, psychotic episodes, papilledema
Focal	*Frontal lobe:* Hemiplegia, expressive aphasia, ataxia, visual field defects, focal seizures
	Parietal lobe: Focal sensory seizures, impaired position sense and two-point discrimination, hemianopia, apraxia, anosognosia, speech disturbances, denial of illness
	Temporal lobe: Convulsions, aphasia/dysphasia, olfactory aura preceding seizures
	Occipital lobe: Hemianopia, flashing light aura preceding seizures
	Brainstem: Hemiplegia, hemianesthesia

Complications

Herniation of the brain can occur when intracranial pressure is expanded beyond compensatory levels. Prompt intervention is required, or the individual will die. Benign tumors that cannot be excised because of their size or location, or both, are generally fatal.

Diagnostic Tests

Clinical Evaluation	Any of above manifestations, particularly headaches and recent onset of seizure activity
Neurological Examination	Focal manifestations, impairment of mental status
CT Scan/ MRI/PET	To detect tumor, midline shifts, and changes in ventricle size
Cerebral Angiography	To determine blood flow and localization of tumor
Eye Examination	To test visual fields and acuity, and detect papilledema
Audiometry	To test hearing

Therapeutic Management

Surgery	Tumor excision; shunting
Medications	Corticosteroids to reduce cerebral edema, anticonvulsants to control seizure activity, chemotherapeutic agents as adjunctive therapy or to treat recurrence; biodegradable wafers impregnated with chemotherapy drugs may be implanted during surgery. Temozolomide is first oral chemotherapy agent that crosses the blood-brain barrier.
General	Radiation for tumor or residual tumor, rehabilitation for neurological sequelae and functional limitations; communication devices for dysphasia

Breast Cancer

Ductal carcinomas account for 75% of all breast cancer, with 15% to 20% of these being ductal carcinoma in situ (DCIS), which present on mammogram as clusters of micro-calcifications. Lobular and nipple carcinomas account for most of the remaining 25%.

Etiology and Incidence

The cause of breast cancer is unknown although estrogen is thought to play some role. More than 50% of women diagnosed with the disorder have none of the known risk factors (see Risk Factors).

Breast cancer is the most common cancer among women in the United States, with more than 212,000 new cases diagnosed each year. The incidence is twice as high for women over age 65 as for those in the 45 to 64 age group. The incidence is rising, particularly among black women and women in their 20s and 30s; however, the mortality rate has remained stable at about 40,000 deaths per year. It is the second leading cause of cancer death in women. Incidence of breast cancer in males is 1% of that in women.

Pathophysiology

Ductal carcinomas originate in the lactiferous ducts, where the cancer cells form a dense fibrotic core with radiating tentacles that invade surrounding breast tissue. The tumor mass is generally solid, nonmobile, irregularly shaped, poorly defined, and unilateral. Lobular carcinomas originate in the breast lobules and are bilateral. Nipple carcinomas originate in the nipple complex and often occur in conjunction with invasive ductal carcinomas. The lungs, bones, brain, and liver are common sites of breast cancer metastasis.

Risk Factors

Familial history of breast cancer (risk is increased if relationship is mother or sister, if disease is bilateral, or if disease developed before menopause)
Abnormalities in *BRCA-1* and *BCRA-2* genes

Personal history of cancer (breast, colon, ovarian, endometrial, thyroid)

Long-term use of oral contraceptives; use of estrogen therapy in menopause

Early menarche (before 11); late menopause (after 52); nulliparity or first child after age 30

Personal history of fibrocystic disease; atypical hyperplasia

Obesity

Exposure to ionizing radiation (particularly if exposure occurs before age 35)

Clinical Manifestations

The most common presenting sign is a lump in the breast. About 50% are found in the upper outer quadrant. Nipple discharge may be present. Pain, tenderness, changes in breast shape, dimpling, and nipple retraction rarely occur until the disease reaches an advanced stage.

Complications

The prognosis dims markedly as the number of involved lymph nodes increases. Pleural effusion, ascites, pathological fracture, and spinal compression can occur with advanced disease. Women treated for stage I tumors and no lymph node involvement have a 10-year survival rate of 80%. Women with stage II tumors have a 10-year survival rate of 60%.

Diagnostic Tests

A mass detected by breast self-examination, physical examination, or mammogram needs further follow-up. Ultrasonography helps distinguish cysts from solid mass. Definitive diagnosis is made by incisional, excisional, fine needle, or stereotactic core biopsy of the mass.

Therapeutic Management

Surgery	Treatment of choice is resection of the lump with removal of a varying amount of surrounding healthy tissue, ranging from a margin of breast tissue to the entire breast, axillary lymph nodes, mammary lymphatic chain, and pectoral muscles; breast reconstruction

Medications   Adjunct systemic multidrug chemotherapy used primarily for premenopausal node-positive women; adjunct hormone therapy (estrogens, androgens, progestins) used primarily for postmenopausal node-positive or receptor-positive women; antiestrogen therapy (tamoxifen, Femara) as first line therapy; biological therapy with trastuzumab (Herceptin) used in select patients for treatment of metastatic disease. Bone marrow/stem cell transplants are under investigation for advanced metastatic disease.

General   Radiation used as adjunct after surgery and for palliation in advanced disease; counseling for altered body image; recovery support groups; good-fitting breast prosthesis if needed

Prevention/ Promotion   Annual mammogram and clinical breast exam for women age 40 and older and those at risk

Clinical breast exam every 3 years for women under 40

Regular breast self-exams

Education   Education about lymphedema risks and prevention and/or reduction if lymph nodes excised or radiated; importance of long-term follow-up

Bronchiectasis

> An irreversible dilation of the tracheobronchial tree, with destruction of the bronchial walls

Etiology and Incidence

Bronchiectasis is caused by conditions that repeatedly damage the bronchial walls and interfere with clearance of bronchial secretions, such as cystic fibrosis (CF), immunodeficiency diseases, repeated respiratory tract infections, tuberculosis (TB), inhalation of noxious gases, repeated aspiration pneumonia, and complications of measles and pertussis. Rare congenital anomalies may also be a cause. The incidence has declined dramatically since the introduction of antibiotics. Children are most vulnerable, and the incidence is highest among Alaskan Native Inuit and New Zealand Maori populations of the world.

Pathophysiology

Repeated inflammatory and infectious processes slowly alter the structure of the bronchial walls, diminishing cilia and impairing the ability to clear secretions, increasing mucus production, reducing elasticity and muscular response, and causing permanent dilation of various areas in the tracheobronchial tree.

Risk Factors

Smoking
Respiratory irritation
Repeated upper respiratory infections
Underlying disease (e.g., CF, immune deficiency, TB)

Clinical Manifestations

The individual is often asymptomatic early in the disease. A chronic cough with sputum production is the most common presenting sign. Hemoptysis and recurrent pneumonia are also common, as are dyspnea, wheezing, and fatigue. Fever, night sweats, weight loss, fetid breath, and hemoptysis may also be seen.

Complications

Pulmonary hypertension, right ventricular failure, and cor pulmonale are common complications with long-standing disease.

Diagnostic Tests

Clinical Evaluation	Chronic cough, mucopurulent sputum, hemoptysis, moist crackles in lung bases
Sputum	Foamy with sediment; large number of WBCs
Radiology	Chest x-ray shows increased markings, honeycombing, tram tracking
CT Scan	Detect cystic lesions and rule out neoplastic obstruction
Bronchography	Visualization of bronchiectatic areas used only when surgery contemplated
Pulmonary Function	Decreased vital capacity and decreased expiratory flow

Therapeutic Management

Surgery	Bronchial resection for confined disease unresponsive to conservative therapy
Medications	Mucolytics to clear secretions; antibiotics to treat bacterial infection; bronchodilators to reduce dyspnea; influenza and pneumonia vaccines for prophylaxis
General	Chest physiotherapy with postural drainage to clear secretions; increase fluids and use vaporizer to liquefy secretions
Prevention/ Promotion	Avoid respiratory infections and air pollution; smoking cessation; flu and pneumonia vaccines in vulnerable or chronic populations

Bronchiolitis/Respiratory Syncytial Virus (RSV)

Acute viral infection of the lower respiratory tract causing respiratory distress

Etiology and Incidence

The major viral pathogens are respiratory syncytial virus and parainfluenza-3 virus. This disease generally affects children under age 2 and often is epidemic in nature. Eighty percent of the cases occur in the first year of life, with cases extremely rare after the age of 5. Boys are one and a half times more likely to be affected than girls. About 10% of the cases require hospitalization, with RSV infection accounting for more than 50% of those cases. RSV is extremely contagious and is transmitted through direct contact with respiratory secretions. The virus may live for hours on tissue, dishes, and countertops.

Pathophysiology

The infecting virus spreads to the medium and small bronchioles in the lower airway and attacks the epithelial cells. This causes edema of the ciliated cells, which protrude into the lumen, losing cilia and fusing with adjacent cells to form a giant cell. These cause edema of the bronchial mucosa and production of exudate, resulting in partial obstruction and trapping of air in the alveoli.

Clinical Manifestations

The illness is usually preceded by an upper respiratory infection, followed by rapid onset of respiratory distress with tachypnea, tachycardia, and a hacking cough. As the disease advances, deepening chest retractions and audible wheezing, lethargy, vomiting, and dehydration develop.

Complications

Atelectasis and pneumonia are common complications. Respiratory failure is also possible.

Diagnostic Tests

Definitive diagnosis is made by isolating the virus or by immunofluorescence or enzyme-linked immunosorbent assay (ELISA).

Radiography   Chest x-rays show hyperaeration and consolidation

Therapeutic Management

Surgery	None
Medications	Ribavirin may be used to treat RSV in specialized cases
General	Oxygen mist, vaporizer, adequate fluid intake, rest
Prevention/ Promotion	Prophylaxis with RSV immune globulin or palivizumab in high- risk children (preterm infants, immunodeficient children, or children with chronic lung disease) in the fall. Scrupulous hand washing to prevent spread

Bronchitis, Acute

B

A self-limited inflammation of the tracheobronchial tree

Etiology and Incidence
The condition is caused either by irritants (e.g., dust, noxious fumes, or smoke) or by a viral or bacterial infection. It often occurs in conjunction with other disease processes, such as influenza, bronchiectasis, emphysema, or tuberculosis (TB). It is more common in the winter months and is generally mild.

Pathophysiology
Congestion of the mucous membranes is followed by desquamation and edema of the submucosa. This interferes with the functioning of the cilia, phagocytes, and lymphatics, resulting in production of a sticky exudate, which lines the tracheobronchial tree until it is coughed up. The exudate is an excellent medium for secondary infection.

Risk Factors
Chronic respiratory irritation
Repeated upper respiratory infections
Smoking
Underlying disease (e.g., asthma, emphysema, bronchiectasis, influenza, TB)

Clinical Manifestations
Acute bronchitis is often preceded by an upper respiratory infection. The most common presenting sign is a dry, hacking cough that increasingly produces viscous mucus. Other symptoms include low-grade fever, substernal pain, and fatigue.

Complications
Pneumonia is the most common complication. Acute respiratory failure occurs in some individuals with underlying pulmonary disease.

Diagnostic Tests

Diagnosis is usually made from the type of cough and sputum. Chest x-rays are taken to rule out other disorders. Arterial blood gases are monitored when underlying chronic disease is present, and sputum is cultured for evidence of superimposed infection.

Therapeutic Management

Surgery	None
Medications	Inhaled bronchodilators for wheezing; expectorants for cough; antipyretics for fever. Antiinfective drugs used only with concomitant chronic obstructive pulmonary disease (COPD) or superimposed infection.
General	Rest, increased fluids, steam vaporizer, smoking cessation

Bronchitis, Chronic

An obstructive pulmonary disorder characterized by a chronic and recurrent productive cough

Etiology and Incidence

Bronchial irritants (e.g., cigarette smoke) in conjunction with a genetic predisposition are thought to be the chief cause. More than 14 million cases of chronic bronchitis are reported annually in the United States. Most cases occur in those under age 45. The incidence is higher in women, individuals living in the South, and those living in heavily polluted areas. More than 3000 deaths from chronic bronchitis occur each year.

Pathophysiology

Chronic irritation leads to hypersecretion and hypertrophy of the bronchial mucous glands and an increase in the size and number of goblet cells. These goblet cells invade the terminal bronchioles and damage the cilia, which results in increased sputum, bronchial congestion, and narrowing of the bronchial lumen. As the disease progresses, leukocytes invade the secretions, increasing edema production and causing tissue necrosis. Granulated squamous epithelium replaces ciliated epithelium and forms fibrous tissue, leading to tissue scarring, stenosis, airway obstruction, and a severe ventilation-perfusion imbalance.

Risk Factors

Chronic bronchial irritants, such as cigarette smoke
Improper or nonuse of respirators in occupational settings
Occupational exposure to airborne particulates

Clinical Manifestations

Chronic bronchitis may be asymptomatic for years. A productive cough with copious mucopurulent sputum, peripheral cyanosis, and variable dyspnea are typical presenting signs. The cough becomes increasingly progressive and the sputum production more copious; several attacks per year are common. Wheezing, tachypnea, and tachycardia may also be present.

Complications

Frequent bouts of cor pulmonale, pulmonary hypertension, right ventricular hypertrophy, and respiratory failure are common complications.

Diagnostic Tests

Clinical Evaluation	Any of the above manifestations; history of chronic lung irritation (e.g., smoking, occupational exposure)
Radiology	Cardiac enlargement, normal or flattened diaphragm, congested lung fields, thickened bronchial markings
Pulmonary Function	Residual volume increased, forced vital capacity and forced expiratory volume decreased, compliance and diffusion normal
Arterial Blood Gases	PaO_2 decreased, $PaCO_2$ increased
Sputum	Culture of multiple microorganisms and neutrophils

Therapeutic Management

Surgery	None
Medications	Antiinfective drugs for infection; bronchodilators to reduce dyspnea; corticosteroids to reduce inflammation; flu and pneumonia vaccines for prophylaxis
General	Removal of irritant; chest physiotherapy to loosen secretions; vaporizer and increased fluids to liquefy secretions; oxygenation for hypoxia; consistent exercise to improve ventilatory and cardiac function; smoking cessation
Prevention/ Promotion	Smoking cessation and/or prevention; proper use of respirators in work place when exposed to respiratory irritants

B

| Education | Education, including disease process, medication administration (schedule, use of spacer), home use of oxygen, chest physiotherapy program, effective coughing, exercise program, nutrition plan to decrease weight if indicated, importance of long-term follow-up |

Bulimia Nervosa

An eating disorder characterized by recurrent episodes of binge eating followed by purging, which is brought about through self-induced vomiting or use of laxatives, emetics, or diuretics. Most individuals maintain a normal or near-normal body weight.

Etiology and Incidence

The etiology is unknown, but societal focus on dieting and thinness and associated negative images of obesity are thought to play a role. The incidence of bulimia is highest among adolescent females in affluent circumstances. The estimated prevalence in the United States is 5% of all young women in high school and college. The disorder is also more often seen in individuals whose occupation necessitates stringent weight control (e.g., jockeys, amateur wrestlers, models, actresses, and ballerinas). Persons with bulimia are highly resistant to treatment.

Pathophysiology

Vomiting causes fluid and electrolyte imbalances, which lead eventually to renal damage and cardiac arrhythmias.

Risk Factors

Adolescence/young adulthood
Affluent households
Female gender
Occupations that necessitate stringent weight control

Clinical Manifestations

Excessive concern about weight, evidence of eating binges, evidence of purging activities (e.g., smell of vomit, laxatives, emetics, and diuretics in residence), rapid weight fluctuations, hypokalemia, swollen parotid glands, dental erosion, esophagitis, scars on knuckles from inducing vomiting.

Complications

Esophageal stricture, rupture, and hemorrhage are common complications. Aspiration pneumonia is possible, particularly in concert with use of alcohol and recreational drugs. Sudden death from ventricular dysrhythmia is possible.

Diagnostic Tests

The diagnosis is made by reconstructing a clinical history of binge-purge behavior that occurs at least twice a week for at least 3 months; manifestations of persistent overconcern with body shape and weight, and feelings of powerlessness during binge cycles

Therapeutic Management

Surgery	Treatment of esophageal stricture/rupture
Medications	Antidepressants (selective serotonin reuptake inhibitors [SSRIs]) for depression
General	Psychotherapy; family therapy; nutritional counseling, food diaries, and meal planning to counter abnormal eating patterns; hospitalization for complications such as electrolyte imbalances, esophageal damage, aspiration pneumonia, cardiac involvement

Burns

Tissue injury, protein denaturation, edema, and loss of intravascular fluid resulting from exposure to or contact with a causative agent, such as heat, electricity, chemicals, or friction

Etiology and Incidence

Causes include (1) exposure to, contact with, or inhalation of the products of thermal agents such as fire, radiation, or hot liquids; (2) contact with an electrical current; or (3) contact with or inhalation or ingestion of chemical agents (e.g., acids, alkalis, phenols, cresols, mustard gas, or phosphorus). In the United States, more than 2.5 million persons are burned each year; more than 100,000 require hospitalization, and 12,000 people die. Burns are the second leading cause of death among young children.

Pathophysiology

Thermal and chemical injury disrupts the normal protective function of the skin, causing local and systemic effects. The extent of these effects depends on the type, duration, and intensity of exposure to the causative agent. Immediately after the injury, blood flow increases in the area around the wound. The burned tissue releases vasoactive substances, which increase capillary permeability. This creates a fluid shift from the intravascular compartment to the interstitial space, which causes edema. Damaged cells swell and platelets and leukocytes collect, causing ischemia and escalating tissue damage. Systemic effects caused by the vascular changes and tissue loss include hypovolemia, hyperventilation, increased blood viscosity, and suppression of the immune system. The severity of the burn determines the extent of local and systemic effects. The severity of a burn is judged by the depth and size of the injury. Superficial partial thickness burns (first degree) affect the epidermis only; deep partial thickness burns (second degree) affect the epidermis and dermis; full thickness burns (third degree) affect all skin layers and extend to subcutaneous tissue, muscle, and nerves; and fourth degree full thickness burns involve all skin layers plus bone. The percentage of body surface area (BSA) system of the American Burn Association classifies size as follows:

Minor burns: Full thickness burns over less than 2% of BSA, partial thickness burns over less than 15% of BSA

Moderate burns: Full thickness burns more than 2% to 10% of BSA, partial thickness burns over less than 15% to 25% of BSA

Major burns: Full thickness burns more than 10% BSA, partial thickness more than 25% BSA; any burn to face, head, hands, feet, or perineum; inhalation and electrical burns; burns complicated by trauma or other disease processes

The extent of the burn is calculated as a percent of total body surface (TBSA) and can be calculated using a Rule of Nines or Lund-Browder chart.

Clinical Manifestations

The following signs and symptoms can be expected within the first 24 hours:

Local	*Superficial:* Wound is red, sensitive to touch, painful, and moist; surface blanches to light pressure
	Deep partial thickness: Blistering likely
	Full thickness: Surface is white and pliable with no blanching, or black, charred, and leathery; hypoesthetic or anesthetic; hairs are easily dislodged from follicles
Systemic (First 24 to 48 Hours)	Hypovolemic shock and dehydration with thready pulse, tachycardia, rapid respirations, decreased blood pressure, clammy skin, intense thirst, and minimal urine output; hypothermia with shivering and cyanosis; anxiety; possible disorientation
	With inhalation injury: Respiratory obstruction or respiratory failure, or both

Complications

Massive hypovolemia, cardiac arrhythmias, acute tubular necrosis and renal failure, infection, pneumonia, respiratory failure, and contractures are all potential complications with severe burns. The prognosis depends largely on the severity and location of the burns, preexisting health status, and expertise of the burn management team.

Diagnostic Tests

Clinical Evaluation	To determine the severity of the injury (degree and BSA) and the causative agent
Baseline Laboratory Studies	CBC, serum electrolytes, blood urea nitrogen, creatinine, arterial blood gases, bilirubin, alkaline phosphatase, urinalysis
Bronchoscopy	To determine extent of airway damage

Therapeutic Management

Partial thickness burns, less than 20% BSA

Surgery	None
Medications	Analgesics for pain, prophylactic antibiotics to prevent infection, tetanus toxoid for immunization, topical antiinfective drugs
General	Cleaning with soap and cold water; débridement of blisters, splinting, and positioning of involved joints; elevation of affected area

Full thickness burns, greater than 20% BSA

Surgery	Surgical débridement; escharotomy to relieve contractures caused by scarring; fasciotomy with some electrical burns; skin grafting; amputation of severely burned extremities; reconstructive and plastic surgery to correct deformity
Medications	IV narcotic analgesics and sedatives for pain control; tetanus immunization; topical antimicrobial agents; IV antibiotics; vitamin and iron supplements

General   Airway maintenance, humidification, and oxygen in inhalation injuries; IV fluid replacement; cleansing of wound; urinary catheter; nasogastric tube; central venous line; mechanical débridement; hydrotherapy; dressing changes; dietary calories and protein increased; parenteral nutrition; physiotherapy; hypertrophic scar management with pressure garments; long-term psychological support; vocational counseling

Education   Instruction in scar management, itching, and chronic pain management; instruction for long-term adaptations to heat and cold intolerances, chemical sensitivities, and skin fragility. Teach to avoid temperature extremes, limit exertional activities; manage fluid balance, use sun protection for sun exposure, exercise regimen with range of motion and stretching exercises, prompt treatment of injuries to skin-grafted skin

Bursitis

An acute or chronic inflammation of a bursa

Etiology and Incidence

The etiology of most bursitis is unknown, although trauma, overuse, arthritis, gout, and infection have been implicated.

Pathophysiology

Exposure to an etiological agent causes irritation of the bursal sac, which becomes inflamed, edematous, enlarged, and tender.

Clinical Manifestations

Localized pain, redness, heat, swelling, and tenderness around a bony prominence (most often the shoulder) accompanied by limited range of motion (ROM).

Complications

Repeated inflammation leads to a chronic condition marked by adhesions and calcifications in the bursal sac, permanent muscle atrophy, adhesion capsulitis, and reduced ROM.

Diagnostic Tests

The diagnosis depends on clinical evaluation and a pattern of the aforementioned symptoms or a history of trauma, repetitive motion, gout, or arthritis. With chronic bursitis, x-rays may show calcifications.

Therapeutic Management

Surgery	Needle aspiration of fluid in sac, excision of calcium deposits, removal of bursal sac
Medications	Nonsteroidal antiinflammatory drugs (NSAIDs) for pain and inflammation, corticosteroid injections into bursa and surrounding tendons
General	Ice for acute trauma; rest and immobilization of joint; passive ROM exercises as pain subsides

Cancer

A cellular malignancy in which the affected cell displays unregulated growth and division and lack of differentiation as it invades adjacent tissue and proliferates. The altered cells, which form solid or diffuse tumors, are classified by the tissue from which they arise and are described according to a histogenetic system. (Specific malignancies are listed in alphabetical order by body site.)

Etiology and Incidence

The transformation of normal cells into cancer cells (carcinogenesis) appears to be a multistep process involving many factors. Thus far, no single theory of causation has satisfactorily explained this process. Causative agents have been identified for some forms of cancer, and others are being investigated. Cancer is the second leading cause of death in the United States. Each year, more than 550,000 persons die of cancer, and 1.35 million new cases are diagnosed. Although various forms of cancer strike different societal subgroups, it is a universal disease seen across cultural, racial, gender, age, and socioeconomic groups. Approximately 77% of all cancers are diagnosed in people age 55 and older. In the United States, males have a 1-in-2 and females a 1-in-3 risk of developing some form of cancer in their lifetime.

Pathophysiology

Cancer occurs when certain cells proliferate without organization and with little or no differentiation. It has been theorized that certain stimuli, as yet to be definitively identified, initiate this proliferation by overpowering the normal mechanisms controlling growth. The result is uninhibited growth, uncontrolled function, and rapid motility, permitting spread of the cancerous cells to other parts of the body through invasion of adjacent tissue or migration via the blood or lymph system. The migration process is commonly called *metastasis*. The primary site of a malignancy (cancer cell growth) is the site of original growth; a secondary site is created when cells migrate to and colonize an additional body site.

Clinical Manifestations

The American Cancer Society lists seven warning signs of cancer that require immediate attention from a physician: (1) a change in bowel or bladder habits; (2) a sore that does not heal; (3) unusual bleeding or discharge; (4) a thickening or lump in the breast or elsewhere; (5) indigestion or difficulty swallowing; (6) an obvious change in a wart or mole; and (7) a nagging cough or hoarseness.

Complications

The prognosis generally declines as the disease stage advances (with evidence of lymph node involvement or metastasis). If the condition goes untreated, the cancer cells continue to proliferate and eventually death results. ◑ Cardiac tamponade, pleural effusion, and paraneoplastic syndromes, which are all complications that can occur with various malignancies, are oncological emergencies.

Diagnostic Tests

Cancer screening is an important tool in the early detection and diagnosis of cancer. The following chart summarizes the American Cancer Society's screening recommendations for asymptomatic individuals of average risk.

Examination	Gender	Age	Frequency
Stool blood test	M/F	>49	Annually
Sigmoidoscopy	M/F	>49	Every 5 years
Colonoscopy	M/F	>49	Every 10 years
Barium enema	M/F	>49	Every 5 years
Digital rectal examination	M/F	>39	Annually
Prostate exam and prostate-specific antigen test	M	>49	Annually
Pap smear and pelvic exam	F	Sexually active or by age 21*	Annually
Endometrial tissue sample	F	Menopause or high-risk individual†	Menopause

Breast self-examination	F	>19	Monthly
Clinical breast examination	F	>20-39	Every 3 years
		>39	Annually
Mammography	F	>39	Annually
Health counseling and cancer evaluation‡	M/F	20-40	Every 3 years
		>40	Annually

*Women over age 30 with three normal Pap smears in a row may go to an every 2- to 3-year schedule; women over 70 with three normal smears in 10 years may choose to cease Pap smears. Pap smear after hysterectomy and removal of cervix is not necessary unless removal is because of cervical cancer.

†History of infertility, obesity, failure to ovulate, abnormal uterine bleeding, or estrogen therapy

‡Counseling on use of tobacco, sun exposure, diet, risk factors, sexual practices, and environmental and occupational exposures

If screening techniques and the clinical evaluation indicate the possibility of cancer, a definitive diagnosis is made through histopathological evaluation of tissue obtained by aspiration cytological techniques or by excisional, endoscopic, or bone marrow biopsy. If an unequivocal diagnosis is made, staging is done for prognostic information and to guide treatment decisions. A comprehensive system known as the TNM system has been developed. It involves assessment of three basic components: the size of the primary tumor (T); whether regional lymph nodes (N) are involved; and whether distant metastases (M) are present.

Therapeutic Management

Surgery	Removal of primary tumor with or without lymph nodes and adjacent structures; palliative procedures to relieve symptoms
Medications	Chemotherapeutic agents, hormones to reduce size of tumor and induce remission; immunotherapy or biological response modifiers to strengthen immune function
General	Radiation therapy to reduce size of tumor and check metastasis; bone marrow transplant

See the following:

Bladder Cancer
Bone Cancer, Primary
Brain Tumor, Primary
Breast Cancer
Cervical Cancer
Colorectal Cancer
Esophageal Cancer
Hodgkin's Disease
Kaposi's Sarcoma
Kidney Cancer
  (Renal Cancer)
Leukemia
Liver Cancer, Primary

Lung Cancer
Lymphoma, Non-Hodgkin's
Multiple Myeloma
Oral and Oropharyngeal Cancer
Ovarian Cancer
Pancreatic Cancer
Prostate Cancer
Skin Cancer
Stomach Cancer (Gastric Cancer)
Testicular Cancer
Thyroid Cancer
Uterine Cancer (Endometrial
  Cancer)

Cardiac Tamponade Ⓘ

A collection of blood or fluid in the pericardial sac causing compression of the heart and decreased cardiac output that may be acute or chronic in nature

Etiology and Incidence

Acute tamponade is caused by blunt or penetrating chest trauma, aortic dissection, myocardial rupture from use of thrombolytics or heparin, open-heart surgery, and central line or pacemaker insertions. Chronic causes are usually associated with underlying disease, such as metastatic cancer, pericarditis, uremia, tuberculosis (TB), scleroderma, rheumatoid arthritis, and myxedema. It may also be caused by external beam radiation to the chest area. The incidence is rare.

Pathophysiology

Normally the pericardial sac holds 30 to 50 ml of fluid. In cardiac tamponade, fluid or blood fills the pericardial space, causing compression and pressure on the heart. As the blood or fluid accumulates, the excessive extracardiac volume restricts blood flow in and out of the ventricles, causing decreased cardiac output and eventual systemic cardiac compromise.

Risk Factors

Blunt or penetrating trauma to the chest or heart

Underlying disease (cancer, pericarditis, uremia, TB, scleroderma, rheumatoid arthritis, and myxedema)

Medical/surgical procedures (thrombolysis, heart surgery, central venous catheter [CVC] insertion, pacemakers, radiation)

Clinical Manifestations

General	Anxiety, restlessness, and feeling of fullness in the chest; change in mental alertness; decreasing chest tube drainage after cardiac surgery
Cardiovascular	Muffled and distant heart sounds, tachycardia, decreasing blood pressure or pulses; pulses paradoxus, narrowed pulse pressure, jugular venous distention,

	elevated central venous pressure (CVP), and shock.
Respiratory	Dyspnea, shortness of breath

Complications

🔵 Cardiopulmonary arrest and death

Diagnostic Tests

History and clinical evaluation are diagnostic for therapeutic intervention of this life-threatening condition. An echocardiogram or right-sided cardiac catheterization may be used to support the diagnosis.

Therapeutic Management

Surgery	Subxiphoid pericardial draining with catheter placement; limited or total pericardiectomy to drain fluid; thoracotomy is definitive surgical treatment to correct the underlying problem
Medications	Treat underlying cause; avoid drugs that reduce cardiac preload and exacerbate tamponade (e.g., nitrates, diuretics); vasopressors for hemodynamic support
General	🔵 *Emergency intervention:* Immediate needle aspiration of pericardial fluid or blood (pericardiocentesis) to rapidly decompress the pericardial space; IV volume expanders; cardiac monitoring, especially during pericardiocentesis

Cardiomyopathy

C

Any structural or functional abnormality of the myocardium that results in enlargement or ventricular dysfunction and is not attributable to pressure or volume overload or to segmental loss of muscle function secondary to ischemia. The three major classifications are: *dilated* (congestive) cardiomyopathy, *hypertrophic* cardiomyopathy, and *restrictive* cardiomyopathy.

Etiology and Incidence

Cardiomyopathy is idiopathic in origin. However, underlying disease processes and factors may produce symptoms of cardiac involvement that simulate cardiomyopathy and as such are important to consider.

Dilated: Coronary artery disease (CAD); infections; granulomatous diseases; metabolic disorders; neoplasms; connective tissue disorders; hereditary autosomal dominant disorders; pregnancy; drugs and toxins (including alcohol, cocaine, psychotherapeutic drugs, cobalt, and radiation)

Hypertrophic: Familial (gene mapped to chromosome 14q), pheochromocytoma, acromegaly, neurofibromatosis

Restrictive: Amyloidosis, fibroelastosis, systemic sclerosis, hemochromatosis, Gaucher's disease or Löffler's disease, neoplasms

More than 400,000 new cases of cardiomyopathy are diagnosed each year, and it is estimated that 2 million to 3 million persons in the United States suffer from cardiomyopathy. The vast majority (greater than 90%) of these cases are classified as dilated and occur in older adults. Congenitally acquired cardiomyopathy presents in young patients and is the most common genetic cardiovascular disease.

Pathophysiology

Dilated cardiomyopathies are characterized by abnormal systolic pump function, gross dilation of the heart, and damage to the myofibrils. The cardiac valves and coronary arteries remain grossly normal.

Hypertrophic cardiomyopathies are characterized by disordered diastolic function and reduced distensibility, and a marked pattern of hypertrophy involving a thickened interventricular septum and a reduced ventricular cavity size. Rigid ventricular walls impede blood flow to left atrium and ventricular ejection.

Restrictive cardiomyopathy is marked by abnormal diastolic filling and excessively rigid ventricular walls. Contractility is relatively unimpaired, and systolic emptying is normal.

Clinical Manifestations

Dilated Type	Exertional dyspnea, fatigue, peripheral edema, neck vein distention, rapid pulse, narrowed pulse pressure, and crackles (symptoms usually are chronic)
Hypertrophic Type	Chest pain, syncope, palpitations, exertional dyspnea, fatigue
Restrictive Type	Exertional dyspnea, fatigue, edema, narrowed pulse pressure, distended neck veins

Complications

Complications include mural thrombus formation, pulmonary embolus, severe heart failure, and sudden death. The prognosis is poor in all categories of disease.

Diagnostic Tests

Chest X-ray	*Dilated:* Enlarged cardiac silhouette, pleural effusion *Hypertrophic:* No enlargement *Restrictive:* No or mild cardiac enlargement
Electrocardiography	*Dilated:* Sinus tachycardia, atrial and ventricular dysrhythmias, ST segment and T-wave changes, conduction disturbances *Hypertrophic:* Left ventricular (LV) hypertrophy, ST segment, and T-wave changes; deep septal Q-waves, atrial and ventricular dysrhythmias *Restrictive:* Low voltage; conduction disturbances
Echocardiography	*Dilated:* LV dilation, abnormal diastolic mitral valve motion, decreased ejection fraction *Hypertrophic:* Narrow LV outflow tract, thickened septum, systolic anterior motion of mitral valve, decreased LV chamber *Restrictive:* Increased LV thickness and mass, pericardial effusion
Radionuclide Studies	*Dilated:* LV dilation, hypokinesis, reduced ejection fraction

	Hypertrophic: Hyperdynamic systolic function, reduced LV volume, increased muscle mass, ischemia
	Restrictive: Myocardial infiltration
Cardiac Catheterization	*Dilated:* LV enlargement and dysfunction, mitral and tricuspid regurgitation, elevated diastolic filling pressures, reduced cardiac output
	Hypertrophic: Decreased LV compliance, mitral regurgitation, hyperdynamic systolic function, LV outflow obstruction
	Restrictive: Decreased LV compliance, elevated diastolic filling pressures, normal systolic function

Therapeutic Management

Surgery	*Dilated:* Cardiac transplantation; implantation of ventricular assist device
	Hypertrophic: Myotomy, myomectomy; selective septal infarction; pacemaker implantation
	Restrictive: Excision of fibrotic endocardium
Medications	*Dilated:* Symptoms direct intervention (e.g., angiotensin-converting enzyme (ACE) inhibitors, beta-blockers, diuretics, digitalis, with congestive heart failure, anticoagulants to prevent mural thrombus formation, antidysrhythmics for dysrhythmias)
	Hypertrophic: Beta-adrenergic blockers and calcium antagonists to decrease ventricular contractility and increase ventricular volume and outflow. Antiinfectives as prophylaxis against endocarditis if mitral valve regurgitation is present,
	Restrictive: Drugs to treat underlying disorders
General	Hemodynamic or cardiac monitoring, cardioversion for atrial fibrillation, intraaortic balloon pump to sustain severely depressed ventricular function, restriction of fluid and sodium intake, oxygen therapy, rest, exercise restrictions

Carpal Tunnel Syndrome

Tingling sensation and decreased functioning in the wrist, hand, and fingers resulting from compression of the median nerve

Etiology and Incidence

The exact cause is unknown, but highly repetitive flexing motions of the wrist are thought to cause swelling and thickening of the protective tendon sheaths, which causes increased pressure to the median nerve. Conditions that cause edema (e.g., diabetes, pregnancy, congestive heart failure, and renal failure) also have been suggested as causes. The incidence of carpal tunnel syndrome has increased dramatically over the past decade; it is one of the three leading occupation-related conditions in the United States and occurs most often in women.

Pathophysiology

The median nerve in the volar aspect of the wrist is compressed between the longitudinal tendons of the forearm muscles that flex the hand and transverse superficial carpal ligament. This causes paresthesias in the thumb, forefinger, middle finger, and half of the ring finger.

Clinical Manifestations

Pain, weakness, clumsiness, heaviness, numbness, burning, and tingling in one or both hands are the usual manifestations. The pain may be worse at night and lessen during the day unless the person's activities necessitate repetitive wrist flexion. The pain may radiate to the shoulder and forearm.

Complications

If left untreated, carpal tunnel syndrome can cause permanent nerve damage with loss of sensation, movement, and function of the hand.

Diagnostic Tests

Clinical evaluation with characteristic signs such as inability to make a fist; positive Tinel's sign (tingling and burning produced by light tapping over the tendon sheath on the ventral surface of the wrist); positive Phalen's sign (pain or numbness after 30 seconds of wrist flexion); wasting around fingernails; history of repetitive use; underlying disease; last trimester of pregnancy; electromyography and nerve conduction studies may detect weakness and conduction defects; wrist x-rays may detect associated abnormalities

Therapeutic Management

Surgery	Release of carpal ligament for decompression of nerve if conservative measures are ineffective
Medications	Nonsteroidal antiinflammatory drugs (NSAIDs), oral corticosteroids, local corticosteroid injections into tendon sheath to reduce inflammation
General	Restriction of repetitive wrist flexion; cock-up splints at night to reduce nerve pressure and relieve pain
Prevention/ Promotion	Relieve awkward wrist positions, repetitive hand movements, and hand tool vibrations in the workplace. Modify workstation layouts, rotate workers among jobs, alternate work and break cycles; redesign tools and tool handles
Education	Workplace training programs to increase worker awareness of prevention methods and symptoms of the syndrome

Cataract

A congenital or degenerative opacity of the lens that leads to a gradual loss of vision

Etiology and Incidence

Cataracts are associated primarily with aging (senile cataracts) and chemical changes in lens proteins. Trauma, toxins, systemic disease, and intraocular inflammation are also causes. Congenital cataracts, which are rare, are the result of inborn errors of metabolism, exposure of a first-trimester fetus to rubella or toxins, and congenital anomalies. Cataracts are the third leading cause of blindness in the United States, and cataracts would develop in virtually everyone if they lived long enough. More than 50% of those over age 65 and 90% of those over age 85 demonstrate lens opacities.

Pathophysiology

Senile cataracts form as a result of a chemical change in the gelatinous lens protein encapsulated behind the iris. As a result, the protein coagulates, the lens gradually clouds, and normal lens fibers swell and migrate within the lens. Because of these changes, a blurred image is cast on the retina. If the condition goes untreated, the opacity eventually becomes complete and blindness results.

Clinical Manifestations

Symptoms include progressive, painless blurring and distortion of objects, glare from bright lights, and gradual loss of vision. Signs include a gray or white coloring on the pupil and myopia.

Complications

The primary complication is blindness.

Diagnostic Tests

Cataracts are identified by ophthalmoscopic or slit lamp examination.

Therapeutic Management

Surgery	Intracapsular (rare) or extracapsular removal of the lens; follow-up laser surgery to remove secondary membrane that often forms
Medications	Topical antiinfective drugs, mydriatic-cycloplegics, and hyperosmotic agents are used preoperatively; corticosteroids and mydriatics are used postoperatively
General	Corrective lenses, lens implants, and eyeglasses to correct farsightedness

Cellulitis

A diffuse, spreading, acute inflammation and infection of the skin and subcutaneous tissue

Etiology and Incidence

The most common cause of cellulitis is infection with *Streptococcus pyogenes* or *Staphylococcus aureus* after a break in the skin. It also can be caused by infection of gram-negative bacilli associated with diabetic foot ulcers or various bacteria introduced by animal or insect bites. Cellulitis is seen most frequently in people with diabetes, in people with venous or lymphatic compromise, or in immunocompromised hosts.

Pathophysiology

A break in the skin caused by trauma, ulceration, or lymphedema is invaded by a pathogen, setting up an inflammatory and infectious process. The infection spreads because the pathogen produces enzymes capable of breaking down the cellular components that usually wall off and contain the inflammation.

Clinical Manifestations

Local redness, swelling, and tenderness—usually of the lower extremities—are the most common presenting symptoms. The skin is hot to the touch and may have an orange peel–like appearance and texture. Red streaks may extend from indistinct borders, and purulent discharge may be present. Occasionally, systemic manifestations develop, such as chills, fever, headache, and tachycardia.

Complications

Rare complications include severe necrotizing subcutaneous infection with gangrene and permanent damage to the lymphatic system.

Diagnostic Tests

The diagnosis is made by clinical evaluation.

Therapeutic Management

Surgery	Incision and drainage of abscesses; debridement of necrotic tissue
Medications	Antiinfective drugs to treat infection; analgesics for pain
General	Immobilization and elevation of affected area to reduce edema; cool, wet dressings to relieve pain

Cerebral (Intracranial) Aneurysm

A localized dilation, bulging, or ballooning of the wall of an artery in the brain. Aneurysms are classified as saccular (berry), fusiform, or mycotic.

Etiology and Incidence

Cerebral aneurysms come from congenital defects in the vessel wall coupled with secondary factors such as atherosclerosis, head trauma, arterial hypertension, infection, and polycystic disease. They are the fourth leading cerebrovascular disorder in the United States, with 24,000 new cases diagnosed annually. The peak incidence is between ages 35 and 60, and women are affected slightly more often than men. More than 95% of ruptured aneurysms are saccular.

Pathophysiology

Saccular aneurysms are small, berrylike sacs that protrude outward in a pouch formation on cerebral arteries, primarily at bifurcations or branches of major arteries in the circle of Willis. A weakness in the vessel wall allows the intima to bulge outward, creating a sac that fills with blood to the point of rupture. Rupture occurs when pulse pressure creates a hole in the sac, leading to subarachnoid hemorrhage and irritation of the cranial nerves and underlying cortex. The damage depends on the severity of bleeding.

A *fusiform aneurysm* involves the entire circumference of the artery. It develops over time as the elastic fibers undergo degenerative changes, smooth muscle is replaced by fibrous tissue, and cholesterol deposits build up on the intima. These aneurysms usually form at the trunk of the basilar artery and rarely rupture.

Mycotic aneurysms, which are rare, occur as a result of a systemic infectious process that causes arterial necrosis and leads to the formation of multiple aneurysms along the distal branches of the anterior or middle cerebral arteries.

Risk Factors

Family history

History of autosomal dominant polycystic kidney disease or aneurysmal subarachnoid hemorrhage

Intracranial neoplasm
Cigarette smoking
Cocaine, alcohol use
Use of contraceptives
Head trauma

Clinical Manifestations

Most aneurysms cause no symptoms until they rupture. At that point, typical symptoms include severe, abrupt-onset headache; stiff neck; nausea; vomiting; steadily increasing neurological deficits; seizures; and loss of consciousness. The extent of the symptoms depends on the location of the aneurysm and the severity of the bleeding. Ruptures are divided into five grades. Grade I ruptures involve minimal bleeding, no neurological deficit, and no loss of consciousness. The person is alert, and the only symptoms may be a slight headache and a stiff neck. Grade II ruptures involve mild bleeding, and the person displays mild neurological deficits (e.g., weakness) in addition to headache and nuchal rigidity. With grade III (moderate) bleeding, the person is confused or drowsy (or both) and has a severe headache, nuchal rigidity, and mild focal neurological deficits. Grade IV (severe) bleeding produces stupor, mild hemiparesis, and possibly decerebrate posturing. Grade V bleeding produces coma and decerebrate posturing.

Complications

Rupture often leads to residual neurological deficits, a permanent vegetative state, or death.

Diagnostic Tests

CT Scan/ MRI	To detect blood in subarachnoid space and displaced cerebral structures
Angiography	To determine whether aneurysm is intact
Lumbar Puncture	**Contraindicated** with any sign of increased intracranial pressure (ICP)
Skull X-rays	Calcification of aneurysm wall
EEG	Shifts in cerebral structures

Therapeutic Management

Surgery	Resection, clipping, ligating, or wrapping of intact or remaining aneurysm after bleeding; ventriculostomy to treat increased ICP; ventriculoatrial shunt to treat hydrocephalus; evacuation of blood clots; endovascular placement of microwire coil to occlude aneurysm.
Medications	Anticonvulsants to control seizures, antihypertensives to control elevated blood pressure, corticosteroids to reduce cerebral edema; drugs such as calcium channel blockers to control vasospasms, stool softeners to prevent constipation and straining that can increase ICP, analgesics for pain, chlorpromazine for shivering, antifibrinolytic agents to prevent bleeding in individuals who are not candidates for surgery
General	Ventilatory support; seizure precautions; antiembolic stockings; monitoring of neurological, cardiovascular, and hemodynamic systems; safety precautions; prevention of disuse syndrome; rehabilitation for residual neurological deficits or coma stimulation; instruction in how to avoid straining at stool
Prevention/ Promotion	Magnetic resonance angiography sometimes employed in high risk populations (autosomal dominant polycystic kidney disease; aneurysmal subarachnoid hemorrhage; two or more family members with aneurysm) Smoking cessation Treatment for alcohol or cocaine abuse

Cerebral Palsy (CP) (Congenital Static Encephalopathy)

A broad classification encompassing nonprogressive motor disorders caused by prenatal, perinatal, or postnatal central nervous system damage and characterized by impaired voluntary movement and possible perceptual, intellectual, and language deficits, and convulsive seizures. The four major categories of CP are spastic, dyskinetic, ataxic, and mixed CP.

Etiology and Incidence

A variety of prenatal, perinatal, and postnatal factors, alone or together, contribute to the development of CP. Prenatal causes, which are implicated in 44% of cases, include genetic factors, chromosomal abnormalities, teratogens, malformations in the brain, intrauterine infection, and fetal or placental transport malfunction. Perinatal causes (27% of cases) include prematurity, preeclampsia, sepsis, birth trauma, and asphyxia. Postnatal causes (5% of cases) include meningitis, head injury, and toxins. The cause is unknown or not readily apparent in 24% of diagnosed cases.

Among infants and children in the United States, the incidence of CP is about 2 in 1000. CP is the most common cause of permanent disability in children, and the incidence is rising.

Pathophysiology

CP has no characteristic pathological picture. Neurological damage varies widely and is manifested in a number of ways. Anoxia seems to play a major role, but that role is ill defined. Spastic syndromes (70% of cases) involve the upper motor neurons. Dyskinetic syndromes (20% of cases) involve the basal ganglia. Ataxic syndromes (10% of cases) involve the cerebellum or cerebellar pathways, or both.

Clinical Manifestations

Clinical signs and symptoms evolve as the damaged nervous system matures. The signs and symptoms vary according to the location and severity of the neurological damage.

General	Gross motor delays, abnormal motor performance, alteration of muscle tone, poor head and trunk control, poor balance, excessive docility or irritability, persistence of primitive reflexes
Spastic Type	Weakness, paralysis, muscle wasting, and spasticity involving one to four limbs; scissors gait; toe walking; weakness of oral and lingual muscles with dysarthria; tongue thrusting; difficulty swallowing; abnormal posture; sudden rigid extension of body while sitting; opisthotonic posturing
Dyskinetic Type	Slow, involuntary writhing movements of the trunk, mouth, and limbs that increase with stress and cease during sleep; abrupt, jerky movements of distal extremities; severe dysarthria; drooling; choking and coughing while feeding
Ataxic Type	Weakness; incoordination; intention tremor; wide-based, ataxic gait; rapid, repetitive movements; disintegration of movement in upper extremities when reaching
Associated Problems	Intellectual, auditory, and visual impairments; language deficits; seizures; hyperactivity; short attention span

Complications

Aspiration and aspiration pneumonia may occur because of swallowing and choking with feeding. Hip dislocations, scoliosis, and joint contractures may occur because of hypertonicity or tone imbalance. Dental problems (e.g., malocclusion, gingivitis, caries, enamel defects) occur secondary to drooling, spasticity, and inadequate oral hygiene. Constipation is common. Skin breakdown and pathological fractures can result from disuse syndrome.

Diagnostic Tests

Because the clinical signs of CP emerge as the neurological system matures, it is rarely possible to detect CP in early infancy. Specific categorization of the syndrome may be impossible before age 2, and other progressive neurological disorders must be ruled out. A thorough neurological examination and history are the primary diagnostic tools in CP. Gross motor delays; motor abnormalities; and altered muscle size, function, and tone are crucial diagnostic indicators. Moro reflex persisting after the age of 4 months and tonic neck reflex persisting after the age of 6 months are also useful indicators. High-risk children should be monitored closely.

Therapeutic Management

Surgery	Correction of hip displacement, release of contractures, lengthening of heel cord to prevent tiptoe stance, spinal instrumentation for scoliosis, implantation of intrathecal pump to deliver medication for spasticity, dorsal rhizotomy (rare) to control spasticity; gastrostomy to facilitate feeding
Medications	Muscle relaxants and antianxiety agents to reduce spasticity and facilitate movement, anticonvulsants for seizure activity, stool softeners or suppositories for constipation
General	Long-term medical monitoring by neurologists, orthopedists, and pediatricians
	Physical therapy to reduce spasticity; maintain ROM; prevent contractures; promote head and trunk control; and improve balance, sitting, standing, and ambulation
	Occupational therapy to improve oral motor skills (sucking, chewing, swallowing) and facilitate activities of daily living (ADLs)
	Speech therapy to improve language and communication skills
	Adaptive equipment to assist mobility (wheelchairs, braces, scooter boards, standers); communication (communication boards, computers, switch controllers, power pads); recreation (adapted toys); and ADLs (bath aids, environmental control units, feeding aids)
	Counseling for child and family to adapt to disability

	Education under provisions of the Americans with Disabilities Act (ADA)
	Case management to provide support and to coordinate efforts by health care team
	Respite care to aid primary caregiver
Prevention/ Promotion	Careful monitoring during pregnancy; use of ultrasound; avoidance of alcohol and drugs; use of prenatal vitamins and iron supplements; sound management of labor and delivery
Education	Long-term family support with access to ongoing resource materials such as those available from United Cerebral Palsy Association

Cerebrovascular Accident (CVA) (Stroke)

C

Impairment of one or more vessels in the cerebral circulation caused by thrombosis, embolus, stenosis, or hemorrhage, which interrupts the blood supply and results in ischemia of brain tissue

Etiology and Incidence

Seventy to 80% of CVAs are caused by occlusion of a cerebral vessel, and 20% to 30% are hemorrhagic. Most occlusions occur secondary to atherosclerosis or hypertension (HTN), or a combination of the two. Other risk factors are diabetes mellitus, myocardial infarction (MI), bacterial endocarditis, rheumatic heart disease, aneurysms, head trauma, sick sinus syndrome, and a history of previous stroke or transient ischemic attacks (TIAs). CVA is the second most common cause of neurological disability and the third most common cause of death in the United States. More than 750,000 cases of CVA are diagnosed each year, and of those diagnosed there are more than 163,000 deaths. The incidence increases with age, with adults age 65 or older at greatest risk. Incidence is 30% higher in males.

Pathophysiology

The general pathophysiology of a CVA involves occlusion of a cerebral vessel, which leads to ischemia of the brain tissue supplied by that vessel. If the obstruction is not removed, the affected tissue infarcts and dies, causing permanent neurological deficit or death. The severity of the CVA depends on the location and extent of the obstruction, the degree of collateral circulation, and the promptness of diagnosis and treatment.

Thrombotic strokes account for approximately 40% of ischemic cerebrovascular disease. The occlusion develops slowly over time as the atherosclerotic plaque builds up in the large-vessel walls. A TIA is a common precursor. Symptoms often evolve over hours or even days and are noticed when the person awakens in the morning. Damage from a CVA is generally extensive because of the large vessels involved and the likelihood that collateral circulation is diminished or absent.

Emboli, which cause 30% of strokes, arise when platelets, cholesterol, fibrin, or other miscellaneous hematogenous material break off from the arterial walls or the heart and travel to and block a cerebral vessel. The onset of symptoms is generally sudden and usually occurs in small distal cortical vessels, affecting cortical functions.

Lacunar strokes, which account for 20% of all CVAs, occur where small perforating arterioles branch off large cerebral vessels in the basal ganglia, internal capsule, and brainstem. The small subcortical arterioles are exposed to the constant high-pressure flow of the large branch arteries. Over the years the smaller vessels become thickened, thrombosed, and then obstructed. The resulting damage is distinctive, and these strokes are often labeled "pure motor" or "pure sensory" strokes.

Intracerebral hemorrhage accounts for 10% of all strokes and is the most catastrophic type of stroke. The onset is sudden, often occurs during exertion, and is triggered by bleeding that obstructs and ruptures the small subcortical arterioles in the deep brain. The pathology of the bleeding is not well understood, although some research indicates that it may be precipitated by microaneurysms that cause arteriolar necrosis.

Risk Factors

History of TIA or recent MI

Underlying disease processes, such as HTN, diabetes, cardiovascular disease, blood dyscrasias

Personal history of previous CVA, aneurysm, rheumatic fever, or heart valve replacement

Familial history of arteriovenous malformation, premature vascular disease

Elevated serum cholesterol, lipoproteins, and/or triglycerides

Atrial fibrillation

Use of medications such as sympathomimetics or oral contraceptives

Use of tobacco products, cocaine

Clinical Manifestations

The signs and symptoms of a stroke depend on the site and size of the obstruction. They typically include altered mental status, hemiparesis or hemiplegia, receptive or expressive aphasia, dysarthria, dysphagia, apraxia, hemianopsia, urinary and/or bowel incontinence, and emotional lability. Headache, seizures, stupor, and marked HTN may also be present.

Complications

Coma and death are the most severe consequences of CVA. Permanent neurological deficits (e.g., paralysis, impaired intellectual capability, speech defects, loss of short-term memory, impaired judgment and problem-solving abilities, reduced impulse control) are common residual complications.

Diagnostic Tests

Clinical Evaluation	Any of the above clinical manifestations, particularly in individuals with identifiable risk factors, decreased carotid pulse, or carotid bruit
CT Scan/MRI	To identify area of infarct or bleeding and extent of injury
Ultrasonography	To identify diminished blood flow in vessels
Angiography	To detect occlusion of large vessels, aneurysm, or malformation
PET	To assess extent of tissue damage
EEG	To detect focal slowing around a lesion
Brain Scan	To detect diminished blood flow, infarction, blood clots, or arteriovenous malformation

Therapeutic Management

Surgery	Evacuation of hematoma or clot; placement of intracranial pressure (ICP) monitor; endarterectomy to remove atherosclerotic plaques; cerebral artery bypass surgery to increase blood flow to the brain; balloon angioplasty with intraarterial shunt to open stenosed vessels; extracranial-intracranial bypass for individuals with TIA
Medications	Thrombolytic enzymes, such as tissue plasminogen activator (TPA), streptokinase, or urokinase to break up the thrombus or

embolus and help restore blood flow to the brain

Drugs must be given within 4 (TPA) to 8 (urokinase) hours of the incident. These drugs are not used for hemorrhagic strokes.

Anticoagulants during stroke evolution to prevent further thrombosis; antihypertensives to control blood pressure; diuretics to reduce edema in the brain; anticonvulsants to control seizures; long-term aspirin, clopidogrel, or ticlopidine therapy to prevent future stroke

General　　Monitoring and support of vital functions; prevention of decubitus ulcers, thrombosis, and pneumonia; rehabilitation (e.g., occupational therapy for adapting activities of daily living (ADLs), physical therapy to increase strength, range of motion and endurance; gait training to improve ambulation; cognitive therapy to improve memory and problem solving; speech therapy to improve communication; counseling for poststroke depression and altered sexual functioning; vocational retraining; support groups for patient and family

Prevention/　Smoking cessation
Promotion　　Control of HTN, hyperlipidemia, diabetes

Regular exercise and nutritionally sound diet

Low-dose aspirin therapy for those at risk

Education　　Educate about warning signs of stroke (headache, dizziness, numbness, TIAs, visual disturbances)

Instruction to patient and caregiver related to home care (exercise regimens, dietary requirements, medication routines, medical and therapy follow-up, available support services)

Cervical Cancer

Cancer of the cervix, predominantly squamous cell carcinoma (90% of cases). The remaining 10% are adenocarcinomas and are thought to be related to in utero exposure to diethylstilbestrol.

Etiology and Incidence

Cervical cancer is now generally considered a sexually transmitted disease (STD). Probable agents are the human papilloma viruses, with the herpes simplex virus a possible co-factor. Cancer of the cervix is the third most common malignancy of the female reproductive tract, with more than 12,200 cases of invasive cervical cancer diagnosed annually in the United States. In addition, 65,000 cases of carcinoma in situ (preinvasive) are diagnosed each year. Incidence is higher in minority women (e.g., black, Hispanic, and Native American). More than 4,100 deaths from cervical cancer occur annually in the United States. Cervical cancer is the leading cause of cancer death in underdeveloped nations, particularly Latin America, Africa, India, and Eastern Europe.

Pathophysiology

Cervical cancer begins as a neoplastic change in the cervical epithelium and eventually involves the full thickness of the epithelium. An invasive tumor forms in a cauliflower shape, with a friable texture and a hard, nodular edge. The bladder, rectum, and lungs are common sites of invasion and metastasis.

Risk Factors

Onset of intercourse before age 20
Multiple sex partners
Teenage and/or multiple pregnancies
Smoking
History of genital warts or other STDs
History of immune deficiency disease

Clinical Manifestations

Cervical cancer has no characteristic or typical symptoms. Bleeding, which begins as a blood-tinged discharge and progresses to spotting and frank bleeding, is the only significant sign. The bleeding is caused by ulceration of the epithelial surface; however, some tumors spread without ulceration and thus without bleeding. Other possible indicators include prolonged menstrual periods or an increase in number of periods and bleeding immediately after intercourse.

Complications

The prognosis with carcinoma in situ and noninvasive tumors is excellent, with survival rates approaching 100%. The prognosis with advanced disease has been poor (5-year survival is 58%), and complications arise from spread to the bowel, bladder, and pelvis and metastasis to the lung. Recent clinical trials using a combination of chemotherapy and radiation in advanced disease have improved the 5-year survival rates to 73%.

Diagnostic Tests

If a Pap smear of the cervix reveals atypical cells, a definitive diagnosis is obtained by colposcopy or biopsy. Cervicography may aid in staging of the tumor.

Therapeutic Management

Surgery	Conization, cryotherapy, electrocautery, or laser ablation to treat carcinoma in situ; hysterectomy to treat tumors with no parametrial invasion; pelvic exenteration to treat advanced disease
Medications	Chemotherapy in combination with internal radiation for treatment of advanced disease
General	Combination of chemotherapy and radium implants to treat invasive disease and recurrences, external radiation as a palliative measure, counseling for body image and changes in sexual function
Prevention/ Promotion	Pap smear annually for early detection Safe sexual practices, including use of condoms

Chickenpox

An acute, viral, communicable disease characterized by clusters of maculopapular skin eruptions that become vesicular and produce a granular scab

Etiology and Incidence

The cause is the varicella-zoster virus, which invades the body through the respiratory membranes. Chickenpox is a common childhood illness, with susceptibility typically extending from the age of 6 months to the time the disease is contracted. Epidemics occur in the winter and early spring in 3- to 4-year cycles. Immunity is produced after a course of the disease. More than 100,000 cases are reported annually in the United States.

Pathophysiology

The virus enters the body by means of direct droplet contact through the respiratory system. The incubation period is 2 to 3 weeks before localized and systemic signs and symptoms appear. The person is considered infectious from the time of exposure until the final lesions crust over. After recovery, the virus is believed to remain in the body in a dormant or latent state in the dorsal root ganglia. Reactivation of the infection in adulthood manifests itself as shingles.

Clinical Manifestations

The first signs and symptoms are mild headache, low-grade fever, malaise, and anorexia, which occur about 24 hours before the first rash appears. The initial rash, which is maculopapular, appears on the head and mucous membranes and evolves within hours to itching, teardrop-shaped vesicles containing a clear fluid. The vesicles break and crust over within 6 to 8 hours. New lesions erupt in successive crops on the trunk and in sparse sprinkles on the extremities. The acute phase of the disease lasts 4 to 7 days, and new lesions seldom appear after the fifth day. All lesions are generally healed in 2 to 3 weeks.

Complications

The disease may be severe in adults, in individuals whose T-cell immunity is depressed, or in those who are taking corticosteroids or undergoing chemotherapy. Complications include conjunctival ulcers, encephalitis, meningitis, thrombocytopenia, secondary abscesses, cellulitis, pneumonia, sepsis, Guillain-Barré syndrome, and Reye's syndrome. Scratching of the lesions may cause scarring and disfigurement.

Diagnostic Tests

Diagnosis depends primarily on clinical evaluation of the characteristic lesions. Giemsa-stained scrapings from the lesions will show multinucleated giant cells, and a culture of vesicular fluid will grow the varicella-zoster virus.

Therapeutic Management

Surgery	None
Medications	Antihistamines, topical steroids to relieve itching; acyclovir at earliest signs of disease in healthy nonpregnant individuals; varicella-zoster immune globulin (VZIG) in infants in whom the disease develops; *no salicylates* (aspirin-containing drugs)
General	Baking soda paste or calamine lotion on lesions to relieve itching, isolation until lesions crust, trimming of nails and use of mittens to prevent scratching of lesions, cool room and distractions to lessen focus on itching
Prevention/ Promotion	Varicella vaccine after first birthday; vaccine recommended for all children and adults who have not had chickenpox and are not immunocompromised (protection lasts at least 6 years); VZIG for prevention in immunocompromised individuals

Chlamydia trachomatis Infections

C

A constellation of sexually transmitted infections comprising urethritis, cervicitis, salpingitis, and lymphogranuloma venereum

(See also Pelvic Inflammatory Disease and Sexually Transmitted Diseases.)

Etiology and Incidence

The cause is the *C. trachomatis* bacterium, which is transmitted during intercourse with an infected individual. Newborns of infected mothers may contract associated otitis, conjunctivitis, and pneumonia during passage through the birth canal. In countries with endemic areas, the disease can be spread through close contact within households. More than 4.5 million people in the United States contract chlamydial infections each year, and these infections are the most common source of sexually transmitted diseases (STDs) worldwide. Chlamydial infections also are the leading cause of infant blindness in underdeveloped countries.

Pathophysiology

After intimate contact with an infected individual, the *Chlamydia* bacterium attaches to and is then ingested by the columnar epithelial cells in various receptacle sites, where it multiplies in the host cell. Common sites are the urethra and prostate in men and the urethra and cervix in women. The rectum and pharynx are sites for both genders. Sites for infants and children include the conjunctiva and respiratory tract.

The pathogenesis after this point is unclear, but most likely an immune response is triggered, producing a patchy, inflammatory response in the submucosa. This is spread by the lymphatics to such sites as the epididymis in men and the fallopian tubes in women. Inflammatory exudate is eventually replaced by fibrous tissue, leading to strictures in the urethra, epididymis, and fallopian tubes and scarring of the conjunctivae.

Lymphogranuloma venereum produces a localized, nodular lesion that spreads regionally via the lymph system (primarily the inguinal nodes), producing other nodular lesions, which mat together and form large abscesses. If the condition is left untreated, abscesses form throughout the lymph system and often rupture through epithelial surfaces, creating draining sinuses and fistulas.

Risk Factors

Unprotected sexual contact (vaginal, anal, oral) with an infected partner

Multiple sex partners

Direct contact with mucous membranes of infected person

Vaginally delivered infants of infected mothers

Clinical Manifestations

Manifestations vary, depending on the mucous membrane initially involved and the infecting strain of *C. trachomatis.*

Urethritis/ Cervicitis	Often asymptomatic; urinary pain and frequency; scanty mucoid urethral discharge (men), mucopurulent vaginal discharge (women); pain in scrotum with epididymitis; flank tenderness with salpingitis
Lymphogranuloma	Early sign is lesion on penis, labia, vagina, cervix, or rectum; men then have lymphadenopathy; systemic signs include fever, chills, severe headache
Pharyngeal Infection	Asymptomatic or sore throat; red, dry tongue
Rectal Infection	Bloody diarrhea, purulent discharge
Trachoma and Conjunctivitis	Purulent discharge from eyes

Complications

Complications from untreated disease include urethral and rectal strictures, pelvic inflammatory disease, sterility, epididymitis, Reiter's disease, fistulas, elephantiasis, blindness, and pneumonia.

Diagnostic Tests

The primary diagnostic tools are a clinical evaluation, with a history of exposure to an infected partner or multiple partners, and a culture of infected cells (not purulent discharge) that tests positive for *C. trachomatis.* A simultaneous culture should be done for *Neisseria gonorrhoeae.* Less expensive and easier to perform nonculture tests are now available and include enzyme immunoassay, direct fluorescent antibody, and deoxyribonucleic acid (DNA) amplification.

Therapeutic Management

Surgery	None
Medications	Antiinfective drugs sensitive to *C. trachomatis* following treatment guidelines for type and dosage issued by the Centers for Disease Control and Prevention (CDC)
General	Reculture and/or retest after therapy completion; trace all potentially exposed sex partners
Prevention/ Promotion	Screen of high-risk populations to treat infected individuals and reduce the reservoir
Education	Caution patient to refrain from sexual activity until he or she is free of disease; information about STDs; safe sex practices such as condom use

Cholecystitis, Cholelithiasis, and Choledocholithiasis

Acute or chronic inflammation of the gallbladder (cholecystitis) usually associated (95%) with gallstones (cholelithiasis), which lodge in the cystic duct. Choledocholithiasis is the obstruction of the common bile duct by gallstones.

Etiology and Incidence

Chronic cholecystitis is caused by repeated acute episodes. The cause of cholelithiasis is not clear, although abnormal metabolism of cholesterol and bile salts plays a crucial role. Most cases of acute cholecystitis (95%) are caused by gallstones lodged in the cystic duct. Five percent of cases are associated with trauma, burns, infection, prolonged anesthesia, or critical illness. Choledocholithiasis results when gallstones lodge in the common bile duct.

An estimated 35 million people in the United States have cholelithiasis, and 1 million new cases are diagnosed each year. Gallstones occur more often in women and in certain ethnic groups, such as Native Americans. The incidence increases with age.

Pathophysiology

Gallstone formation begins with supersaturation of bile with an insoluble solute, such as cholesterol or calcium bilirubinate. Rapid precipitation of cholesterol crystals occurs through some as-yet-unexplained process involving mucin glycoproteins. The precipitates grow under static conditions (i.e., reduced gallbladder motility or contractility) and form macroscopic stones. When the stone obstructs a cystic duct, the gallbladder distends and the wall becomes edematous and compresses capillaries and lymphatic channels, producing inflammation of the mucosa. The inflamed, ischemic mucosa allows reabsorption of bile salts, which sets up further damage. If the condition goes unchecked, the wall becomes friable and necrotic and is susceptible to perforation. When a stone obstructs the common bile duct, it often causes extrahepatic obstructive jaundice, infection, pancreatitis, or liver disease.

Risk Factors

Native American, Asian American, or African American population

Female

Obesity

Rapid weight loss

Lack of exercise

Underlying disease processes such as diabetes mellitus, regional enteritis, acquired immunodeficiency syndrome (AIDS), or blood dyscrasias

Use of medications such as birth control, estrogen supplements, and/or cholesterol-lowering drugs

Multiple pregnancies

Familial history of gallbladder disease

Clinical Manifestations

Acute Cholecystitis	Colicky pain in right upper quadrant and right lower scapula; nausea, vomiting; low-grade fever
Chronic Cholecystitis	Anorexia, flatulence, nausea, fat intolerance, episodic or diffuse abdominal pain, heartburn
Cholelithiasis	Asymptomatic in 80% of people
Choledocholithiasis	Asymptomatic; jaundice and pain

Complications

Necrosis and perforation of the gallbladder with generalized peritonitis, cholangitis with or without septic shock, pancreatitis, biliary cirrhosis, and bowel obstruction with perforation and peritonitis are all complications of biliary disease.

Diagnostic Tests

Ultrasonography	To visualize gallstones
Endoscopic Retrograde Cholangiopancreatography (ERCP)	Visualization of gallbladder, cystic duct, common hepatic duct, and bile ducts; obtain bile cultures
Biliary Scintigraphy	If common bile duct is obstructed, gallbladder cannot be visualized on scan

Transhepatic Cholangiography	To visualize stones in common bile duct

Therapeutic Management

Surgery	Laparoscopic cholecystectomy to remove gallbladder, endoscopic procedure to remove stones by balloon or basket, ERCP with or without stent placements or sphincterotomy to extract ductal stones, laparotomy with cholecystectomy and T-tube placement in some cases when other methods are not appropriate
Medications	Oral ursodiol to dissolve stone; methyl terbutyl ether instilled directly into gallbladder via percutaneous transhepatic catheter to dissolve stone; antiinfective drugs; analgesics; anticholinergics and/or antispasmodics; fat-soluble vitamins and bile salts
General	Lithotripsy delivers external shock waves to pulverize stones; diet low in polyunsaturated fats after treatment
Prevention/ Promotion	Avoid polyunsaturated fats in diet; exercise program; maintain normal weight (any weight loss needs to be slow to prevent sludgy bile)
Education	Instructions that stones can recur and medical follow-up necessary

Chronic Fatigue Syndrome
(Immune Dysfunction Syndrome)

A poorly understood illness characterized by pervasive, chronic, and incapacitating fatigue

Etiology and Incidence

The etiology is unknown, although popular theories propose a viral link and/or an overactive immune system. Prevalence in the United States is 100 to 300 per 100,000 people and occurs most frequently in young and middle-aged adults. The syndrome is diagnosed in women twice as often as in men. Cases are increasingly diagnosed in children.

Moderate to complete recovery occurs in 22% to 60% of patients within a year.

Pathophysiology

The cause is unknown, but a viral infection (e.g., herpesvirus, retrovirus, or enterovirus) in interaction with a dysfunctional immune response is suspected.

Clinical Manifestations

The primary symptom is persistent or relapsing debilitating fatigue that does not respond to bed rest and reduces normal activity levels by 50% or more for 6 months or longer. Other signs and symptoms include low-grade fever; sore throat; pharyngitis; painful, palpable cervical or axillary lymph nodes; myalgia; arthralgia; sleep disturbances; depression; and inability to concentrate.

Complications

None known

Diagnostic Tests

No definitive tests exist. The Centers for Disease Control and Prevention (CDC) has set forth the following criteria:

Major—unexplained, persistent, or relapsing chronic fatigue; fatigue is not because of ongoing exertion, unsubstantially relieved by rest, and results in substantial reduction of normal function.

Minor—substantial short-term memory impairment/loss of concentration; sore throat; tender cervical/axillary lymph nodes; muscle pain; multijoint pain without swelling or tenderness; new headaches; unrefreshing sleep; postexertional malaise more than 24 hours.

Diagnosis is based on inclusion of all major criteria and four or more minor criteria that have persisted or recurred for 6 consecutive months. Fibromyalgia or rheumatologic conditions may coexist with chronic fatigue. Tests to rule out other disorders (e.g., leukemia, lymphoma, or underlying psychiatric disorders) are important.

Therapeutic Management

Surgery	None
Medications	Nonsteroidal antiinflammatory drugs (NSAIDs) for headache, fever, muscle and/or joint aches; selective serotonin reuptake inhibitor (SSRI) antidepressants for mood and sleep disturbances
General	Supportive measures, balanced regimen of exercise and rest cycles, counseling for depression, support groups
Prevention/ Promotion	Carefully graduated exercise program to preserve strength and improve symptoms
Education	Education to develop reasonable goals and expectations about long-term functional abilities

Chronic Obstructive Pulmonary Disease (COPD)

An umbrella term encompassing a cluster of diseases, including bronchitis, bronchiectasis, and emphysema in which recurrent obstruction of airflow is a prominent feature.

(See also Bronchiectasis; Bronchitis, Acute; Bronchitis, Chronic; and Emphysema.)

Etiology and Incidence

Causes are discussed under the specific disease processes; however, smoking, air pollution, and industrial exposure are major risk factors. More than 15 million persons in the United States are estimated to have some type of COPD. This disease constellation is the fourth leading cause of death in the United States with more than 124,000 deaths reported annually.

Risk Factors

Use of or exposure to tobacco products
Occupational exposure to pulmonary toxins such as cadmium
Atmospheric pollution
Recurring respiratory infection
Alpha-1-antitrypsin deficiency (seen in rare form of hereditary emphysema)

For **Pathophysiology, Clinical Manifestations, Diagnostic Tests,** and **Therapeutic Management,** see the specific disease.

Cirrhosis

A chronic, degenerative disease of the liver characterized by destruction of the hepatic parenchymal cells, which are replaced by regenerative nodules surrounded by fibrotic tissue

(See also Esophageal Varices)

Etiology and Incidence

The etiology is not fully understood, but several factors play important roles, including alcohol abuse; malnutrition; infectious processes (e.g., hepatitis, schistosomiasis, syphilis); toxins (e.g., arsenic, carbon tetrachloride, phosphorus); drugs (e.g., chlorpromazine, methyldopa, methotrexate, tolbutamide, isoniazid, amitriptyline); genetic disorders (e.g., galactosemia, Wilson's disease, alpha-antitrypsin deficiency); congenital malformations (e.g., biliary atresia); and vascular disorders (e.g., portal vein thrombosis, Budd-Chiari syndrome, chronic heart failure). Other factors remain unknown.

In the United States, most cirrhosis develops secondary to alcohol abuse and is the twelfth leading cause of death, with more than 26,500 deaths reported annually. Hepatitis C infections are causing a rapid increase in cirrhosis incidence. In Africa and Asia, cirrhosis secondary to chronic viral hepatitis B is a major cause of death.

Pathophysiology

Cirrhosis is the end-stage disease that begins with one of the many etiological factors. The development and progression of cirrhosis are tied to the severity of the injury and the liver's response. A severe, acute injury may be involved, as in hepatitis, or a moderate chronic injury may be the cause, as in alcohol abuse. When an injury causes destruction of parenchymal cells, the initial response is fibrosis, as the liver attempts to repair itself. Fat-storing cells proliferate and are transformed into myofibroblasts, which alter the secretion, synthesis, and degradation of collagen. This results in deposition of excessive connective tissue, which alters normal lobular structures, interferes with cellular nutrition, obstructs hepatic blood flow, and forms anastomotic channels that shunt arterial blood away to efferent hepatic veins. The regenerative attempts continue as long as an injury is present. The resulting changes in the intrahepatic circulatory pathways make the system less efficient and eventually lead to an increase in portal vein pressure. The change in or destruction of lobular architecture interferes with various liver functions, such as metabolism, detoxification, storage, and blood and bile formation.

Risk Factors

Excessive chronic alcohol ingestion
Malnutrition
History of infectious diseases (e.g., hepatitis, schistosomiasis, syphilis); biliary disease; vascular disorders (e.g., portal vein thrombosis, Budd-Chiari syndrome, chronic heart failure) genetic disorders (e.g., galactosemia, Wilson's disease, alpha-antitrypsin deficiency)
Use of hepatotoxic drugs
Exposure to hepatotoxic chemicals or toxins

Clinical Manifestations

Early	Often asymptomatic; otherwise, abdominal pain, diarrhea, nausea, vomiting, fatigue, fever
Midcourse	Chronic dyspepsia, constipation, anorexia, weight loss, pruritus, easy bruising, bleeding gums, nosebleeds, upper gastrointestinal bleeding, enlarged liver
Late	Telangiectasis, spider angiomas, enlarged breasts, testicular atrophy, jaundice, impotence, enlarged spleen, depression, abdominal vein distention, ascites, encephalopathy, peripheral neuropathy

Complications

Complications include bleeding esophageal varices, which can lead to massive hemorrhage; hepatorenal syndrome, which leads to renal failure; and hepatic encephalopathy, which leads to coma and death.

Diagnostic Tests

Liver Biopsy	Definitive histological changes
Serum Albumin	Decreased
Prothrombin Time	Prolonged
Liver Function Studies	Elevated alkaline phosphatase; elevated aminotransferase; elevated alanine aminotransferase
CBC	Evidence of anemia, leukopenia, thrombocytopenia
Blood Glucose	Decreased
Ultrasonography	Hepatosplenomegaly, enlarged portal veins
Liver Scans	Reduced liver uptake

Therapeutic Management

Surgery	Liver transplantation for advanced disease, portosystemic shunt to treat resistant esophageal varices, peritoneovenous shunt for ascites
Medications	Diuretics to reduce edema, digestants to promote fat digestion, supplemental vitamins, stool softeners
General	Elimination of toxic agents, such as alcohol or drugs; diet high in protein, carbohydrates, and calories and low in sodium; blood and blood products, gastric lavage, esophageal balloon for bleeding varices
	Transjugular intrahepatic portosystemic shunt (TIPS) to divert portal blood from liver
	Variceal sclerosis via endoscopy to treat esophageal varices
	Abdominal paracentesis for ascites
	Renal dialysis for renal failure
Prevention/ Promotion	Cease chronic heavy alcohol consumption
	Eliminate chemical or drug exposure

Cold, Common (Upper Respiratory Infection)

A self-limiting, acute viral infection of the upper respiratory tract. The resulting inflammation involves the nasal passages, throat, sinuses, trachea, and bronchi.

Etiology and Incidence

The common cold can be caused by one of many viruses. The rhinovirus group causes about 40% of cases. Spring and summer colds are often caused by picornaviruses, fall colds by parainfluenza viruses, and winter colds by coronaviruses. The mechanisms of spread are not clearly defined and may vary somewhat by viral type. Direct contact is implicated in rhinovirus colds; airborne infection by droplet is probably the mechanism in other viral strains. Upper respiratory infections are the leading cause of acute morbidity in the United States. More than 65 million cases are reported annually.

Pathophysiology

The pathogenesis of colds is still uncertain. The virus is deposited in the nasopharynx, where it moves to the adenoids and a rich bed of viral receptors. An inflammatory reaction is evoked, resulting in vasodilation, mucus production, coughing, and sneezing about 16 hours after initial infection. The virus spreads to the ciliated epithelial cells in the nasal passages, and symptoms continue for 4 to 10 days. The virus is active for about 3 weeks and may affect the trachea and bronchi, particularly in individuals with chronic respiratory disease.

Clinical Manifestations

Typical symptoms include nasal congestion and discharge, sore throat, sneezing, coughing, headache, and fatigue. Febrile reactions occur in infants and young children but are uncommon in older children and adults.

Complications

The most common complications are the secondary overlay of a bacterial infection with purulent sinusitis or otitis media and the triggering of bronchospasms in people with asthma.

Diagnostic Tests

The diagnosis is made by clinical evaluation, while ruling out secondary bacterial sinusitis, otitis media, and streptococcal pharyngitis.

Therapeutic Management

Surgery	None
Medications	Nonsteroidal antiinflammatory drugs (NSAIDs) and first generation antihistamines for sneezing, runny nose, decongestion, malaise, and headache; oral decongestants for nasal obstruction, expectorants for cough; saline gargles, lozenges, or topical anesthetics for sore throat; *no aspirin for infants or children, no antibiotics*
General	Rest for comfort and to minimize spread; proper hand washing and careful handling of items in the environment to minimize viral contact by others; adequate fluids for hydration
Prevention/ Promotion	Avoid exposure; careful hand washing; avoidance of finger-face contact

Colorectal Cancer

C

Most colorectal tumors (95%) are adenocarcinomas, which originate as benign, adenomatous polyps in the rectum or colon.

Etiology and Incidence

No definitive etiological factors have been identified, although environmental and dietary factors have long been suspected. The incidence of colon cancer in the United States ranks behind breast and lung cancer in women and prostate and lung cancer in men. Each year colorectal cancer is diagnosed in more than 147,500 persons, and it is the second leading cause of cancer deaths, with an overall rate of more than 57,000 deaths annually. In 93% of cases, the disease is diagnosed after age 50, and the incidence is equally distributed across gender lines, although women more often have cancer of the colon and men cancer of the rectum.

Pathophysiology

Over a period of 5 years or longer, the adenomatous polyps degenerate into malignant tumors, which are most often located in the rectum or lower colon. The tumor spreads by direct extension through the bowel wall and by intraluminal, hematogenous, and regional lymph node metastases. The liver and lungs are common sites of distant metastasis. Five-year survival rates are 62%.

Risk Factors

Familial history of colorectal cancer and/or polyposis syndromes

Personal history of inflammatory bowel disorders and/or bowel polyps

History of cholestectomy

Diet high in animal fat and red meat (fried or broiled) and low in fiber, calcium, and vitamin D

Alcohol abuse

Smoking

Clinical Manifestations

Cancer of the bowel is largely asymptomatic during the early stages. The most common presenting sign is rectal bleeding on defecation. Changes in bowel patterns, excessive gas, bloating, and cramping may also occur. Pain is unlikely until advanced stages of the disease.

Complications

The chance of survival falls below 50% for patients with regional node involvement, and more than half of these individuals have node involvement at the time of diagnosis. Bowel obstruction or perforation, paralytic ileus, hemorrhage, and liver failure occur with advancing disease.

Diagnostic Tests

A history of risk factors, positive result on occult fecal blood test, or palpable lesion on rectal examination indicates a need for follow-up. Visualization of a lesion by colonoscopy or barium enema evaluation or an elevated carcinoembryonic antigen level indicates the need for tissue biopsy, which is the only definitive mode of diagnosis.

Therapeutic Management

Surgery	Excision of well-differentiated rectal tumors, resection of the colon around the tumor with removal of the associated lymphatic drainage system, colostomy, laser or bypass surgery for inoperable obstructing tumors
Medications	Adjunct systemic chemotherapy of 5-fluorouracil (5-FU) and irinotecan; oxaliplatin and 5-FU followed by levamisole for metastasis
General	Radiation plus chemotherapy when four or more positive nodes are found and for palliation; endoscopic polypectomy for certain qualifying tumors; support groups; counseling for altered body image

Prevention/ **Promotion**	Reduce animal fat in diet; alcohol in moderation
	Starting at age 50 or those at risk: annual fecal occult blood; flexible sigmoidoscopy or double contrast barium enema every 5 years; a colonoscopy every 10 years
Education	Education about effects and side effects of treatments; information about resources and support groups; instruction in ostomy care

C

Congestive Heart Failure (CHF)

A complex clinical syndrome that results when the heart is unable to pump an adequate supply of blood to meet the body's metabolic needs, leading to inadequate tissue perfusion; vascular, cardiac, and pulmonary congestion; diminished functional capacity

Etiology and Incidence

CHF can have a number of causes, which can be classified as either decreasing myocardial motility or increasing myocardial workload. Causes that decrease motility include coronary artery disease (CAD), myocarditis, cardiomyopathy, tumors, lupus erythematosus, and scleroderma, and drugs such as beta-blockers and calcium antagonists. Hypertension (HTN), valvular heart disease, intracardiac shunting, anemia, hyperthyroidism, and arteriovenous fistulas increase workload. Pericarditis, tamponade, and cardiac dysrhythmias interfere with ventricular filling. The incidence of CHF is increasing as the population ages. It is estimated that 4.7 million persons in the United States have CHF, and it is the most common hospital discharge diagnosis for individuals over age 65.

Pathophysiology

When the heart is unable to pump a sufficient supply of blood to meet the body's demands, three primary compensatory mechanisms attempt to maintain cardiac function: (1) the sympathetic nervous system response increases, with increased catecholamine discharge, in an effort to increase myocardial contractility, which in turn causes vasoconstriction that increases peripheral resistance and cardiac workload; (2) cardiac fluid volume increases in an effort to stretch the fibers in the ventricles and increase the force of the contraction; (3) the myocardium hypertrophies in an attempt to increase the amount of contractile tissue available and thus increase contractility.

When these compensatory mechanisms are insufficient or when they are active over extended periods, they become ineffective and eventually contribute to failure of the pump. Pump failure usually begins with the left ventricle and progresses to the right ventricle. It may be either acute or chronic, depending on the cause.

Risk Factors

Underlying disease processes (e.g., CAD, HTN, diabetes)
Smoking
Obesity
Elevated cholesterol and/or lipid levels

Clinical Manifestations

Left Ventricle Failure	Tachycardia, fatigue, and dyspnea on exertion; intolerance to cold; cough; blood-tinged sputum; restlessness; paroxysmal nocturnal dyspnea; insomnia; crackles and wheezes in the lungs; ventricular and atrial gallops
Right Ventricle Failure	Fatigue, fullness in the neck and abdomen, ankle swelling, distention of neck veins, weakness, anorexia, nausea, liver enlargement, nocturia, ascites, tricuspid murmur

Complications

🔴 Acute pulmonary edema occurs with acute heart failure and is manifested as extreme dyspnea, cyanosis, hyperpnea, and plunging oxygen saturation. Death occurs if the condition is not treated immediately. Myocardial infarction, cardiac arrhythmias, hepatomegaly, and renal failure are other complications of CHF.

Diagnostic Tests

Blood Chemistry	Elevated BUN, creatinine, and glucose; decreased potassium and sodium; elevated aspartate aminotransferase, bilirubin; prolonged partial thromboplastin time
Arterial Blood Gases	Decreased oxygen saturation

CBC	Decreased Hgb and Hct with anemia
Chest X-ray	Cardiomegaly; engorged pulmonary vasculature
Echocardiography	To visualize increased or decreased chamber dimensions, decreased wall motion
Cardiac Catheterization	Definitive diagnosis of cause and extent of damage

Therapeutic Management

Surgery	Heart transplantation for end-stage failure, intraaortic balloon pump to provide circulatory assistance, left ventricular assistive device for those awaiting transplantation
Medications	Diuretics to reduce edema and ventricular filling volume; vasodilators, antihypertensives, or alpha-adrenergic blocking agents to dilate vessels and reduce venous filling pressure and peripheral resistance; beta blocking agents to increase contractility; inotropics (digitalis, dobutamine, milrinone) to increase contractility; angiotensin-converting enzyme inhibitors to reduce angiotensin II in individuals with advanced CHF
General	Bed rest with head elevated; oxygenation; low-salt diet; fluid restriction; daily weights; monitoring and support of vital functions; pacemaker for chronic failure and intraventricular conduction delay; prevention of thrombosis, pneumonia, and skin breakdown; stress reduction
Prevention/ Promotion	Balanced nutrition Exercise Maintain normal weight Smoking cessation

Education   Instruction in functional adaptation to chronic
disease; dug therapy regimen; signs of
digitalis toxicity and monitoring of pulse for
those on digitalis preparation; dietary
regimen; balance of rest-activity; importance
of seeking care for any signs of exacerbation
(shortness of breath [SOB] on exertion or
lying flat, hacking cough, fatigue, nausea
with abdominal pain, dizziness, rapid weight
gain of 3 to 5 pounds)

Conjunctivitis

An inflammation or infection of the conjunctiva of the eye

Etiology and Incidence

Causes include viruses, bacteria, airborne or contact allergens, and environmental irritants (e.g., sun, wind, dust, smog, smoke, and noxious gases). Conjunctivitis is common and is easily spread when bacterial or viral in nature. Peak incidence is in the fall.

Pathophysiology

The severity varies by exposure and cause. The causal agent comes in contact with and irritates the conjunctiva, setting up an inflammatory response. Recurrent inflammation leads to thickening of the conjunctival layer and lid margins.

Clinical Manifestations

Bacterial Type	Purulent drainage, lid swelling, moderate discomfort, redness of conjunctiva
Viral Type	Clear discharge, swollen preauricular node, tearing, redness, moderate discomfort, light sensitivity
Allergen or Irritant	Clear discharge, profuse tearing, feeling of something in the eye, intense itching (allergen), severe swelling of the lid, generalized redness of the eye, moderate burning feeling

Complications

If left untreated, infection may spread from conjunctiva to cornea and cause ulceration, perforation, and blindness.

Diagnostic Tests

Smears and cultures of discharge are done to determine if viral or bacterial agent is present. Conjunctival scrapings are used to rule out inclusion conjunctivitis, trachoma, and vernal conjunctivitis. Vision, intraocular pressure, cornea, iris, pupil, and pupillary response are all normal.

Therapeutic Management

Surgery	None
Medications	Topical antiinfective drugs for bacterial cause, topical corticosteroids or mast cell stabilizers for allergens
General	Saline irrigation for discharge and comfort, warm compresses for inflammation and cool compresses for itching, careful hand washing
Prevention/ Promotion	Avoidance of irritants and contact allergens

Corneal Ulcer

A local necrosis of corneal tissue that ultimately leads to scarring and reduced visual acuity

Etiology and Incidence

The most common cause is infection after trauma or contact lens overwear. Other causes include herpes simplex infection, chronic blepharitis, conjunctivitis, gonorrhea, trachoma, chemical burns, prolonged exposure to air in the absence of a blink reflex, and severe vitamin A or protein depletion resulting from malnutrition. Prevalence is high in the United States.

Pathophysiology

The cornea usually becomes infected or inflamed through an outside agent or chronic irritant, and a dull, grayish lesion forms and then necroses and suppurates, creating an ulcer. The ulcer may or may not infiltrate deeper layers of tissue. The deeper the penetration, the more severe the signs, symptoms, and complications. As the ulcer heals, it is replaced by fibrous tissue, which causes opaque scarring and reduced vision.

Clinical Manifestations

Pain, tearing, and photophobia are the most common manifestations. Bloodshot eyes and pus in the anterior chamber behind the cornea may be present in chronic cases.

Complications

Perforation of the cornea, with a prolapse of the iris and eventual destruction of the eye, is the major complication.

Diagnostic Tests

A fluorescein stain turns green and readily delineates the ulcerated area. A slit lamp examination allows inspection of the eye's surface and the deeper layers of the cornea to determine the extent of ulceration. Cultures identify the infectious organism.

Therapeutic Management

Surgery	Repair of any laceration or removal of foreign object; removal of prolapsed tissue; corneal transplantation for severe scarring or perforation
Medications	Topical anesthetics for pain; topical and systemic antibiotics, antifungals to treat infection; mydriatics to dilate pupil with increased intraocular pressure; cycloplegics to restrict eye movement and reduce pain
General	Warm compresses for lid swelling; irrigation to cleanse eye; bilateral pressure dressings to aid reepithelialization; dark glasses for photophobia
Prevention/ Promotion	Avoid finger to eye contact Follow guidelines for contact lens wear; avoid contaminated contact solution; avoid practices such as cleaning or wetting contact lens with saliva

C

Coronary Artery Disease (CAD)

A disorder that impedes the blood flow in the arteries serving the myocardium of the heart
(See also Angina Pectoris and Myocardial Infarction)

Etiology and Incidence

The primary causes of CAD are arteriosclerotic and atherosclerotic processes, which narrow and occlude the vessel lumen and thicken the arterial walls.

Vascular disease (CAD and cardiovascular accident [CVA]) is the leading cause of death in the United States. The incidence of CAD increases with age, with men up to five times as susceptible as women, until menopause, when risk equalizes for men and women. CAD is much more prevalent in western societies than in other areas of the world.

Pathophysiology

The exact pathological mechanisms that induce atherosclerosis are not well understood. Current hypotheses are (1) the lipid hypothesis, in which an elevation of plasma low-density lipoprotein penetrates the arterial wall and causes a lipid buildup in the smooth muscle cells, and (2) the endothelial injury hypothesis, which suggests that a mechanical or chemical injury to the endothelial barrier sets up a tissue response, with platelet adhesion and aggregation. In either case, atherosclerosis is marked by changes in and thickening of the intimal lining of the arterial vessel. Lipids, smooth muscle cells, and connective tissue form a plaquelike substance on the lining. This process is slow and may occur over a lifetime. Arteriosclerosis causes hypertrophy and subintimal fibrosis, resulting in intimal thickening and loss of elasticity of the vessel wall, which widens the pulse pressure and increases the systolic pressure. Atherosclerotic processes reinforce this loss of elasticity. Arterial lumens become increasingly narrow and may become obstructed, causing ischemia of the myocardium. The plaque may harden, calcify, and undergo fissure or rupture, simulating a thrombosis or embolus that is rapidly occluding a lumen.

Risk Factors

Underlying disease processes (e.g., hypertension or diabetes)
Familial hyperlipidemia
Gender (males ages 35 to 55, females after menopause)
Smoking
Elevated serum lipids
Sedentary lifestyle
Obesity
Stress
Use of birth control pills or estrogen in women under age 50

Clinical Manifestations

CAD is asymptomatic until myocardial ischemia occurs. The two major manifestations of ischemia are chest pain (angina) and myocardial infarction. (See Angina Pectoris and Myocardial Infarction for diagnosis and treatment options.)

Crohn's Disease (Regional Enteritis)

A nonspecific chronic inflammatory disease of the gastrointestinal system most commonly affecting the distal ileum and the colon

Etiology and Incidence

The etiology is unknown, and research examining the causal role of immune factors, infectious agents, and dietary factors has proved fruitless. An estimated 30 to 50 cases occur per 100,000 persons, and the incidence is rising in underdeveloped countries—among blacks and Hispanics—and in Western and Northern European and Anglo-Saxon populations. The disease is equally distributed across gender lines, is most common among the Jewish population, and occurs primarily between ages 15 and 30.

Pathophysiology

Crohn's disease begins with lymphedema in the gastrointestinal (GI) submucosa and microscopic focal ulcerations of the mucosa. The inflammation spreads slowly and progressively, involving all layers of the intestinal wall, which thicken with extensive fibrosis and granulomas as patchy ulcerations form on the mucosa. This process creates a characteristic cobblestone appearance of the mucosa. As the disease progresses, the mesentery becomes edematous and thickens, and mesenteric fat extends onto the serosal surface of the bowel, causing serositis with adhesion of bowel loops to one another. Mesenteric lymph nodes enlarge, and abscess and deep sinus tracts and fissures are formed. Eventually the lumen of the intestine severely narrows or becomes obstructed. This process often affects one segment of the intestine, skips over normal tissue, and then repeats the obstructive process in another segment (i.e., forming skip lesions).

Clinical Manifestations

Symptoms may be abrupt or insidious in onset and are characterized by exacerbations and remissions. The most common presenting features are chronic diarrhea with urgency and incontinence; abdominal pain and cramping, often in the lower right quadrant; fever; anorexia; and weight loss. However, some individuals have acute abdominal pain resembling that caused by appendicitis.

Complications

Complications of Crohn's disease can be either intestinal or systemic. An anal fistula or perianal abscess caused by chronic diarrhea is the most common complication. Other fistulas may form to the bladder, vagina, or skin. Malabsorption, obstruction, perforation, and cancer of the colon are other intestinal complications. Systemic complications include arthritis, episcleritis, stomatitis, erythema nodosum, pyoderma gangrenosum, ankylosing spondylitis, sacroiliitis, uveitis, and sclerosing cholangitis.

Diagnostic Tests

Barium Series	Linear ulcerations, skip lesions, thickening of wall, narrowing of lumen
Colonoscopy	Cobblestone mucosa
Biopsy	To aid in differentiation of disease
Laboratory Studies	Nonspecific; may include decreased Hgb and Hct, serum albumin, and folic acid; elevated erythrocyte sedimentation rate

Therapeutic Management

Surgery	Bowel resection with failure to respond to conservative therapy, colectomy with ileostomy when disease is limited to colon, strictureplasty to open obstructions
Medications	Sulfasalazine, corticosteroids, and metronidazole to treat inflammation and ulceration; anticholinergics for diarrhea; fat-soluble vitamins, folic acid, iron, calcium magnesium, and zinc for replacement; immunosuppressive agents for intractable disease; infliximab for tumor necrosis

General   Adequate rest; nutrition; NPO in acute phase to rest bowel, followed by total parenteral nutrition or restricted diet low in fiber; emotional support for anxiety and depression; referral to source of information and support group; follow up with monitoring of liver enzymes and B_{12} levels on annual basis

Education   Instruction in chronic relapsing nature of disease and medication effects and side effects; strategies in rest, dietary management, perianal care

Croup

A general term applied to an acute viral symptom complex characterized by inflammation of the upper and lower respiratory tracts, hoarseness, a "barking" or "brassy" cough, respiratory distress, or stridor most commonly heard on inspiration

Etiology and Incidence

A host of viruses, including parainfluenza viruses (most common), influenza A and B, adenovirus, and respiratory syncytial virus cause croup. Croup is a commonly occurring disease seen primarily in children 1 to 6 years of age and peaking in 2 year olds. Most cases occur in late fall or early winter. Males are considered to be more susceptible than females. Croup accounts for 10% to 15% of lower respiratory tract infections in young children in the United States.

Pathophysiology

The infecting virus causes inflammation of the larynx, trachea, bronchi, bronchioles, and the lungs themselves. Airway obstruction, if it occurs, is in an area of the trachea just below the glottis (the subglottal region). As airway obstruction increases, the work of breathing and breathing distress increase and the child tires.

Clinical Manifestations

The child often has an upper respiratory infection but can have no symptoms at all. The child is put to bed and awakens with respiratory distress including a "barking" or "metallic" cough, hoarseness, noisy inspirations, and restlessness. Often the child is frightened and anxious. Fever may or may not be present. The child's fright and alarm on the part of the parents only make the child more anxious and make the symptoms worse. Most commonly with symptom management and calm parents, the attack subsides within a few hours and by the next day, the child appears well.

Complications

Hospitalization is necessary for 1% to 15% of children with croup. Airway obstruction, pneumonia, dehydration, and otitis media are possible complications.

Diagnostic Tests

Croup must be differentiated from other noninfectious causes of stridor (foreign body) and from epiglottitis or acute tracheitis by clinical evaluation and x-rays of soft tissue of the neck. Tissue cultures may be used to identify the causative agent.

Therapeutic Management

Surgery	None
Medications	Racemic epinephrine, nebulized and systemic steroids used in severe cases
General	Mildly ill children (no stridor at rest) may be managed at home. The child should be kept comfortable and well hydrated. Rest is important. Crying and/or agitation may cause fatigue and increase respiratory distress. Use cold-steam vaporizers or humidifiers with fine mist. If vaporizer and/or humidifier not available, child may be exposed to cool night air, or placed in front of an open freezer.
	If hospital admission is necessary, use cool-mist humidification; rest; fluids; humidified oxygen if PaO_2 is less than 60 mm Hg. Endotracheal intubation and ventilatory support may be necessary if the child's $PaCO_2$ is greater than 45 mm Hg.
Prevention/ Promotion	Avoid exposure, wash hands thoroughly
Education	Reassurance to parents about self-limiting nature of disease, instructions in use of humidifier, cool-mist vaporizer

Cushing's Syndrome (Hypercortisolism)

Hypersecretion of glucocorticoids by the adrenal gland, which produces a characteristic constellation of clinical abnormalities, including a moon face and truncal and neck fat pad deposits. It is classified into adrenocortico-tropic hormone (ACTH)-dependent (75%) and ACTH-independent (25%) forms. ACTH-dependent forms are also referred to as *Cushing's disease.*

Etiology and Incidence

The most common cause is iatrogenic from chronic administration of glucocorticoids. ACTH-secreting tumors (pituitary adenoma, ectopic) cause ACTH-dependent Cushing's syndrome. Other causes include adrenal cancer, adrenal adenoma, and micronodular adrenal disease. Overall incidence of Cushing's syndrome is rare and is most common in women of childbearing age.

Pathophysiology

Increased glucocorticoid production is triggered by one of the causal agents. The increased glucocorticoids act as a sort of antianabolic, creating a mediated antagonism in insulin action that results in biochemical energy deprivation. This leads to protein wasting, glucose intolerance, fragility of the vascular system, and reduced effectiveness of the immune system.

Clinical Manifestations

General	Muscle weakness and wasting; fragile and thinned skin; purple striae; easy bruising; poor wound healing; moon face; buffalo hump; heavy trunk; thin extremities; back pain; kyphosis; edema; hypertension; mood swings
Children	Precocious puberty, cessation of linear growth
Women	Masculinization (hirsutism, atrophy of breasts, clitoral enlargement, deepening voice, and temporal baldness); menstrual irregularities

| Men | Feminization (breast enlargement, higher voice, lighter beard); testicular atrophy and impotence |

Complications

Potential complications include osteoporosis, pathological fracture, peptic ulcer, diabetes mellitus, congestive heart failure, and psychoses.

Diagnostic Tests

24-hour Urine	Increased urinary-free cortisol greater than 250 μg/day
Dexamethasone Suppression	Dose of dexamethasone is given at night; positive test result shows reduced plasma cortisol levels next morning (less than 50% of baseline)
Metyrapone, ACTH Stimulation, Corticotropin-Releasing Hormone Tests	To determine etiology
CT Scan/MRI	To detect adrenal tumors

Therapeutic Management

Treatment is directed at the underlying cause.

Surgery	Transsphenoidal pituitary resection of the tumor; resection of ectopic tumors, adrenal adenomas, adrenal carcinoma; bilateral adrenalectomy for treatment-resistant pituitary tumor and micronodular adrenal disease
Medications	Glucocorticoid and mineralocorticoid lifelong replacement when bilateral adrenalectomy is performed; adrenal inhibitors or ketoconazole used when ectopic tumor cannot be removed; chemotherapy with mitotane for inoperable adrenal carcinomas

| General | Irradiation of the pituitary when surgery cannot be tolerated in treating a pituitary tumor; gradual withdrawal from steroids when cause is from steroid therapy |
| Education | Education that recovery can take a year or longer and that treatment initially makes the patient feel worse; instruction in drug effects, side effects, adjusting replacement hormones as needed |

Cystic Fibrosis (CF)

An inherited disease of the exocrine glands that results in multisystem involvement primarily by affecting the respiratory and gastrointestinal systems. It typically is characterized by chronic obstructive pulmonary disease (COPD), abnormally high loss of electrolytes through the sweat glands, and pancreatic enzyme insufficiency, leading to digestive impairments and malabsorption syndrome.

Etiology and Incidence

CF is caused by defective genes that are inherited from both parents as an autosomal recessive trait. One gene is responsible for encoding a membrane-associated protein called *cystic fibrosis transmembrane conductance regulator (CFTR)*. The exact function of CFTR is unknown, but research shows that it is closely tied to chloride transport. Current research focuses on the causes of seemingly unrelated multisystem effects.

CF is the most common lethal genetic disease among white children and young adults in the United States, with an incidence of 1 in 2500 to 3500 live births. Blacks also are affected, but the rate is about 1 in 17,000 births. CF is rare in Asians and Native Americans. Median survival rate is 30 years.

Pathophysiology

With CF, the exocrine glands are affected in one of three ways: (1) they produce and become obstructed by thickened, sticky mucus; (2) they produce excess normal secretions; (3) they secrete excess sodium and chloride. The lungs are normal at birth, but bronchioles and bronchi soon become clogged with thick mucous plugs, leading to associated opportunistic infections and overinflation of the lungs. Bronchial walls thicken and airways remain filled with purulent secretions, leading to fibrosis and atelectasis. Chronic hypoxemia leads to hypertrophy of the pulmonary arteries, which leads to pulmonary hypertension (HTN) and right ventricular hypertrophy. The pancreatic ducts also become clogged with mucous plugs, which interfere with pancreatic enzyme activity. Digestive enzymes fail to reach the small intestine, and as a result, digestion and absorption of nutrients are markedly impaired, leading to excess fat and protein in the stools. The biliary tracts in the liver become plugged with mucus and fibrose over time. Salivary glands and bile ducts may also become clogged. Sweat glands secrete abnormal levels of sodium and chloride, leading to excessive loss of these electrolytes.

Clinical Manifestations

Signs and symptoms vary widely, involve several systems, and change as the disease progresses. Some children show manifestations at birth, whereas others do not show symptoms for years. Manifestations range from mild to life threatening. The earliest sign is a meconium ileus, seen at birth in about 10% of infants with CF. All children display sweat gland abnormalities, 85% to 90% have pancreatic and gastrointestinal (GI) tract involvement, and 50% show respiratory involvement.

Sweat glands/ Skin	Salty-tasting skin; salt crystals on nose, forehead, and hairline; dehydration; alkalosis in heat or with fever
Pancreas/GI Tract	Meconium ileus with cramps, nausea, vomiting, and abdominal distention; frequent, bulky, oily, and foul-smelling stools; normal or voracious appetite; weight loss; failure to thrive; pot belly; wasted buttocks; thin extremities; sallow skin; anemia; easy bruising; rectal prolapse
Respiratory Tract	Wheezing; dry cough; rhinitis; gagging; dyspnea; intercostal retractions; use of accessory muscles to breathe; barrel chest; digital clubbing; cyanosis; repeated episodes of upper respiratory infection (URI); bronchial pneumonia
Reproductive System	Delayed onset of puberty; amenorrhea; viscous cervical secretions that block sperm entry in women; sterility in men

Complications

Complications are numerous and can include biliary cirrhosis, esophageal varices, portal HTN, diabetes mellitus, pneumothorax, cor pulmonale, congestive heart failure, peptic ulcer, intestinal obstruction, intussusception, pancreatitis, cholecystitis, and cardiac arrhythmias. CF is a terminal disease.

Diagnostic Tests

Clinical Evaluation	Any of the above manifestations, particularly salty skin; failure to thrive; frequent URIs; family history
Quantitative Pilocarpine Iontophoresis Sweat Test	Sodium or chloride concentration more than 60 mEq/L To obtain definitive diagnosis

Therapeutic Management

Surgery	Heart-lung or liver transplantation with advanced disease; treatment of complications (e.g., resection of bowel obstructions, cholecystectomy, portal shunt for esophageal varices)
Medications	Antibiotics to treat pulmonary infections; amiloride HCl (aerosol) to inhibit sodium and water reabsorption in the lungs; DNase and other drugs to thin mucus; alpha-antitrypsin to reduce inflammation; pancreatic enzyme replacements (e.g., pancrelipase); bronchodilators to aid breathing
General	Diet therapy with 50% increase in normal caloric and protein intake, high fat intake, multivitamins, water-miscible vitamin E, sodium supplements, enteral supplementation in severe cases Prophylaxis against respiratory infection with pertussis, measles, influenza, and pneumonia vaccines Chest physiotherapy to increase movement of mucus from lungs (postural drainage, percussion, vibration, and assisted coughing; oxygen therapy for hypoxia; exercise to stimulate mucus movement)

Long-term psychological counseling for individual and family; genetic counseling for parents; support groups; home care and respite care

Cystitis

(See Urinary Tract Infection, Lower)

Cysts (Dermoid, Epidermal, Sebaceous)

A slow-growing, benign cystic tumor found in the subcutaneous tissue below the skin or in the intradermal tissue of the skin

Etiology and Incidence

Cyst formation is commonly caused by inflammation, internal rupture of an acne pustule or whitehead, impaired localized circulation, or trauma. Some individuals may be genetically predisposed to cyst formation.

Pathophysiology

Cysts contain a soft, yellow-white, cheesy substance that is often fetid and that forms when a hair follicle becomes obstructed. The type of cyst determines the contents of the cyst. Dermoid cysts are located deep in the subcutaneous tissue; have walls of keratinizing epidermis containing sweat glands, hair follicles, and sebaceous glands; and are often present at birth. Epidermal cysts (e.g., acne cysts) are found in the epidermis on the face, scalp, neck, and back; they contain laminated layers of keratin. Sebaceous cysts, or wens, occur primarily on the scalp and contain soft keratin, epidermal debris, and greasy material.

Clinical Manifestations

Cysts are found on or under the skin, are generally less than 3 cm in diameter, and are round, firm, globular, and movable to the touch. They are nontender unless infected. Cysts, particularly the sebaceous type, can grow as large as a grapefruit.

Complications

Cysts may become infected.

Diagnostic Tests

A characteristic lesion is seen on clinical evaluation.

Therapeutic Management

Surgery	Excision of the cyst and cyst wall, incision and drainage of infected cysts
Medications	Antibiotics for infected cysts
General/ Education	Instruction not to touch, squeeze, or pick lesions, since this may lead to infection

Cytomegalovirus (CMV) Infection
(Cytomegalic Inclusion Disease Virus)

Various infections that may be congenitally induced or occur at any age. Cases range from subclinical to fulminant.

Etiology and Incidence

CMV infections are caused by the cytomegalovirus, which is a beta herpesvirus. The virus may lie dormant in the system for years and be reactivated if the body is immunosuppressed. The incidence of the virus is very common and up to 70% of the adult population in the United States has been infected and tests positive for viral antibodies. Incidence increases during the perinatal period, with day care exposure, and during reproductive years with sexual activity. Populations at risk for human immunodeficiency virus (HIV) are also at increased risk for CMV infection.

Pathophysiology

CMV is transmitted through exchange of blood or body fluids. Sexually acquired CMV occurs via contact with semen or vaginal discharge, or through blood from mucosal tears in anal intercourse with an infected partner. Congenital transmission occurs via the placenta in utero. Perinatal transmission can occur through maternal vaginal secretions or breast milk. Blood transfusions, shared needles in IV drug use, and transplanted organs can also transmit infection. Once transmitted, the virus establishes itself on a mucosal surface, in the blood, or on an organ surface and replicates setting up cell lysis, inflammation, and infectious processes. The immune response of the host is activated to stop the replication and eliminate the infection. The virus when active is shed in the urine and saliva.

Risk Factors

Unprotected sexual contact (vaginal, anal, oral) with an infected
    partner
Contact with saliva or oral secretions
Fetuses/infants of infected mothers
Organ transplant or allograft bone marrow transplant recipients

Blood transfusion recipients
IV drug users who share needles
Use of systemic steroids
Immunosuppressed individuals (e.g., HIV, acquired immuno-
    deficiency syndrome [AIDS], cancer)
Day care or other institutional living environments (prisons,
    nursing homes)

Clinical Manifestations

General	Frequently asymptomatic; any combination of the following: fever, chills, rash, fatigue, nausea, vomiting, bone pain, diarrhea, jaundice, splenomegaly, dyspnea
Congenital	Asymptomatic cytomegaloviruria, petechial rash, lethargy, respiratory distress, anemia, jaundice, hepato-splenomegaly, hemorrhage, seizures, sensory motor deafness, mental retardation; abortion of fetus, intrauterine growth retardation, or premature birth may also occur
Postnatal	Crouplike symptoms (respiratory distress, barking cough, restlessness, irritability); pharyngitis, bronchitis or pneumonia, CMV mononucleosis
Immunosuppressed	Febrile mononucleosis; retinitis; esophageal, gastric, or bowel ulcerations; pneumonitis; encephalitis; hepatitis; cholecystitis; enterocolitis; esophagitis; CNS damage; dementia; diabetes; adrenalitis
Transplant	Pneumonitis, cough, chills, fever, chest pain

Complications

Fetuses, infants, and immunosuppressed individuals (HIV,
AIDS, cancer, and transplants) are at high risk for severe disease
forms that cause permanent organ damage, disability, and/or
death.

Diagnostic Tests

Clinical Evaluation	Symptom patterns consistent with disease
Serum Labs	Evidence of leukopenia, thrombocytopenia, lymphocytosis
Cultures	Urine, blood, body fluids, or tissue positive for CMV
Biopsy	Used to demonstrate invasive disease
Chest X-ray	If pneumonitis suspected
Endoscopy	If GI involvement suspected
Funduscopy	Retinitis
CT Scan/MRI	If central nervous system (CNS) involvement suspected

Therapeutic Management

Surgery	None
Medications	Ganciclovir, foscarnet, cidofovir for retinitis or pneumonitis; fomivirsen injections into vitreous humor as salvage therapy in retinitis
General	Isolation, bed rest for symptomatic disease
Prevention/ Promotion	Prevention of disease transmission, particularly among high-risk groups; emphasis on elimination of high-risk behaviors, such as unprotected sexual activity and sharing needles when engaging in IV drug use; promotion of safe-sex practices, such as use of latex condoms and/or barriers treated with viricidal spermicides; use of universal precautions by health care workers and family members to prevent transmission; ganciclovir as prophylaxis in transplant recipients and those with HIV; valacyclovir as prophylaxis in bone marrow transplants
Education	Education about prophylaxis, drug effects, side effects

Decubitus Ulcer

(See Pressure Ulcer)

Delirium/Dementia
(Formerly Organic Mental Syndromes)

A constellation of behavioral signs and symptoms associated with transient or permanent dysfunction of the brain and characterized by impaired intellectual functioning, confusion, and agitation

Etiology and Incidence
Delirium is a rapidly developing, reversible, self-limiting condition characterized by a disturbance of consciousness with a reduced ability to maintain attention to or appropriately shift attention among different external stimuli. *Dementia* is a structurally caused, permanent decline in memory, abstract thinking, and judgment.

The primary causes of *delirium* are an underlying medical condition (i.e., acute inflammation of the meninges, infection, hypoxia, metabolic disturbances, central nervous system (CNS) pathology, cerebrovascular events, seizures, or hypertensive crisis); chemical exposure (medications, recreational drugs, toxins); and abrupt chemical withdrawal (i.e., alcohol, barbiturates). Environments that produce increased or decreased stimuli such as isolation, recovery, or intensive care units and factors such as sleep deprivation, pain, anxiety, stress and/or aging in conjunction with a medical condition can also precipitate delirium.

The most common cause of *dementia* is Alzheimer's disease (see Alzheimer's Disease). Other causes include vascular disease, human immunodeficiency virus (HIV) infection, CNS infection, severe head injury, toxic metabolic disturbances, normal pressure hydrocephalus, underlying neurological disease (Parkinson's disease, Huntington's chorea, multiple sclerosis

(MS), and Pick's disease), and drug, alcohol, or nutritional abuse.

Delirium affects from 10% to 30% of people hospitalized for a medical condition. Those in certain high-risk populations have even higher incidences (i.e., 30% to 40% of hospitalized HIV patients; 50% of postoperative patients, and up to 60% of skilled care residents over 75 years old). More than 1 million persons in the United States have *dementia,* and the elderly are at greatest risk. The incidence of dementia rises steadily with age, with 25% of those over age 80 displaying severe symptoms of dementia. The incidence of acquired immunodeficiency syndrome (AIDS) also contributes to an increase in the incidence of dementia. Dementia develops in an estimated 50% of individuals with end-stage AIDS.

Pathophysiology

The pathophysiology of *delirium* is not yet understood, but there are a number of competing hypotheses, including neurotransmitter abnormalities, inflammatory response resulting from increased cytokines, changes in the permeability of the blood-brain barrier, and abnormalities of chemical messenger systems. In *dementia*, pathological changes vary by causation and in Alzheimer's-related dementia include atrophy of brain tissue with wide sulci and dilated ventricles, senile plaque formation, and neurofibrillary tangles. Vascular disease–induced dementia is characterized by multiple cerebral infarcts. In AIDS-related dementia, the neurons are infected with HIV, and in hydrocephalus, cerebrospinal fluid (CSF) circulation and absorption are impeded.

Risk Factors

Delirium	Dementia, disease (particularly involving CNS, renal, or hepatic systems), major medical illness, multiple medical conditions, multiple medications, recent major surgery, history of psychiatric disorder and/or substance abuse, toxin exposure, age over 65, malnourished state, abrupt withdrawal of alcohol or drugs, sensory impairments (hearing or visual), sleep deprivation, and environments that induce sensory deprivation or sensory overload

Dementia   Familial tendencies, cortical disease states
              (Pick's, Lewy body), movement disorders
              (Parkinson's, Huntington's), neoplasms,
              demyelinating diseases, head trauma,
              metabolic encephalopathies, chronic alcohol
              or drug abuse, and chronic malnourishment

D

Clinical Manifestations

Delirium   Rapid onset: Acute change in mentation,
              fluctuating levels of consciousness,
              disorientation, including loss of self-
              recognition in some instances, impaired
              memory, inability to maintain or shift
              attention, irritability, agitation, restlessness,
              hyperactivity, perceptual disturbance,
              hallucinations, delusions, rambling and
              fragmented speech, impaired sleep-wake
              cycle, lucid intervals with symptoms worse
              at night, duration of about 1 week on
              average

Dementia   Symptoms vary widely, but the overall
              picture is a slow, insidious disintegration of
              personality and intellect with impaired
              insight and judgment, and loss of affect.
              Memory impairment is often the most
              prominent initial symptom. Others include
              increasing rigidity of thought, restricted
              interests, easy distractibility, lack of
              initiation, speech disturbances, loss of
              impulse control, change of former traits or
              exaggeration of those traits (e.g., a neat
              person becomes slovenly or becomes
              obsessively preoccupied with orderliness),
              and depression.

Complications

Delirium places medically ill individuals at greater risk for medical complications (pneumonia, decubitus) and is associated with functional decline and institutional placement. Delirium may lead to dementia. Dementia (except that caused by trauma) is progressive; the individual eventually becomes totally oblivious to his or her surroundings and ultimately dies. Individuals with dementia are more susceptible to accidents and infection.

Diagnostic Tests

Delirium	There are four DSM IV diagnostic criteria for delirium: (1) disturbance of consciousness with reduced awareness and diminished abilities to focus and to maintain or shift attention; (2) a change in cognition, such as disorientation, memory loss, or language disturbance; (3) the disturbance develops over a period of hours to days and fluctuates during the day; (4) evidence from clinical evaluation and/or lab findings that the disturbance is caused by physiological consequences of a medical condition.
Dementia	A diagnosis of dementia is warranted with demonstrable impairment of long- and short-term memory and demonstrable disturbances in abstract thinking, judgment, personality, or other higher cortical functions that interfere with social activities and relationships. Attention and arousal tend to be normal in dementia, and manifestations are relatively stable, worsening over time. A definitive diagnosis is available only on autopsy.

Therapeutic Management

Surgery	None
Medications	*Delirium:* Withdrawal of toxic agents (alcohol, barbiturates) and IV sedation with

antianxiety agents for agitation, seizure
activity, and tremors

Dementia: Treatment of underlying disorders;
antianxiety agents as disease progresses to
relieve anxiety and frustration (see also
Alzheimer's Disease)

D

General   *Delirium:* Adequate fluid and electrolytes,
seizure precautions, safety precautions (e.g.,
prevent wandering, climbing over bedrails),
support and orientation, environmental
control (adequate lighting, familiar objects,
clear space, removal of hazards, avoidance
of sensory extremes; allowance for adequate
sleep, use of glasses, hearing aids, and
dentures, consistency of caretakers), family
involvement, removal of underlying etiologic
agent

Dementia: Kept in familiar surroundings with
minimal environmental changes; use of
frequent orientation devices (clocks,
calendars, schedules, memory books, name
tags); encouragement to do familiar
repetitive routines; safety precautions to
prevent wandering; use of adult day care,
respite care, or home care to relieve
caregiver; family support groups and
counseling; prevention of disuse syndrome in
end-stage disease

Prevention/   Moderate use of alcohol
Promotion   Avoid etiologic agents
Education   *Dementia:* Emphasize to caregiver ways to
create safe environment, use of orientation
and cueing, importance of support and
respite care to prevent caregiver burnout

Depression, Major

Depression is an abnormal mood state in which a person characteristically has a sense of hopelessness, helplessness, worthlessness, despair, morbid thoughts, and psychomotor retardation or agitation. Many adults have experienced "blue" or down days. These feelings are situational and transitory. However, clinical depression is a mood state that lasts longer and causes the individual to become dysfunctional.

Etiology and Incidence

The cause of clinical depression is unknown but is thought to have genetic links with multiple precipitating or triggering factors. It is the most frequently occurring psychiatric condition in the general population. It is estimated that the prevalence of major depression ranges from 8% to 10% in women and from 2.5% to 5% in men. Women are particularly susceptible in the postpartum period. The predominant age is usually between 25 and 44 years of age, but it may be seen at any age.

Pathophysiology

The two subsets of clinical depression are exogenous or reactive and endogenous. *Reactive depression,* also referred to as *secondary depression,* is precipitated by something outside the person such as loss of a loved one, environmental catastrophe, divorce, or a serious medical condition. *Endogenous* depression is primary or biological. It arises within the individual and may be caused by genetic or biochemical factors, such as neurotransmitter functioning. Of the two, endogenous depression is often more severe and difficult to treat. All types of major clinical depression cause changes and abnormalities in the body's biochemical functioning including corticotropin, acetylcholine, dopamine, noradrenaline, and gamma-aminobutyric acid. Changes occur in structural brain images and reduced metabolism in the frontal cortex. Many individuals exhibit abnormalities in sleep electroencephalograms (EEGs) and alterations in the neurotransmitters.

Risk Factors

Women at 2 : 1 higher risk
Familial tendencies

Stressful life events, prolonged stress, lack of social support
Introverted or anxious temperament
Prior episodes of depression
Substance use/abuse
Isolation
Chronic illness

Clinical Manifestations

Mild	Unpleasant feeling about self; self-sacrificing, especially in relation to giving in to others; inhibition of normal pleasurable activities or spontaneous behavior; difficulty concentrating; preoccupation with trivial things; pessimistic outlook toward life; irritability toward self for not living up to an ideal standard; dependence on others for gratification; somatic symptoms
Severe	Utter despair and hopelessness, sense of emptiness, unrelieved sense of guilt and feelings of worthlessness, severe immobility or agitated behavior, catastrophic expectations and outlook, lack of interest in self and environment, retarded thought process, retarded body processes, preoccupation with self, delusional thinking, loss of contact with reality

Complications

Untreated depression may migrate into recurrent or chronic depression. Individuals with major depression are at increased risk for suicide. The suicide rate secondary to depression is approximately 15% to 20%.

Diagnostic Tests

Clinical Evaluation	Interviewing, history taking, and clinical evaluation are important forms of diagnostic evaluation of depression.
Suicide Screening	If the individual is clearly depressed, suicide screening and potential for lethality should be determined.

Blood Tests	Conduct tests to screen for general medical causes and to rule out problems such as thyroid abnormalities.

Therapeutic Management

Surgery	None
Medications	Antidepressants for depression and dysthymia; monoamine oxidase inhibitors (MAOIs) if other antidepressants fail; antipsychotics for psychotic depression/delusions
General	*Mild:* Establish trusting, supportive relationship, therapy, and/or support group; assess strengths and coping strategies; encourage occupational and recreational therapy; provide support to family
	Severe: Assess for suicidal thoughts and self-destructive behaviors; provide protective environment as indicated; establish trusting, supportive relationship; assess strengths and coping strategies; encourage occupational and recreational therapy; provide support to family; intermittent supportive psychotherapy for acute depressive episodes; hospitalization for severe acute episodes, psychosis, severe functional deficits, or high suicide potential
	Electroconvulsive therapy may be indicated if individual does not respond to other therapies.
	Transcranial magnetic stimulation and vagal nerve stimulation are being investigated for treatment of depression.
Education	Education about disorder and cyclic nature, effects and side effects of medications, and importance of not stopping antidepressants abruptly

Dermatitis (Eczema)

A superficial inflammation of the skin with redness, edema, vesicles, crusting, scaling, and sometimes itching; common types include atopic, contact, nummular, or seborrheic dermatitis, all of which may be acute or chronic in nature

Etiology and Incidence

The cause of atopic dermatitis is unknown, but overproduction of immunoglobulin E (IgE) antibodies, defective cell immunity, and T-lymphocyte activation are thought to play a major role. The condition is genetically determined, hereditary, and often associated with other atopic diseases, such as allergic rhinitis, asthma, or hay fever. Incidence is between 5 and 25 cases per 1000 persons with the highest incidence reported in children. Contact dermatitis, which can be irritant or allergic in nature, is caused by contact with various biological or chemical irritants, such as acids, alkalis, dyes, detergents, latex, metals, plant oils, and solvents. The cause of nummular dermatitis is unknown, but the condition is associated with increased stress and winter weather and is most commonly seen in middle age. The cause of seborrheic dermatitis is also unknown; this condition is associated with hereditary factors and underlying neurological disease and can be seen in neonates, children, and adults.

Pathophysiology

The histological agent causes inflammatory changes in the skin, including vasodilation, edema, mononuclear cell infiltration into the dermis and epidermis, and breakdown of the epidermal cells. This leads to the visible changes on the skin's surface (e.g., redness, swelling, oozing, crusting, scaling, and itching). If the process is repeated over a period, the epidermis thickens, producing hyperkeratosis and a chronic scaly appearance.

Clinical Manifestations

Atopic Type	Constant itching that sets up an itch-scratch-rash-itch cycle; red, scaly papules that coalesce

	into plaques that ooze and crust; common sites are hands, face, and flexural areas
Contact Type	Transient redness to bulla formation; itching is common; weeping, crusting
Nummular Type	Sharply circumscribed, moist, oozing discoid plaques that later become dry and scaly
Seborrheic Type	Dry, diffuse scaling of scalp; oozing, crusted, red-yellow scalp lesions or scaly plaques that recur; may be found in external ear canals, eyebrows, and nasolabial folds and on sternum

Complications

Secondary infection is the most common complication. Chronic dermatitis, which appears on the hands or feet, can restrict function and become crippling.

Diagnostic Tests

Clinical evaluation with characteristic manifestations; detailed history to locate possible source of contact rash; patch test may isolate allergens; immunofluorescence shows elevated IgE in atopic dermatitis.

Therapeutic Management

Surgery	None
Medications	Antipruritics for itching; topical/systemic corticosteroids, pimecrolimus cream or tacrolimus ointment to relieve inflammation; topical keratolytics to reduce scaling
General	Oils on affected areas; removal of irritant in contact dermatitis; daily use of seborrheic shampoos; humidification; cool, wet cloths on open lesions; emollients to relieve dryness; clip nails to decrease abrasion from scratching
Prevention/ Promotion	Avoid triggering factors such as sudden temperature shifts, contact with irritants, foods that provoke exacerbations, stressful situations, allergens, excessive hand washing.

Diabetes Insipidus (DI)

A transient or permanent disturbance of water metabolism that results in excretion of excessive quantities of diluted urine; it may be pituitary (central or neurogenic), renal (nephrogenic), or intake regulated (primary or dipsogenic) in nature

D

Etiology and Incidence

Central DI is the result of a lack of antidiuretic hormone (ADH), which can be caused by brain injury from head trauma, neurosurgery, irradiation of the pituitary, hypothalamic tumors, or infiltrative metastatic diseases. More than half of diagnosed cases are idiopathic.

Nephrogenic DI results when the body is unable to respond normally to ADH. The condition is inherited as an X-linked recessive disorder or acquired in association with disorders such as renal disease, sickle cell disease, fibrosarcoma, granuloma, polynephritis, metabolic disease, polycystic disease, or pregnancy, or with toxic agents that reduce glomerular filtration. *Primary DI* results from excessive water intake caused by psychogenic disorders (e.g., schizophrenia) or dipsogenic disorders (e.g., multiple sclerosis [MS], meningitis, encephalitis, neurosarcoidosis, or tuberculosis [TB]).

Pathophysiology

Central DI begins when some form of brain injury reduces the amount of ADH. This leads to a decrease in the hydroosmotic permeability of the distal collecting tubes in the kidney, allowing the dilute urine formed in the proximal nephrons to be excreted unchanged. The result is a slight dehydration effect, an increase in plasma osmolality, and stimulation of the thirst mechanism. The individual drinks more, and as a result, input and output are balanced, and osmotic pressure in the body stabilizes at an above-normal level. In *nephrogenic DI* the kidneys are rendered ADH resistant and hydroosmotic permeability is reduced, with the same end result as in central DI.

Primary polydipsia is caused by excessive water intake, either because of a severe cognitive dysfunction or because the thirst regulator has been disrupted by disease or trauma. Plasma osmolality is reduced, which causes a decrease in the production of ADH and dilutes the urine, and excretion rises to meet intake. As intake and output are balanced, plasma osmolality stabilizes at below-normal levels.

Clinical Manifestations

The most common presenting signs and symptoms are unquenchable thirst, frequency of urination, polyuria, nocturia, dry skin, slight dehydration, and constipation. The individual typically excretes large quantities of urine (5 to 20 L/day) with a very low specific gravity (less than 1.005).

Complications

A prolonged increase in urine volume and flow can lead to hydroureter and hydronephrosis. An individual who has no thirst mechanism may experience severe dehydration and circulatory collapse.

Diagnostic Tests

Fluid Deprivation Test	*Central and nephrogenic DI:* Urine osmolality remains low
	Primary DI: Osmolality increases
Vasopressin Administration After Fluid Deprivation	*Central DI:* Osmolality rises
	Nephrogenic and primary DI: Osmolality is unchanged

Therapeutic Management

Surgery	None unless related to underlying disease
Medications	*Central DI:* Synthetic pituitary hormone replacement with vasopressin (IV, IM, SC) or desmopressin (IV, oral, or nasal spray); chlorpropamide for control of polyuria in mild cases
	Nephrogenic DI: Thiazide diuretics to reduce urine volume

General	Identification and treatment of any underlying organic cause for DI, reduction of sodium in diet for nephrogenic DI, daily weights
Education	Information about long-term hormone replacement therapy and symptoms of overdose (e.g., nasal irritation, nausea, headache, shortness of breath [SOB]); education about control of fluid balance, prevention of dehydration, monitoring of daily weights, signs of water intoxication

D

Diabetes Mellitus (DM)

A disease complex that is characterized by persistent hyperglycemia caused by insufficient insulin production and/or resistance to the metabolic action of insulin. There are four general classifications of DM: type 1 insulin-dependent, type 2 noninsulin-dependent, gestational diabetes mellitus (GDM), and secondary DM.

Etiology and Incidence

The precise causal mechanisms in DM are unknown, although genetics and a faulty autoimmune response are thought to play major roles in type 1 diabetes. Genetics and obesity are risk factors for type 2 diabetes. GDM manifests during pregnancy, with 90% to 95% of the cases spontaneously disappearing in the postpartum period. However, type 2 DM will develop in almost 50% of these women within 5 years. Secondary DM is caused by an array of underlying primary pathological abnormalities such as pancreatic disease, liver disease, muscle disorders, endocrine dysfunction, or genetic system defects, or as a result of drug side effects.

DM has been diagnosed in more than 10 million persons in the United States and is the sixth leading cause of death, with more than 71,000 deaths annually. It is the leading cause of irreversible blindness and chronic renal failure and plays a large role in the development of cardiovascular disease and stroke. DM is found worldwide, and the incidence is increasing rapidly. Type 1 accounts for 10% to 15% of cases, and the age of onset is primarily in childhood or adolescence. Type 2 accounts for 85% to 90% of cases, and onset generally occurs after age 40, although incidence in children and adolescents is increasing rapidly. GDM complicates 2% to 5% of all pregnancies in the United States and accounts for 90% of all DM during pregnancy. A very small number of cases are secondary DM, and the age of onset varies according to the cause of the underlying primary pathological condition.

Pathophysiology

DM occurs if the body cannot produce insulin (type 1), or if it is unable to use the insulin produced (type 2). In either case, the ultimate result is hyperglycemia and impaired glucose transport. Type 1 diabetes is characterized by a genetic predisposition manifested in one of several human leukocyte antigens (HLAs). Recent research suggests that the genetic predisposition, coupled with an unknown factor (viral or chemical agent), triggers an ongoing autoimmune process that systematically destroys the beta-cells in the pancreas, thereby interfering with the body's ability to produce insulin. Type 2 diabetes involves either a defect in the insulin-release sites in the pancreas or a resistance to the action of insulin stemming from a decrease in the number of receptor sites in the peripheral tissue. This type of DM is often associated with obesity.

In all types of DM, the result is interference with glucose transport across cell membranes in peripheral muscle and adipose tissue, leading to faulty oxidation and energy production. Metabolism of fat, carbohydrate, and protein is impaired, as are storage of glycogen in the muscle and liver, and storage of fatty acids and triglycerides in adipose tissue. Amino acid cell transport is disrupted. Unrestrained gluconeogenic and glycogenolytic processes in the liver cause overproduction of glucose. As the blood glucose level rises, renal tubules fail to reabsorb all the glucose. This produces glucosuria and osmotic diuresis, with water and electrolyte loss through the urine. Hyperglycemia also damages myelin nerve coverings, leading to neuropathy. Glycosylation (attachment of glucose to protein molecules) in the capillaries causes thickening of the capillary membrane and microangiopathy. Atherosclerotic processes are accelerated, and vessel elasticity diminishes.

Risk Factors

Type 1	Faulty autoimmune system, genetic predisposition
Type 2	Obesity, familial tendency, history of gestational DM, aging, sedentary lifestyle, African-American, Hispanic, and Native American
Gestational	Over 30 years of age; obesity; family history of type 2 DM; GDM with previous pregnancy; obstetrical history of stillbirth, miscarriage, polyhydramnios, congenital anomaly, or large infants (more than 9 lb); hypertension (HTN); recurrent monilial vaginitis; glycosuria during pregnancy

Secondary	Presence of underlying primary pathological agent or drug

Clinical Manifestations

Type 1	Abrupt onset with polyuria, polydipsia, polyphagia, weight loss, weakness, fatigue, dehydration
Type 2	Usually asymptomatic in early stages, with pruritus vulvae a common presenting symptom in women; later manifestations include skin infections, cold extremities, fatigue, blurred vision, delayed healing, and polyuria
Gestational	Onset of glucose intolerance that begins during pregnancy

Complications

Diabetic ketoacidosis is a common acute complication in type 2 diabetes. If left untreated, it leads to coma and death. Nonketotic hyperglycemic-hyperosmolar coma is an acute complication in type 2 diabetes. It is often accompanied by seizure activity and has a mortality rate of about 50%. Complications of gestational diabetes include stillbirth, miscarriage, premature birth, cesarean birth, and/or hypertensive disorders associated with pregnancy. Fetal and neonatal complications include macrosomia, shoulder dystocia, birth trauma, hypoglycemia, hypocalcemia, hyperbilirubinemia, thrombocytopenia, polycythemia, and respiratory distress syndrome.

Chronic systemic complications of DM include cardiovascular and peripheral vascular disease, retinopathy, nephropathy, neuropathy, dermopathy, and impotence.

Diagnostic Tests

Fasting Blood Sugar	Greater than 126 mg/dl on two occasions
Glucose Tolerance Test	Greater than 200 mg/dl for 2-hour sample and one other sample after administration of 75 g of glucose

Hemoglobin A_1C	Used to measure blood glucose levels cumulatively over a 3-month period. A value greater than 7% is abnormal. This test is also used to monitor control of DM.
Blood Insulin	Absent in type 1, normal or elevated in type 2
Plasma C-peptide	Absent in type 1, normal or elevated in type 2
Glucola Screen	Used in pregnancy a value of 140 mg/dl is positive and indicates need for further testing with glucose tolerance test

D

Therapeutic Management

Surgery	Recommended only for chronic complications, such as coronary artery grafts and eye surgery Pancreas transplant surgery in conjunction with renal transplant surgery is experimental for type 1 cases
Medications	Insulin for type 1; oral hypoglycemics (sulfonylureas, biguanides, a-glucosidase inhibitors, thiazolidinediones, meglitinides) and/or insulin for type 2 and gestational DM
General	Dietary control aimed at maintaining stable body weight; distributing caloric intake into small, evenly spaced loads; weight reduction with obesity; regular monitoring of blood sugar; regular exercise program; counseling and support for adaptation to long-term disease; intensive fetal biophysical monitoring (nonstress testing) in women with poor glucose control, requiring insulin, with history of HTN or stillbirth; monitor glucose levels every 2 hours during labor; test for carbohydrate intolerance 6 to 12 weeks postpartum or after breast-feeding ceases
Prevention/ Promotion	Healthy adults over age 45 should be tested for DM every 3 years.

High-risk pregnant women should be screened for GDM on first prenatal visit and again at 24 to 28 weeks of gestation.

Education   Education about disease and complications, medications and medication administration, glucose monitoring, diet and exercise; importance of regular medical, ophthalmologic, and podiatric follow-up

Diarrhea

A change in bowel habits marked by frequent passage of loose, watery, unformed stool; diarrhea may be an acute or a chronic condition

Etiology and Incidence

Diarrhea can be caused by a wide range of factors, such as sugar intolerance, use of antacids that contain poorly absorbed salts, laxative abuse, ingestion of large amounts of certain sugar substitutes, bacterial toxins, viral infections, bile acids, drugs, fat, carbohydrate malabsorption syndromes, mucosal disease, and bowel surgery that alters intestinal transit and strictures. Diarrhea is a common symptom that may be transient or may indicate underlying disease.

Pathophysiology

Diarrhea occurs when the amount of fluid absorbed by the body declines; when the amount of fluid produced increases, overwhelming the bowel's absorptive capacities; when motor disturbances affect bowel motility and secretory capacities; or when injury to the bowel mucosa produces blood and mucus in the stool.

Clinical Manifestations

The primary symptom is a change in normal bowel habits that results in frequent, loose, watery, unformed stools that are often accompanied by cramping, abdominal pain, and urgency.

Complications

Hypokalemia, dehydration, and vascular collapse are possible complications with severe or chronic diarrhea. Infants and small children are particularly prone to dehydration.

Diagnostic Tests

The diagnosis is made by clinical evaluation, history, and examination of the stool macroscopically and microscopically. Stool measurements, cultures, microscopic examination, and flexible sigmoidoscopy can help determine the cause.

Therapeutic Management

Surgery	None
Medications	Antidiarrheal drugs that increase intestinal tone (paregorics), reduce peristalsis (anticholinergics), increase bulk (methylcellulose), and absorb fluid (pectin)
General	Treatment of underlying disorder, monitoring and replacement of fluid and electrolytes, perirectal skin care
Education	Education about infection control, hygiene, hand washing; instruction on proper handling, cooking, and storage of food if cause is food related

Diphtheria

An acute, highly communicable disease affecting the mucous membranes of the respiratory tract

D

Etiology and Incidence

Diphtheria is caused by the gram-positive rod *Corynebacterium diphtheriae* and is spread by direct contact with an infected person, carrier, or contaminated articles or surfaces, particularly in crowded and poorly maintained environments. Effective immunization efforts have made this disease rare in many parts of the world. The last culture-confirmed case indigenous to the United States occurred in 1988.

Pathophysiology

The pathogen invades and multiplies in the nasopharynx, producing a toxin that causes necrosis of the epithelial membrane and forms a patchy, grayish-green pseudomembrane composed of bacteria, fibrin, leukocytes, and necrotic tissue. The toxin is spread systemically by the bloodstream, and lesions form in distant organs, including the lungs, heart, kidneys, and central nervous system (CNS). The individual is communicable from exposure until the bacilli are no longer present (2 to 4 weeks). Cutaneous diphtheria, characterized by skin lesions, is also common.

Clinical Manifestations

The incubation period is 1 to 4 days; the first symptoms include a mild sore throat, nasal discharge, dysphagia, low-grade fever, cough, hoarseness, nausea, vomiting, and chills. A grayish-green membrane forms on the nasal mucosa, soft palate, nasopharynx, larynx, and tonsils. If a respiratory obstruction develops, dyspnea, stridor, retractions, hypoxia, and cyanosis may be evident.

Complications

Severe complications are common without prompt treatment; they include myocarditis, heart failure and sudden death, polyneuritis, encephalitis, renal failure, cerebral infarction, thrombophlebitis, pulmonary emboli (PE), respiratory paralysis, pneumonia, and respiratory failure.

Diagnostic Tests

Clinical evaluation and characteristic clinical signs, particularly the membrane, are used for tentative diagnosis. Definitive diagnosis is made by culture of the causative agent.

Therapeutic Management

Surgery	Tracheostomy for airway obstruction
Medications	Diphtheria antitoxin given promptly on clinical diagnosis; antiinfective drugs to kill the causative gram-negative bacteria; immunization of close contacts, including health care personnel
General	Respiratory isolation; parenteral nutrition with bulbar signs; cardiac pacing with heart block; bed rest progressing to restricted activity; oxygen; fluid replacement if needed; cultures until three negative results are achieved; cultures of close contacts; report of all cases to public health authorities
Prevention/ Promotion	Diphtheria-tetanus-pertussis immunization for all children, with periodic diphtheria-tetanus toxoid boosters through adulthood

Diverticular Disease

Inflammation of acquired, saclike projections (diverticula) that have formed in the gastrointestinal (GI) wall and have pushed the mucosal lining through the surrounding muscle; they may become infected, bleed, or rupture

Etiology and Incidence

Diverticula are thought to be caused by an increase in intraluminal pressure in the bowel, which forms a pouch in weakened areas of the wall. The mechanism that weakens the wall is unclear. However, a highly refined diet lacking fiber is believed to be a contributing factor. Abnormal colonic motility patterns and spastic colon have also been implicated. The formation of diverticula is known as *diverticulosis*. An infection of the diverticula that causes inflammation is *diverticulitis*.

Diverticulosis and diverticulitis are most common in developed Western countries. The incidence of diverticulosis increases with age, and approximately one third to one half of those over age 60 have the disease; of those, 10% to 20% develop diverticulitis. Diverticulitis is more severe in those under age 50, and men are three times more likely than women to be affected in that age group.

Pathophysiology

Diverticulitis occurs when undigested food mixed with bacteria accumulates in a diverticulum, forming a hard mass called a *fecalith*. The fecalith diminishes the blood supply to the diverticulum and an infection ensues, followed by inflammation and a microperforation of the diverticular mucosa, submucosa, and adjacent serosa into the surrounding pericolic fat. A pericolic abscess forms, which may range from microscopic to a large mass. Repeated episodes of diverticulitis lead to scarring, fibrosis, stricture of the bowel wall, and continued narrowing of the lumen.

Clinical Manifestations

Diverticulosis is largely asymptomatic. Complaints of pain and localized tenderness in the lower left abdominal quadrant with a low-grade fever are the typical presenting symptoms of diverticulitis. Nausea, vomiting, and abdominal distention and chills are also seen.

Complications

Intestinal obstruction, fistula formation, and 🔱 perforation of the bowel with peritonitis and hemorrhage are possible complications of recurrent bouts of diverticulitis.

Diagnostic Tests

A history of diverticulosis, complaints of localized abdominal pain, and a possible palpable abdominal mass are highly suggestive. A flexible sigmoidoscopy or colonoscopy may detect orifices of diverticula and thickening of bowel wall (contraindicated during acute attack); a water-soluble contrast enema or CT scan is used to outline diverticula and display effacement of pericolic fat. Laboratory tests reveal a polymorphonuclear leukocytosis with an elevated sedimentation rate.

Therapeutic Management

Surgery	Bowel resection with or without colostomy to treat recurrent attacks or complications
Medications	Analgesics for pain, antibiotics for infection, stool softeners
General	Nothing by mouth (NPO) with bed rest, nasogastric tube and IV hydration for acute attack, high-fiber diet after inflammation resolves
Prevention/ Promotion	Adequate fiber in diet; regular exercise program
Education	Instruction about continuing diet with high-fiber content; bulk laxatives; exercise program; colostomy care instructions

Dysmenorrhea

Pain associated with menstruation

Etiology and Incidence

The cause of primary dysmenorrhea is unknown, but the disorder is thought to be tied to uterine contractions and ischemia mediated by prostaglandin. The most common cause of secondary dysmenorrhea is endometriosis. Dysmenorrhea is a common gynecological complaint, occurring in 50% of menstruating women with a 10% rate of severe symptoms that cause incapacitation for 1 to 3 days a month. It declines in severity with age and childbirth.

Pathophysiology

It is thought that increased sensitivity of the myometrium to prostaglandin causes uterine contractions and ischemia of the uterine muscle, resulting in a cramping pain. Secondary dysmenorrhea is tied to an underlying pelvic disorder that produces similar cramping conditions.

Clinical Manifestations

An aching pain low in the abdomen may radiate to the lower back and legs. The pain begins up to 24 hours before onset of menses, peaks after 24 hours, and typically subsides within 2 days. Headache, nausea, diarrhea, and urinary frequency may also be present.

Complications

None

Diagnostic Tests

With secondary dysmenorrhea, a pelvic examination or laparoscopy or both to rule out underlying disorders is recommended.

Therapeutic Management

Surgery	Laser ablation of endometriosis, dilation and curettage (D&C), hysterectomy for underlying disorders; presacral neurectomy for primary dysmenorrhea that is unresponsive to medication
Medications	Prostaglandin synthetase inhibitors (e.g., ibuprofen, naproxen sodium) to relieve pain; low-dose oral contraceptives if pain continues
General	Regular exercise, adequate rest, no tobacco use, heat to lower abdomen or back

Ebola Virus

Ebola hemorrhagic fever is a severe, often fatal disease in humans and nonhuman primates (monkeys and chimpanzees) that has appeared sporadically since its initial recognition in 1976.

E

Etiology and Incidence

Ebola is a viral hemorrhagic fever caused by the Ebola virus, a member of a family of ribonucleic acid (RNA) viruses known as Filoviruses. Four genetically distinct subtypes of the virus have been identified. The exact origin of the Ebola virus remains unknown, although researchers believe that the virus is animal-borne and is found in African animal hosts. Approximately 600 fatalities have occurred in Africa since an initial outbreak in 1976. People in the United States are at risk only if they have close personal contact with people in Africa who are infected with the Ebola virus.

Pathophysiology

The pathophysiology of this rare yet deadly disease remains speculative. Humans do not "carry" the virus. The manner in which the virus first appears in a human at the start of an outbreak has not been determined. It is thought that the first patient becomes infected through contact with an infected animal. Humans can transmit the virus to each other by direct contact with blood and/or secretions of an infected and unprotected person or by close, personal contact with health care workers working with infected people. The course of the disease remains inconsistent; some individuals recover and others die. It is speculated that those who die usually have not developed a significant immune response to the virus at the time of death.

Risk Factors

Exposure to diseased primates in Africa
Providing care for a diseased individual and not wearing full protective clothing
Contact with an unprotected health care provider who is caring for a diseased individual

Clinical Manifestations

Incubation	3 to 16 days from exposure
Initial	High fever, headache, muscle aches, stomach pain, fatigue, diarrhea followed by conjunctivitis, vomiting, nonbloody diarrhea and abdominal pain, and intensely dry sore throat and chest pain
	A maculopapular rash with desquamation develops in some patients, and some patients display petechiae; hemorrhage, profound lethargy, and expressionless facies
Remission	24 to 48 hours
Late	Normothermia, tachypnea, shock, oliguria, hemorrhage, and hepatitis; severe cases display mucosal bleeding, anuria, hiccups, and encephalopathy with irritability, confusion, delirium, and convulsions

Complications

Cardiopulmonary collapse and death are possible complications. Mortality rates range from 55% to 83%.

Diagnostic Tests

Clinical Evaluation	History of contact with primates or infected individual; red, itchy eyes and skin rash
Laboratory	CBC; antigen-capture Enzyme-linked immunosorbent assay (ELISA) testing; immunoglobulin G (IgG) ELISA; polymerase chain reaction (PCR); blood cultures for malaria and virus isolation; stool culture

Therapeutic Management

Currently no standing treatments exist for Ebola hemorrhagic fever. If the fever is suspected, local and state health departments should be immediately advised.

Surgery	None
Medications	Electrolyte replacement, antiinfectives for secondary infections
General	Support; fluid therapy; oxygenation; strict "barrier technique" isolation, including careful handling of blood and body fluids; use of disposable materials; use of sanitizing solutions
Prevention/ Promotion	If Ebola is suspected, strict isolation of the index case is essential. Biosafety level 4 precautions are to be implemented and local and national health authorities should be notified immediately. All nonhuman primates suspected of disease should be quarantined.

E

Eclampsia

(See Preeclampsia and Eclampsia)

Eczema

(See Dermatitis [Eczema])

Emphysema

A chronic obstructive pulmonary disorder characterized by permanent anatomical alteration of the airway spaces distal to the conducting airways
(See also Chronic Obstructive Pulmonary Disease)

Etiology and Incidence

Any factor that leads to chronic alveolar inflammation can serve as a precursor for the formation of emphysematous lesions. Common precursors are tobacco smoking; air pollution, particularly in an occupational setting; underlying respiratory disease; and severe respiratory infection in early childhood. A rare congenital alpha$_1$-antitrypsin deficiency also is a precursor. Emphysema has been diagnosed in more than 1 million Americans. It is the leading cause of death from respiratory disease in the United States, with more than 16,500 deaths reported annually. The incidence increases with age and is highest in white, male, blue-collar workers in the Midwestern United States.

Pathophysiology

Recurrent alveolar inflammation leads to degradation of elastin in the distal airways because of an imbalance in the elastase-antielastase mechanism. As the degradation proceeds, elastic recoil is lost, the alveolar walls are destroyed, blood vessel density is reduced, the air spaces enlarge, and the peripheral bronchioles collapse; this leads to air trapping and impaired gas exchange.

Clinical Manifestations

Emphysema is thought to begin in early adulthood and remain asymptomatic until middle age. Gradual, progressive, exertional dyspnea is the most common complaint. Skin is pink because of adequate oxygen saturation. Cough and sputum are negligible; wheezing, marked weight loss, and fatigue may also be present. Severe dyspnea, chest retractions, and barrel chest are late signs.

Complications

Alveolar blebs and bullae may form and rupture, leading to ♀ pneumothorax. Cor pulmonale may occur during end-stage disease.

Diagnostic Tests

Clinical Evaluation	History of smoking, occupational exposure
Radiology	Normal in early disease; as the disease progresses, localized radiolucency with decreased vascular markings, flattened appearance of diaphragm, widened intercostal margins
Pulmonary Function	Total lung capacity and residual volume are increased; vital capacity, forced vital capacity, and forced expiratory volume are decreased
Arterial Blood Gases	Decreased PaO_2; normal $PaCO_2$ until late in disease when it increases
CBC	Elevated RBCs, leukocytosis, normal hemoglobin, and hematocrit until late in disease

Therapeutic Management

Surgery	Bullectomy, lung volume reduction, transplantation
Medications	Bronchodilators (ipratropium and β_2 agonists); antiinfective drugs to treat secondary bacterial infection; oxandrolone to stimulate appetite; influenza and pneumonia vaccines for prophylaxis; antitrypsin replacement therapy for individuals with demonstrated deficiency (experimental)
General	Removal of irritants; low-level oxygen to treat hypoxemia, with careful monitoring of blood gases for rise in PaO_2 without rise in $PaCO_2$; consistent exercise to improve ventilatory and cardiac function; counseling for depressive episodes

Prevention/ Promotion	Smoking cessation Eliminate industrial exposure Reduce exposure to air pollution
Education	Education including disease process, medication administration (schedule, use of spacer), home use of oxygen, breathing retraining (pursed lip abdominal breathing), energy conservation (pacing and pursing), exercise conditioning, nutrition plan to increase weight if indicated, importance of long-term follow-up

Encephalitis, Primary

An acute febrile syndrome marked by inflammation of the tissues of the brain and spinal cord that may result in altered neurological function

E

Etiology and Incidence

The cause of primary encephalitis is usually direct invasion by one of several viruses (e.g., arbovirus, enterovirus, adenovirus, herpes virus, mumps virus). The mode of transmission is usually a mosquito bite, but ticks and amebae may also transmit the virus. Some forms of the virus (e.g., herpes virus) may be spread by direct contact with nasal excretions or open lesions. A more rare secondary encephalitis may occur as a complication of another primary viral infection, such as measles, chickenpox, or rubella. Primary encephalitis occurs worldwide and may be sporadic or epidemic. There are about 20,000 cases reported to the Centers for Disease Control and Prevention (CDC) in the United States each year.

Pathophysiology

Within 24 hours of contact, the virus invades the bloodstream, lymph nodes, bone marrow, and most organs. Within 48 hours, there is marked lymphocyte destruction and necrosis of lymph nodes. By day 4, macrophages have replaced the destroyed lymph nodes, bone marrow is depleted, and the cytoplasm and megakaryocyte nuclei are degenerating. The viral titer declines in peripheral tissue and increases in the brain. By day 6, there is extensive involvement of the meninges, brain, and spinal cord, with petechial hemorrhages, lymphocytic perivascular cuffing, gliosis, and neuronal necrosis, causing cerebral dysfunction.

Clinical Manifestations

Subclinical cases of encephalitis do occur and are largely asymptomatic or are accompanied by flulike symptoms, such as fever and general fatigue. Common early signs of encephalitis are fever, severe frontal headache, nausea, and vomiting. If encephalitis is untreated, neurological signs that may manifest 6 to 7 days after initial infection are nuchal rigidity, lethargy, confusion, stupor, coma, seizure activity, and extremity paralysis.

Complications

The likelihood of complications is related to the etiological agent and the person's general premorbid condition. Complications include permanent neurological damage and death.

Diagnostic Tests

Clinical Evaluation	History of exposure, nuchal rigidity, positive Kernig's sign, pathological reflexes, muscle weakness, paralysis
Lumbar Puncture	Elevated pressure; cerebrospinal fluid, WBCs elevated; proteins slightly elevated; glucose normal; occasional isolation of the virus (mobile amebae can be seen on wet mount)
Serology	Increase in antibody titer early in disease
Immunofluorescent Stain of Biopsy Brain Tissue (Rarely Done)	Positive for specific viruses

Therapeutic Management

Surgery	None
Medications	Antiinfective drugs for amebic infections; vidarabine and acyclovir for herpes infections, sedatives for restlessness, anticonvulsants for seizure activity, mannitol and corticosteroids to reduce cerebral edema and inflammation

General	Maintenance of fluid and electrolytes; maintenance of the airway: may need mechanical ventilation; oxygen to maintain blood gases; maintenance of nutritional status: may need nasogastric tube; seizure precautions; rest; neurological assessments; secretion precautions to prevent transmission of some viral agents; rehabilitation for permanent neurological sequelae
Prevention/ Promotion	Secretion precautions to prevent transmission of some viral agents; prevention of spread through mosquito-ant-tick control

E

Endocarditis, Infective

An inflammation and infection of the endothelial layer of the heart and cardiac valves

Etiology and Incidence

Endocarditis is caused by staphylococcal, streptococcal, pneumococcal, enterococcal, and gonococcal organisms. Fungi and diphtheroids have also been implicated. Men are more susceptible, and the mean age is about 55 years. The American Heart Association estimates that there are 10,000 to 20,000 new cases of infective endocarditis annually. The overall mortality rate is about 25%, but it rises to as high as 70% in elderly patients.

Pathophysiology

The bacterial agent travels to the heart via the bloodstream after a transient bacteremia. It is attracted to and colonizes a fibrin-platelet vegetation that forms from previous endothelial damage. The pathogens are resistant to normal host defense mechanisms because the vegetation prevents access of the defense mechanisms to the microorganisms.

Risk Factors

Personal history of rheumatic heart disease, valvular disease, or congenital heart defect
Individuals with prosthetic valves, pacemakers, or arteriovenous shunts
Recent history of invasive cardiac procedures or cardiac surgery
IV drug abusers
Immunosuppressed individuals
Multiple body piercing and tattoos
Recent history of dental or periodontal work
Use of an intrauterine device

Clinical Manifestations

Onset is nonspecific and highly variable. Fever is the common complaint, but it is often intermittent and can be high or low grade. Other early signs include chills, aching, shortness of breath, rigors, weakness, fatigue, and headache. When embolization occurs, petechiae of the skin and mucous membranes, splinter hemorrhages of the fingernails, macules on the palms and soles, retinal hemorrhage, and neurological sequelae are also present.

Late signs include clubbing of the fingers and splenomegaly.

Complications

The course of endocarditis is progressive and fatal without treatment. Complications include stroke, congestive heart failure, renal failure, meningitis, subarachnoid hemorrhage, and heart failure.

E

Diagnostic Tests

Clinical Evaluation	History of symptoms, risk factors, heart murmur
CBC	Anemia, leukocytosis, elevated erythrocyte sedimentation rate
Blood Cultures	To identify causative agent
Echocardiography	To detect vegetations, abscesses, damaged valves, regurgitation
Urinalysis	Proteinuria, hematuria with renal involvement
Rheumatoid Factor	Positive in 50% of individuals with subacute bacterial endocarditis (SBE) of at least 6 weeks' duration

Therapeutic Management

Surgery	Removal of thrombi, valve replacement in cases of uncontrollable sepsis
Medications	Antiinfective drugs targeted at causative agent; aspirin for fever, aches
General	Rest, forcing fluids during temperature elevation, high-calorie supplements, monitoring for complications
Prevention/ Promotion	Antiinfective prophylaxis for high-risk individuals for dental or surgical procedures

Endometriosis

Growth of endometrial tissue outside the uterine cavity, associated with infertility, abnormal uterine bleeding, and pain

Etiology and Incidence

The cause of endometriosis is unclear, but the prevailing hypothesis suggests dissemination and implantation of endometrial cells at local ectopic sites via retrograde menstruation through the fallopian tubes and distant sites via the bloodstream or lymphatics. Sites can be anywhere in the body, but pelvic structures are most common. Another hypothesis suggests transformation of coelomic epithelium into endometrium-like glands. Endometriosis develops in approximately 25% of women. It is seen most commonly during the childbearing years and incidence peaks by age 40.

Pathophysiology

After implantation of endometrial cells, primarily on pelvic structures (e.g., the ovaries, ligaments, oviducts, and peritoneal surface of the uterus), the cells grow to form lesions. These lesions are subject to hormonal cycles and bleed during menstruation, causing irritation and inflammation of the surrounding tissue, leading to fibrosis and adhesions.

Risk Factors

Familial history
Late childbearing or nulliparity
Müllerian duct abnormalities
Cervical or vaginal atresia

Clinical Manifestations

The major symptom is secondary dysmenorrhea, although many individuals are asymptomatic. Other symptoms are abnormal uterine bleeding, dyspareunia, infertility, lower abdominal pain, nausea and vomiting, and pain associated with a full bladder or with defecation.

Complications

The primary complication is infertility or spontaneous abortion. Bowel obstruction or painful urination can occur with formation of extensive adhesions.

Diagnostic Tests

Laparoscopy with biopsy allows visualization and histological confirmation of the lesions.

Therapeutic Management

Surgery	Laparoscopy to remove or vaporize lesions, hysterectomy with bilateral salpingo-oophorectomy for intractable pain and/or extensive disease
Medications	Gonadotropin-releasing hormone agonists, progestins, and antigonadotropic agents to inhibit ovarian function and suppress endometrial growth; prostaglandin synthase inhibitors to relieve dysmenorrhea; estrogen replacement and calcium supplement after removal of ovaries
General	Emotional support for depression, altered body image, and possible infertility

Epididymitis

Inflammation of the epididymis of the testes

Etiology and Incidence

There are many causes of epididymitis, including different kinds of infections or trauma. The most frequent cause is a sexually transmitted disease (STD), specifically, STDs caused by *Neisseria gonorrhoeae* and *Chlamydia trachomatis* among heterosexual men and *Escherichia coli* among homosexual men. Cytomegalovirus (CMV) and *Salmonella* have been identified in individuals with acquired immunodeficiency syndrome (AIDS). Other causes include trauma, urological procedures, prostatitis, toxoplasmosis (in AIDS), urethral structure disease, and seminal vesiculitis. It is the most common of all intrascrotal problems. An estimated 600,000 cases of epididymitis occur each year in the United States.

Pathophysiology

Epididymitis occurs most often unilaterally, when urine is mixed with bacteria or a virus, and refluxes from the posterior urethra, prostate ducts, or seminal vesicles. In the early stages, cellulitis associated with local pain and edema appears. As the condition progresses and becomes acute, the entire scrotum becomes erythematous and painful, often producing an inflammatory hydrocele. Late stages of the disease may cause peritubular fibrosis and occlusion of the epididymis that may result in sterility.

Risk Factors

STDs resulting in urethritis
Prostatitis
Urinary reflux or cystitis
Urological procedures
Strenuous activities

Clinical Manifestations

Scrotum	*Early stages:* Scrotal sac may be reddened, swollen, tender, or hot to touch; varicocele

Late stages: Significant edema; redness; diffuse pain; overlying scrotal skin may be dry, flaky, and without the normal rugated appearance

Testis	The affected side may be enlarged and painful. A mass may be palpated.
Abdomen	Pain on the affected side lower quadrant may be present.
	Nausea and vomiting
	Pain and overall status may cause nausea and vomiting.

Complications

Orchitis is the most common complication of epididymitis. Infertility and sterility are serious long-term complications.

Diagnostic Tests

Blood Tests	WBC count (elevated in acute episodes)
Urinalysis	Evidence of infection; culture may identify causative organism
Urethral Discharge Culture	Culture may identify causative organism, especially gonococcal or chlamydial urethritis
Prostatic Secretion Culture	Evidence of associated prostatitis
Doppler Stethoscope and/or Testicular Radionuclide Scan	To rule out torsion of the testis

Therapeutic Management

Surgery	Aspiration of local abscesses; correction of underlying structural defects when infections recurrent
Medications	Antibacterial or antiinfective agents as appropriate for identified organisms;

	analgesics for pain; antiemetics for nausea and/or vomiting
General	Bed rest; scrotal support either by positioning or by athletic support; Sitz bath, local heat, or ice packs may be used to decrease discomfort
Prevention/ Promotion	Practice of safe sex and careful cleansing after intercourse

Epiglottitis (Acute Supraglottitis)

E

A severe, rapidly progressive infection of the epiglottis and surrounding tissue that causes obstructive airway inflammation

Etiology and Incidence

The organism responsible for epiglottitis is usually *Haemophilus influenzae* type B. This uncommon yet serious disease is seen most often in children between ages 2 and 5 but can occur from infancy to adulthood. It is usually seen in late fall and winter months.

Pathophysiology

The infection, acquired through the respiratory tract, moves and settles in the supraglottic region, causing inflammation, swelling, and cellulitis. ❶ The swelling is rapid and severe, resulting in mechanical obstruction of the airway. Breathing becomes difficult and as the airway swells shut, CO_2 retention and hypoxia result. Clearance of inflammatory secretions is also impaired.

Risk Factors

No *H. influenzae* type B conjugate vaccine

Clinical Manifestations

Often starts with an upper respiratory infection, cold, sore throat. The common history is that the child goes to bed with slight cold-type symptoms and awakens later complaining of sore throat and pain on swallowing with a fever and ill appearance. As airway swelling progresses, child assumes a sitting position, leaning forward with chin thrust forward, mouth open, and tongue protruding outward. Drooling is common because of inability to swallow. The child appears irritable, extremely restless, and frightened. The child is not hoarse, but because of the swelling, has a thick and muffled voice. The child's throat is red and inflamed and a distinctive, large, cherry red edematous epiglottis is visible on careful inspection of the throat. *However, visualizing the throat should not be attempted if emergency airway equipment is not available.*

Complications

❶ The most significant complication of epiglottitis is the loss of airway. Throat inspection should never be attempted unless the child is in the hospital and emergency airway equipment, including endotracheal intubation equipment, is available.

Diagnostic Tests

Direct Visualization of the Epiglottis	Direct visualization of the epiglottitis is diagnostic, but manipulation of the airway may initiate sudden and potentially fatal airway obstruction.
X-ray	Lateral and anteroposterior neck x-rays show enlargement of epiglottis, ballooning of hypopharynx
Cultures	Blood and/or urine and/or epiglottic cultures reveal infective organism

Therapeutic Management

🟢 Speed is vital. An adequate airway is critical and priority above all other care. Care should be taken not to upset the child. If at all possible, keep the parents with the child and keep the child in a sitting position.

Surgery	Tracheostomy if needed for airway maintenance
Medications	Antiinfectives for bacterial infection, corticosteroids to reduce edema
General	Endotracheal intubation with airway support
Prevention/ Promotion	The American Academy of Pediatrics recommends that all children, beginning at 2 months of age, receive the *H. influenzae* type B conjugate vaccine.
Education	Education for parents on expected course of treatment

Epilepsy

(See Seizures)

Epistaxis

Bleeding from the nose

Etiology and Incidence

Epistaxis may be caused by a variety of factors, such as irritation, trauma, underlying coagulation disorders, or localized or systemic infections. At least 10% of the population is thought to have suffered at least one episode of epistaxis. Children and men are more susceptible, and winter is the time of most common occurrence.

Pathophysiology

Bleeding results when damage interferes with the vascular integrity of the superficial vessels in the fragile mucosa of the nasal passages. Most bleeding originates in the anterior portion of the nose from Kiesselbach's plexus, a highly vascular network in the anterior nasal septum. Posterior bleeding usually originates from the turbinates or lateral nasal wall.

Clinical Manifestations

Bleeding from the nostrils

Complications

Pooled blood may cause sinusitis and otitis media. Large blood loss can cause anemia or interfere with cerebral and cardiopulmonary tissue perfusion. In individuals with an altered mental status, aspiration of blood is also a possible complication.

Diagnostic Tests

Inspection with a nasal speculum to determine the site of bleeding
Radiographs to locate fracture if trauma is the cause

Therapeutic Management

Surgery	Reduction and fixation of nasal fractures, ligation of the internal maxillary artery for uncontrolled posterior bleeding, split-

	thickness skin grafts to correct chronic bleeding in Rendu-Osler-Weber syndrome
Medications	Analgesics for pain; if posterior chamber is packed, antiinfective drugs to prevent sinusitis and otitis media; if a large amount of blood was swallowed, nonabsorbable antibiotics to prevent breakdown of blood and ammonia absorption
General	Upright position; pinching of the nose with thumb and forefinger for 5 to 10 minutes (anterior bleeding); endoscopic cauterization of site if pressure fails; packing of nasal cavity to apply pressure (posterior bleeding); blood replacement if anemia is evident

Esophageal Cancer

Squamous cell carcinomas, which account for 60% of esophageal cancer, arise from the surface epithelium, most commonly in the middle and lower esophagus. Adenocarcinomas, which constitute 35%, arise from the gastric fundus and develop in the lower third of the esophageal tract.

Etiology and Incidence

The etiology is not well defined but is associated with chronic esophageal irritation. The incidence is low in the United States (less than 14,000 cases annually), but the disease is endemic in central China and southeast Africa, with reports of as many as 130 cases per 100,000. This cancer is most common in older adults, with blacks affected three times as often as whites and men three times as often as women. Morbidity in the United States is approximately 13,000 persons a year.

Pathophysiology

A squamous cell carcinoma begins as a small mucosal patch that grows, ulcerates, and extends into the esophageal lumen and then the recurrent laryngeal nerve and tracheobronchial tree. Extension to the aorta and other adjacent structures also occurs. Metastasis to local and abdominal lymph nodes and to most body organs follows.

Risk Factors

Smoking and tobacco use (chewing)
Alcohol abuse
Drug abuse (e.g., morphine, opium)
Malnutrition
Environmental carcinogens (e.g., nitrosamines, silica, fungi)
History of cancer of the larynx or pharynx
History of chronic inflammation of esophagus, achalasia (failure of esophageal sphincter to relax), tylosis, or caustic burns to esophagus

Clinical Manifestations

Dysphagia is the most common presenting symptom. Regurgitation and weight loss may also occur.

Complications

The prognosis is poor, with less than 5% long-term survival. Complications of advanced disease include esophageal obstruction, hemorrhage, and perforation.

Diagnostic Tests

The tumor is diagnosed with visualization on esophageal x-ray followed by esophagoscopy with a brush biopsy.

Therapeutic Management

Surgery	Resection of tumor for palliation; esophagectomy with Dacron graft replacement; esophageal dilation or gastrostomy to aid eating
Medications	Preoperative systemic; cisplatin-based chemotherapy
General	Radiation for palliation and to control pain, head of bed propped up on 4-inch blocks to prevent reflux, treatment of esophagitis
Prevention/ Promotion	Smoking cessation
	Treatment for alcohol/drug abuse
	Good oral hygiene
	Adequate nutrition
	Treatment of gastroesophageal reflux disease (GERD)
	Avoidance of esophageal irritants such as silica

Esophageal Varices

Dilated blood vessels in the esophagus

Etiology and Incidence

The cause of esophageal varices is portal hypertension (HTN) in association with cirrhosis, liver parenchymal disease, duodenal ulcer, or acute pancreatitis. Bleeding esophageal varices eventually develop in about 50% of individuals with cirrhosis.

Pathophysiology

Portal veins narrow and become obstructed as a result of the underlying disease process. As the lumen narrows, the venous blood returning to the right atrium from the intestine and spleen seeks new routes through collateral vessels. These collateral vessels enlarge and become tortuous, and the mucosa ulcerates.

Clinical Manifestations

Hematemesis and melena are common. However, bleeding may occur abruptly, with massive hemorrhage accompanied by blood coming out of the mouth.

Complications

Esophageal rupture, with massive hemorrhage and death, is the most common complication. With acute bleeding, the mortality rate is about 50%. Approximately 60% of individuals die within a year of the first episode of bleeding.

Diagnostic Tests

History of underlying disease, plus hematemesis or melena

Hemorrhage with varices confirmed by an upper gastrointestinal (GI) series, and bleeding site confirmed by endoscopy or mesenteric angiography

Therapeutic Management

Surgery	Portacaval, splenorenal, or mesocaval shunt to relieve portal pressure; ligation of bleeders
Medications	Vasopressin or beta-blocker to lower portal HTN, antacids or histamine receptor antagonists to inhibit gastric acid, vitamin K, antibacterial agents
General	Control of acute bleeding through ice water lavage and esophageal tamponade techniques, blood transfusions, fluid replacement, sclerotherapy to thrombose varices, transjugular intrahepatic portosystemic shunt (TIPS) to divert portal blood flow from liver

Esophagitis

(See Gastroesophageal Reflux Disease [GERD])

Fibrocystic Breast Disease

Single or multiple cysts in the breast

Etiology and Incidence

The cause is unclear but is thought to be related to a hormonal imbalance, with an excess estrogen production and a progesterone deficiency during the luteal phase of the menstrual cycle. Fibrocystic disease is the most common breast condition and occurs primarily during the childbearing years. It is estimated to be present in at least half of all women and accounts for half of all breast surgery.

Pathophysiology

The precise process of cyst formation is unknown. However, a wide variety of morphological changes occur in fibrocystic disease, including fibrosis, cyst formation, sclerosing adenosis, and ductal hyperplasia. The cysts may be nonproliferative, proliferative without atypia, or atypically hyperplastic.

Clinical Manifestations

Symptoms typically appear about 1 week before the onset of menstruation and subside about 1 week after menstruation stops. They include lumpy breast tissue; tender, burning, aching, heavy breasts; and nipple discharge.

Complications

Women with atypical hyperplasia have a greater risk of cancer. Infection is another possible complication.

Diagnostic Tests

Clinical evaluation with mammography or ultrasound
Definitive diagnosis made by biopsy and histological examination of tissue

Therapeutic Management

Surgery	Biopsy/stereotactic biopsy of lumps, microcalcifications; aspiration of palpable cysts

Medications	None
General	Support bra, heat compresses to reduce breast pain
Prevention/ Promotion	Regular breast self-examination (BSE), annual clinical evaluation and mammograms for individuals with ductal or lobular hyperplasia

Food Poisoning

Enteric or neural intoxication after ingestion of bacterially contaminated food

Etiology and Incidence

Food poisoning is caused by one of the following organisms: staphylococcal enterotoxins, *Clostridium botulinum*, *Clostridium perfringens*, *Vibrio parahaemolyticus*, or *Bacillus cereus*. The resulting illness is noncommunicable. Occurrence is common and estimates of incidence range from 60 to 80 million in the United States.

Pathophysiology

The causative organism multiplies in the food before ingestion; the pathogenesis is organism specific. Staphylococcal enterotoxins form in foods held at room temperature. They act on the gastric mucosa, producing hyperemia, erosion, petechiae, and purulent exudate. *C. perfringens* reproduces rapidly in cooled and reheated food and acts on the epithelial layer of the ileum, increasing absorption of fluid, sodium, and chloride and inhibiting glucose absorption. *V. parahaemolyticus* multiplies in uncooked seafood and invades the intestinal tissue, producing necrosis, ulceration, and granulocytic infiltration of the mucosa. *B. cereus*, an aerobic spore, multiplies in food held at room temperature and attacks either the gastric or intestinal mucosa. *C. botulinum* forms a toxin in improperly processed foods in anaerobic conditions. It is a neurotoxin that impairs autonomic and voluntary neurotransmission and causes muscular paralysis.

Clinical Manifestations

The signs and symptoms depend on the causative agent.

Staphylococci	Symptoms appear within 7 hours of ingestion: weakness, acute nausea and vomiting, intestinal cramps, diarrhea
Enteric Type (*C. perfringens*, *V. parahaemolyticus*, *B. cereus*)	Symptoms appear within 24 hours of ingestion: nausea, vomiting, abdominal pain, diarrhea

C. botulinum	Symptoms appear within 36 hours of ingestion: dry mouth, diplopia, loss of pupillary light reflex; nausea, vomiting, cramps, and diarrhea precede dysphagia, dysarthria, and progressive descending muscular paralysis

Complications

The complication of enteric manifestations is dehydration; infants and small children are most susceptible. Botulism is fatal in about 10% of cases, usually because of respiratory failure.

Diagnostic Tests

Cultures	Stomach contents, feces, or suspected food for causative organism
Serum	Positive for botulinal toxins

Therapeutic Management

Surgery	Tracheostomy if necessary for airway with botulism
Medications	Trivalent botulinal antitoxin as soon as possible after onset of botulism; antiinfectives
General	*Botulism:* Gastric lavage, mechanical ventilation if necessary, nasogastric tube feedings, fluid and electrolyte replacement, prevention of skin breakdown and contractures during paralysis, minimization of stimuli, precise communication because of altered vision and loss of speech, allaying anxiety about paralysis and treatment
	Other causes: Fluid and electrolyte replacement
Prevention/ Promotion	Avoidance of contaminated food substances
Education	Instruction in prevention (food handling, storage, preparation; hand washing)

Frostbite

Localized cold injury

Etiology and Incidence

Frostbite is caused by exposure to damp cold temperatures around freezing or to dry cold temperatures well below freezing. Susceptibility is increased by dehydration, exhaustion, hunger, substance abuse, impaired circulation, and impaired consciousness. Factors that promote heat loss (e.g., wet clothing, contact with wet metal, wind chill, radiation) increase the severity of injury, as does prolonged exposure to cold. The very young and the elderly are more prone to frostbite as are those from warmer climates who are not acclimated to the cold.

Pathophysiology

Cold exposure can cause cellular injury either by direct formation of ice crystals in the cells or by vascular spasm and occlusion, which result in inadequate tissue perfusion. Cell dehydration leads to vasoconstriction and increased blood viscosity, with sludge and thrombus formation. As thawing takes place, venous stasis occurs at the sites of injury, obstructing the vascular bed and causing edema and tissue necrosis. Tissue damage may range from superficial (skin and subcutaneous tissue) to deep (muscle, tendon, and neurovascular structures).

Risk Factors

Environmental factors	Increased wind chill, temperatures below freezing, prolonged exposure, increased altitude, damp conditions
Host factors	Dehydration, exhaustion, hunger, substance abuse, impaired circulation, skin damage, impaired consciousness, underlying central nervous system (CNS) or cardiovascular disease, anemia, hypothyroid.

Clinical Manifestations

Superficial	Injured area is white, waxy, soft, and numb while still cold; as thawing occurs, area becomes flushed, edematous, and painful, and may become mottled and purple.
	In 24 hours, large blisters form and remain about 2 weeks before turning into a hardened eschar, which remains for about a month before separating—leaving painful, sensitive new skin that often sweats excessively.
Deep	Injured part remains hard, cold, mottled, and blue-gray after thawing; edema forms in entire limb and may remain for months.
	Blisters may or may not form after a delay of several weeks; after several weeks, dead tissue blackens and sloughs off; a line demarcates dead from live tissue.

Complications

Loss of digits, ears, nose, and extremities is possible, as is secondary infection.

Diagnostic Tests

Diagnosis is made by physical examination plus a history of exposure to cold.

Therapeutic Management

Surgery	Escharotomy; sympathectomy for severe vasospasm; debridement after retraction of viable tissue (3 to 4 months after injury); amputation of nonviable extremities (several months after injury)
Medications	Immunological agents (tetanus) and antiinfective drugs for prophylaxis; analgesics for pain; plasma expanders to reduce sludge and thrombus formation

General	Rapid rewarming by immersion in water (37.8° C to 43.3° C [100° F to 110° F]); fluid and electrolyte replacement; whirlpool baths; precautions with injured area to prevent dislodgment of eschar and further damage; counseling for altered body image from loss of limbs; exercise to prevent joint restriction
Prevention/ Promotion	Avoidance of cold temperatures without adequate protection (layered clothing, head covering)
	Carrying supplies in car when driving in cold weather, ice, snow (extra clothing, coats, blankets, fluids, high-carbohydrate foods, cell phone, hazard markers)

F

Gastritis

An acute or chronic inflammation of the gastric mucosa

Etiology and Incidence

Many factors can cause acute gastritis, including alcohol ingestion; drugs (e.g., aspirin, nonsteroidal antiinflammatory agents [NSAIDs], corticosteroids, cytotoxins, antimetabolites); ingested poisons (e.g., DDT, ammonia, mercury, or carbon tetrachloride); ingestion of corrosive agents; *Helicobacter pylori* infection; trauma; burns; and endotoxins. Acute gastritis occurs five times more often in those who abuse alcohol than in the general population. Chronic gastritis is associated with peptic ulcer disease, renal disease, alcoholic cirrhosis, ulcerative colitis, and diabetes mellitus. Chronic use of NSAIDs, radiation treatments, genetics, diet, prolonged emotional stress, and gastrectomy may also be predisposing factors in chronic gastritis.

Pathophysiology

In acute gastritis, the stomach mucosa, which protects the stomach tissue, breaks because of one or more predisposing irritants. Hydrochloric acid then erodes the mucosa, resulting in edema, possible hemorrhage, and inflammation. Spontaneous remission occurs if the irritant is removed. Chronic gastritis results from repeated episodes of acute gastritis. There is progressive gastric atrophy as chronic alterations in the mucosa cause death of the hydrochloric acid (HCL)–secreting cells so there is decreased and/or lack of acid production.

Risk Factors

Ingestion of alcohol, aspirin, nonsteroidal antiinflammatory drugs (NSAIDs), steroids, cytotoxins, antimetabolites, dichlorodiphenyltrichloroethane (DDT), ammonia, mercury, or carbon tetrachloride

Cigarette smoking

Radiation exposure

Presence of *Helicobacter pylori, Salmonella, Staphylococcus* organisms

Underlying conditions producing critical illness such as burns, renal disease, sepsis, peptic ulcers, ulcerative colitis, diabetes mellitus (DM), cirrhosis

Endoscopic procedures, nasogastric (NG) tube suctioning, mechanical ventilation

Emotional or physiological stress

Clinical Manifestations

Acute	Rapid onset of epigastric pain, indigestion, feeling of early fullness, anorexia, weight loss, cramping, nausea, vomiting, hematemesis, melena, general malaise
Chronic	Often asymptomatic; dyspepsia, flatulence, diarrhea, intolerance of spicy and fatty foods, no relief from antacids

Complications

Pernicious anemia often develops in individuals who have gastric atrophy. Untreated gastric disease can lead to obstruction, perforation, and peritonitis. Individuals with metaplasia have a higher risk of gastric cancer.

Diagnostic Tests

Clinical Evaluation	History of exposure to one or more predisposing factors or agents
	Endoscopy with biopsy/cytology To visualize lesions, erosions, and bleeding sites, and to rule out carcinoma
Stool Guaiac	Positive
Urea Breath Test	Positive for *H. pylori*
Nasogastric Aspiration	Frank blood

Therapeutic Management

Surgery	Partial or total gastrectomy, pyloroplasty, vagotomy for major uncontrollable bleeding associated with acute gastritis

Medications	Proton pump inhibitors, antacids, histamine-2 receptor blockers and vasoconstrictors for acute gastritis; vitamins C and B_{12} for chronic gastritis with accompanying pernicious anemia; antibacterial agents for *H. pylori* infection
General	Removal of causative agents; ice water lavage to control bleeding; laser therapy by endoscopy; blood transfusions; for acute gastritis: nothing by mouth (NPO), then diet that eliminates irritants
Prevention/ Promotion	Avoidance of mucosal irritants such as alcohol, NSAIDs, trigger foods Smoking cessation
Education	Education about long-term medication protocols, lifestyle changes for individuals with chronic gastritis

Gastroenteritis

A self-limiting, acute inflammation of the stomach and small intestine caused by ingestion of food, water, or feces contaminated with pathogenic agents, parasites, or toxins

Etiology and Incidence

Causative agents include bacterial and viral pathogens, such as *Campylobacter coli, Escherichia coli, Salmonella* and *Shigella* organisms, Norwalk virus, and rotavirus; parasites, such as *Ascaris, Enterobius,* and *Trichinella* species; and toxins, such as poisonous plants or toadstools, arsenic, lead, and mercury. Inability to digest and absorb carbohydrates has also been implicated as a cause, although it is rare, and the mechanism is poorly understood. Various forms of gastroenteritis are common manifestations worldwide and are often mistaken for food poisoning. Bacterial, parasitic, and viral types of gastroenteritis are infectious and can be transmitted directly or indirectly.

Pathophysiology

The pathological conditions depend on the causative agent. Toxicogenic agents, such as some *E. coli* and *Shigella* strains, release an exotoxin that impairs intestinal absorption. Invasive pathogens, such as some *Shigella* and *Salmonella* species and *E. coli,* penetrate the mucosa of the small bowel, causing cellular destruction, necrosis, ulceration, bleeding, and exudation of protein-rich fluid. Pathogens, such as rotaviruses, attach to the mucosal wall and destroy cells in the intestinal villa, causing malabsorption of electrolytes. Parasites and toxins also interfere with intestinal functioning. The general result of all pathogenic agents is increased gastrointestinal (GI) motility and increased secretion of fluids and electrolytes.

Clinical Manifestations

The onset is often sudden, with abdominal pain and cramping, nausea and vomiting, diarrhea with or without blood and mucus, anorexia, general malaise, and muscle aches. Dehydration, hypokalemia, and hyponatremia occur with persistent vomiting and diarrhea.

Complications

Dehydration, shock, vascular collapse, and renal failure, in rare instances leading to death, are complications of gastroenteritis. Infants, small children, the elderly, and debilitated individuals are at greatest risk.

Diagnostic Tests

Diagnosis relies on identification of the causative agent through stool and blood cultures, Gram's stain, and direct swab rectal cultures.

Therapeutic Management

Surgery	None
Medications	Antidiarrheal agents for all types; antiemetics, except for viral or bacterial gastroenteritis, in which impairment of GI motility is avoided; antiinfective agents for bacterial gastroenteritis with systemic involvement (not generally recommended for simple gastroenteritis because these drugs may prolong the carrier state and contribute to the emergence of drug-resistant organisms)
General	Rest, increased fluid intake, electrolyte replacement, bland diet

Gastroesophageal Reflux Disease (GERD)

Esophageal, laryngeal, or pulmonary inflammation and injury related to repeated reflux of gastrointestinal (GI) contents; esophageal inflammation is often called *esophagitis*

Etiology and Incidence

Reflux (backflow of gastric and intestinal contents into the esophagus) is the result of an incompetent lower esophageal sphincter. Factors that contribute to this incompetence include pyloric surgery; prolonged nasogastric tube intubation; drugs, alcohol, nicotine, or fatty foods, which lower intrinsic sphincter pressure; conditions or positions (lying down) that increase intraabdominal pressure. GERD is one of the most prevalent disorders of the GI tract. Nearly 7% of the U.S. population experiences daily heartburn, and nearly 60% of the population experiences intermittent heartburn. It is particularly prevalent during pregnancy.

Pathophysiology

Gastric secretions and bile salts are belched back into the esophagus from the stomach, causing esophageal irritation, inflammation, corrosion, and the formation of patchy, superficial lesions. As the disease progresses, the lesions spread to the entire esophagus. After the mucosal tissue necroses, the normal cells are replaced with basal cells, causing narrowing and branching of papillae—leading to esophageal hyperplasia. With chronic reflux, the normal squamous epithelium is gradually replaced by columnar epithelium, and the esophagus eventually becomes scarred, develops strictures, and is shortened.

Risk Factors

Pyloric surgery

Prolonged nasogastric tube intubation

Ingestion of certain drugs (calcium channel blockers, beta-blockers, anticholinergics), alcohol, or foods (chocolate, peppermint) that lower pressure on lower sphincter

Tobacco, alcohol abuse

Underlying conditions such as hiatal hernia, incompetent lower sphincter, and delayed gastric emptying

Clinical Manifestations

Early	Heartburn (particularly with spicy or fatty meals, exercise, and recumbent positions) that is relieved by antacids
Midcourse	Heartburn accompanied by high epigastric and substernal pain, regurgitation, dysphagia
Late	Bleeding, dysphagia, disappearance of heartburn

Complications

Complications include obstruction, hemorrhage, and tearing or esophageal perforation from strictures. If the gastric contents are refluxed and then aspirated, the larynx, trachea, and lungs are damaged. Repeated aspiration may lead to chronic pulmonary disease. Infants, children with brain injuries, and adults in a vegetative state are particularly susceptible to pulmonary complications from repeated reflux and aspiration. Individuals with long-standing disease have a greater risk of esophageal cancer.

Diagnostic Tests

Esophageal Acidity Test	To confirm reflux
Esophageal Manometry	To determine sphincter competence
Acid Perfusion Test	To confirm esophagitis
Endoscopy With Biopsy	To evaluate extent of disease

Therapeutic Management

Surgery	Fundoplication to eliminate reflux is performed in patients with severe complications, particularly recurrent aspiration pneumonia
Medications	Antacids for pain, proton pump inhibitors to inhibit hydrogen ion production, histamine-receptor blockers to decrease hydrochloric acid (HCL) secretion; antisecretory drugs to reduce gastric secretions, gastrokinetics to

	stimulate salivation and improve sphincter pressure; *anticholinergics are contraindicated* because they lower sphincter pressure
General	Head of bed elevated; avoidance of food or drink that stimulates acid production (e.g., coffee, alcohol) or lowers sphincter pressure (e.g., smoking, chocolate, fats); many small meals; no food at least 2 hours before bedtime or remain upright 2 hours after eating; increased fluid intake; esophageal dilation to manage strictures
Prevention/ Promotion	Periodic endoscopic evaluation for cancer
	Avoidance of alcohol, tobacco
	Avoid drugs or foods that decrease sphincter pressure
	Elevate head of bed on 4-inch blocks
	Eating frequent small meals
	Weight reduction if obese
Education	Instruction on lifestyle changes for chronic reflux

G

Genital Warts (Condyloma Acuminatum)

A highly contagious, sexually transmitted viral disease of the genitalia and perianal regions characterized by multiple fleshy, painless growths
(See also Sexually Transmitted Disease [STDs])

Etiology and Incidence

Genital warts are caused by various strains of the human papilloma virus (HPV) and are transmitted by sexual contact. Worldwide the incidence has been increasing rapidly. An estimated 20 million individuals in the United States are currently infected with HPV.

Pathophysiology

The HPV invades superficial layers of the epidermis, infects cells in the stratum spinosum, and stimulates cell division, causing excessive cell proliferation and formation of the wartlike projections on the penis, vagina, cervix, vulva, perineum, rectum, and anus and in the perianal regions; they may also be seen on oral mucosa. Laryngeal warts have been seen in vaginally delivered infants born to infected mothers.

Risk Factors

Unprotected sexual contact with an infected partner
Multiple sex partners

Clinical Manifestations

Soft, moist, fleshy pink-to-brown projections, which appear in clusters on genital, perianal, or oral mucosa

Complications

Secondary infections, giant condylomata that destroy large segments of penile tissue, and malignant transformation are all possible complications.

Diagnostic Tests

The diagnosis is made by clinical evaluation and confirmed by a biopsy. A biopsy is also performed to rule out carcinoma and the condylomata seen in late-stage syphilis.

Therapeutic Management

Surgery	Removal by curette, cryotherapy, laser, or electrosurgery
Medications	Topical application of trichloroacetic acid/podophyllin/5-fluorouracil (5-FU) cream to warts; interferon injections into lesions
General	Refraining from sexual activity until clear of disease
Prevention/Promotion	Examination and treatment of all potentially exposed sex partners Use of condoms to prevent spread of infection and/or reinfection
Education	Instruction about sexually transmitted diseases, the importance of completing treatment regimens, and the importance of regular examinations for genital and cervical carcinoma; instruction that treatment does not cure and that relapse is common

G

Glaucoma

A disorder in which increased intraocular pressure leads to eventual vision impairment and possible degeneration of the optic nerve. It may occur primary and secondary to other ocular disease. Glaucoma is classified as open or closed angle.

Etiology and Incidence

The cause of primary glaucoma is unknown, but predisposing factors include heredity, hyperopia, and vasomotor instability. Glaucoma is the second leading cause of permanent blindness in the United States. An estimated 15 million individuals have glaucoma, with more than 1.5 million displaying loss in visual fields. African Americans, diabetics, and those with a family history are most susceptible. Ninety percent of primary glaucoma cases are the open-angle type, which occurs most often after age 65.

Pathophysiology

Increased intraocular pressure (IOP) is related to an imbalance in the production, inflow, and outflow of aqueous humor. Inflow occurs through the pupil and outflow through the meshwork at the juncture of the iris and cornea. In secondary glaucoma the meshwork becomes clogged by blood, fibrin, or inflammatory cells produced by an underlying ocular disorder. Primary open-angle glaucoma is marked by degenerative changes to the meshwork that block outflow. In primary closed-angle glaucoma, the anterior chamber is shallow, the filtration angle is narrow, and the iris obstructs the meshwork at Schlemm's canal. Sometimes dilation of the pupil or trauma pushes the iris forward, narrowing the angle and resulting in obstruction in an acute attack. Primary or secondary glaucoma may be congenital; the condition is hereditary (primary) or is caused by fetal defects in the ocular structure or by underlying congenital systemic disorders (secondary).

Clinical Manifestations

Open-angle Glaucoma	Often asymptomatic, frequent changes in prescription for glasses, mild headaches, vague visual disturbances, halos around lights, difficulty adjusting to darkness
Closed-angle Glaucoma	Severe pain in and around eye, tearing, colored rainbow halos around lights, recurring episodes of blurring and impaired vision, mild dilation of pupils, hazy cornea, possible nausea and vomiting

G

Complications

Untreated glaucoma leads to progressively diminishing vision, degeneration of the optic nerve, and blindness.

Diagnostic Tests

Tonometry	To measure elevation in IOP
Visual Field Studies	To detect impairment in central and peripheral visual fields
Gonioscopy	To detect cellular debris or adhesions and differentiate open-angle from closed-angle type
Ophthalmoscopy	To visualize optic nerve

Therapeutic Management

In secondary glaucoma, treatment focuses on the underlying disease process in conjunction with mydriasis.

Surgery	*Open-angle:* Laser/external trabeculoplasty to improve drainage if medications fail
	Placement of filtering devices if trabeculoplasty fails
	Closed-angle: Laser iridotomy/peripheral iridectomy to push iris back and increase angle
	Ocular implants for some complex forms of glaucoma

Medications	*Open-angle:* Beta-adrenergic blockers and diuretics to reduce production of aqueous humor, miotics to reduce pressure, and adrenergics to increase aqueous outflow
	Closed-angle: ☻ Acute attack—use hyperosmotic agents, carbonic anhydrase inhibitors, and miotics to reduce intraoccular pressure; narcotic analgesics for pain
Prevention/ Promotion	Glaucoma screening (annual tonometry) recommended for adults over age 35 for early detection
	Smoking cessation
Education	*Open-angle:* Instruction in avoidance of tobacco products, fatigue, emotional upset, and large quantities of fluid; instruction in instillation of eye drops; long-term use of medications and their side effects

Glomerulonephritis, Acute

A primary or secondary autoimmune renal disease involving the glomerulus in the kidney and classified as postinfectious, rapidly progressive (crescentic), or immunoglobulin A (IgA) nephropathy

Etiology and Incidence

Postinfectious glomerulonephritis is caused by a bacterial, viral, or parasitic pathogen. Acute poststreptococcal glomerulonephritis (APSGN), the prototypic postinfectious disease, is caused by a streptococcal infection that occurs elsewhere in the body, such as in the respiratory tract or skin. The incidence of APSGN is dropping rapidly in developed countries. It is most common in boys ages 3 to 7 years but can occur at any age. It has a rapid onset and usually resolves spontaneously.

Rapidly progressive (crescentic) glomerulonephritis is either idiopathic, related to the production and deposition of the antiglomerular basement membrane antibody, or occurs as part of multisystem disease. This type of glomerulonephritis is rare and is most often seen in men.

IgA nephropathy is idiopathic and is usually a primary disease, although it can be secondary. It is common in children and young adults, affects males six times as often as females, and is particularly prevalent in Asia.

Pathophysiology

Acute glomerulonephritis occurs when antigens from the causal agent provoke an antibody response, which results in antigen-antibody complexes that are deposited in the glomerular capillary walls. The deposits can be the continuous type or the more common discontinuous granular form. They cause a cascade of inflammatory changes in the glomeruli, resulting in vasoconstriction, a marked decrease in plasma flow, and a decrease in the filtering surface; this in turn reduces the glomerular filtration rate (GFR). A compensatory mechanism increases the synthesis of prostaglandins and the hydrostatic pressure in other glomeruli to increase flow and maintain the filtration rate. If acute glomerulonephritis is progressive, the compensatory mechanisms eventually induce glomerular damage through thickening and scarring of the filtration membrane.

Clinical Manifestations

APSGN	Onset of symptoms occurs 1 to 6 weeks after infection; symptoms include hypertension (HTN), headache, edema, oliguria, dark urine, reduced urine output, flank pain, weight gain, fever, chills, nausea, and vomiting; about half of cases are asymptomatic.
Crescentic Type	Similar to APSGN but the onset is more insidious and weakness, fatigue, and fever are the predominant symptoms.
IgA Nephropathy	Similar to APSGN but the onset usually occurs 1 to 2 days after upper respiratory infection (URI) or enteral illness and is often accompanied by hematuria.

Complications

Complications include congestive heart failure (CHF), acute or chronic renal failure, and end-stage renal disease.

Diagnostic Tests

Urinalysis	Hematuria (microscopic or gross), proteinuria, sediment, RBC casts
Blood Chemistry	Increased BUN, serum creatinine, serum lipid, decreased serum albumin
Renal Biopsy	Obstruction of glomerular capillaries
Antistreptolysin O (ASO) Titers	Positive in APSGN
IgA Serum	Elevated in 50% of IgA nephropathy cases
IgA-Fibronectin	Elevated aggregates with IgA nephropathy

Therapeutic Management

Therapy focuses on treating symptoms and preventing complications.

Surgery	Renal transplantation for end-stage renal disease
Medications	Antihypertensives for HTN, diuretics for edema, antiinfective drugs if infection is still present, Kayexalate for hyperkalemia, phosphate-binding agents, corticosteroids for crescentic glomerulonephritis
General	Bed rest; fluid, potassium, and sodium restrictions; reduced protein intake if uremia is present; hemodialysis or peritoneal dialysis for renal failure
Prevention/ Promotion	Omega-3 fatty acids to prevent slow loss of renal function in IgA nephropathy
	Early diagnosis and treatment of sore throat and skin lesions to prevent APSGN

G

Gonorrhea

An acute, sexually transmitted infection of the epithelium of the genitalia, perianus, and pharynx
(See also Sexually Transmitted Disease [STDs])

Etiology and Incidence

Gonorrhea is caused by *Neisseria gonorrhoeae*. It is the second most frequently occurring STD, with an estimated 600,000 new infections occurring annually. The peak incidence occurs between 20 and 24 years of age. Infants born to mothers infected with the disease can contract gonococcal ophthalmia during the passage through the vagina.

Pathophysiology

After intimate contact, the gonococcus attaches to and penetrates the columnar epithelium, producing a patchy inflammatory response in the submucosa with resultant exudate. In men, affected areas include the urethra, prostate, Littre's and Cowper's glands, and seminal vesicles. In women, affected areas include the urethra, cervix, and Bartholin's and Skene's glands. The rectum, pharynx, and conjunctivae are vulnerable in both genders. Direct extension of the infection occurs through the lymphatic system to the epididymis and fallopian tubes. The inflammatory exudate is replaced by fibroblasts, producing fibrous tissue and strictures of the lumen of the urethra, epididymis, or fallopian tubes.

Risk Factors

Unprotected sexual contact (vaginal, anal, oral) with an infected partner
Multiple sexual partners
Vaginally delivered infants of infected mothers
History of STDs

Clinical Manifestations

Male Genitalia	Urethral pain; dysuria, purulent discharge; urinary frequency and urgency

Female Genitalia	Usually asymptomatic; urinary frequency
Pharynx	Sore throat; dry, red tongue
Perianal	Anal itching, burning, and bleeding; pain on defecation; diarrhea; rectal discharge
Conjunctivae	Purulent discharge

Complications

Complications arise with untreated disease and include pelvic inflammatory disease (PID) in women and epididymitis and urethral stricture in men. Both genders may have disseminated disease, with pustular skin lesions, septicemia, endocarditis, meningitis, and arthritis.

Diagnostic Tests

The primary diagnostic tools are the clinical evaluation, a history of exposure to an infected partner, and a culture of the exudate that is positive for the organism.

Therapeutic Management

Surgery	None
Medications	Antiinfective drugs sensitive to the organism, following treatment guidelines of the Centers for Disease Control and Prevention (CDC)
General	Refrain from sexual activity until free of disease; reculture after treatment
Prevention/ Promotion	Examination and treatment of all potentially exposed sex partners
	Use of condoms to prevent spread of infection and/or reinfection
Education	Instruction about STDs, the importance of completing treatment regimens, and the importance of follow-up exam and reculture 4 to 7 days after completion of treatment

Gout

A primary or secondary recurrent, acute arthritis of the peripheral joints, particularly the great toe, associated with hyperuricemia

Etiology and Incidence

Hyperuricemia and gout develop from excessive uric acid production and/or a decrease in renal excretion of uric acid. Gout occurs most often in men (95% of the cases) and is rare in women before menopause. In postmenopausal women, gout is often linked to diuretic use. The incidence of gout is increasing in developed countries.

Pathophysiology

A factor triggers an overproduction or undersecretion of uric acid. The plasma becomes supersaturated with uric acid, and a crystal urate precipitate is formed and deposited in avascular tissue (e.g., cartilage, tendons, and ligaments of peripheral joints) and cooler tissue (e.g., ears). Through an undefined mechanism, the crystals are released at various times, causing an acute inflammatory reaction in the joint with extension to the periarticular tissue. Repeated acute attacks lead to chronic arthritis and deformed joints.

Risk Factors

Genetic Factors	Hyperactivity of hypoxanthine-guanine phosphoribosyltransferase, superactivity of phosphoribosyl pyrophosphate, fructose intolerance
Environmental Factors	Ethanol abuse, foods high in purines, diuretic use, severe muscle exertion
Underlying Disease Processes	Diabetes mellitus (DM), polycythemia, hypertension (HTN), renal disease, leukemia, sickle cell anemia
	Evolutionary absence of the enzyme uricase

Clinical Manifestations

Acute pain, redness, swelling, tenderness, and heat at the affected joint are typical presenting features. Fever, chills, and malaise may also be present. Limited motion is present in the affected joint or joints.

Complications

Complications include infection of ruptured deposits, renal involvement with formation of renal calculi, secondary degenerative arthritis, and joint deformity.

G

Diagnostic Tests

A tentative diagnosis is made by clinical evaluation and elevated serum uric acid levels and confirmed with needle aspiration of synovial fluid, which is positive for urate crystals.

Therapeutic Management

Treatment is aimed at terminating the acute attack and preventing future attacks by lowering uric acid levels and resolving existing deposits.

Surgery	Removal of large crystal deposits (tophi)
Medications	Colchicine, nonsteroidal antiinflammatory drugs (NSAIDs) to reduce inflammation in acute attack; steroids used if NSAIDs and/or colchicine not effective or contraindicated; colchicine, antihyperuricemic drugs for those with frequent attacks or chronic disease to reduce uric acid levels or increase excretion of uric acid (lifelong treatment); sodium bicarbonate to alkalize urine in patients who form calculi
General	Rest of joint; avoidance of alcohol and purine-rich foods, weight reduction if necessary to reduce wear and tear on joints, increased fluid intake
Prevention/ Promotion	Prophylaxis with colchicine in those prone to attacks
Education	Instruction in long-term use of medications and their side effects

Guillain-Barré Syndrome (GBS)

A rapidly progressive, acute inflammatory demyelinating polyneuropathy characterized by muscle weakness and paralysis of the extremities and possible respiratory paralysis with abnormal sensation and loss of reflexes

Etiology and Incidence

The cause is unknown, but GBS is hypothesized to be an autoimmune disorder involving sensitization of peripheral nerve myelin. It is thought to be connected to a previous nonspecific infection and has been associated with inoculation for swine influenza. *Campylo-bacter jejuni* infection often precedes GBS. The incidence of GBS in the United States is 1 to 2 cases/ 100,000 individuals annually, and the disorder occurs across age and gender lines.

Pathophysiology

Mononuclear cells infiltrate the peripheral nervous system and set up an inflammatory response in the blood vessels of the cranial and spinal nerves. Demyelination of the peripheral nerves results, causing muscle weakness that begins in the lower extremities and ascends through the body in a symmetric fashion. Respiratory paralysis and facial weakness occur in 30% to 40% of cases. In some cases axonal destruction can cause atrophy in distal muscles and permanent neurological impairment.

Risk Factors

Infection (human immunodeficiency virus [HIV], *Campylobacter jejuni,* Epstein-Barr, cytomegalovirus [CMV], mycoplasma, hepatitis B virus [HBV])
Upper respiratory infection (URI)
Hodgkin's lymphoma
Pregnancy
Immune system stimulation from factors such as viral immunizations, trauma, surgery

Clinical Manifestations

The first sign is symmetric muscle weakness in the distal extremities accompanied by paresthesia. This weakness spreads upward to the arms and trunk and then to the face. This ascension usually peaks about 2 weeks after onset. Deep tendon reflexes are absent. Difficulty chewing, swallowing, and speaking may occur, and respiratory paralysis may develop. Bladder atony, postural hypotension, tachycardia, and heart block may be seen. Deep, aching muscle pain is also common.

G

Complications

About 5% of affected individuals die of respiratory failure. Another 10% have permanent residual neurological deficits. About 90% of survivors make a full recovery, but the recovery time may be as long as 3 years.

Diagnostic Tests

The diagnosis is based on history and clinical presentation.

Lumbar Puncture	Cerebrospinal fluid (CSP) shows an increase in protein without an increase in lymphocyte count
Electromyography (EMG)/Nerve Conduction Studies	Markedly abnormal with reduced nerve conduction velocity

Therapeutic Management

Surgery	Tracheostomy to provide ventilation in the event of respiratory failure
Medications	Immunoglobulin given IV to counteract neurological defect, narcotic analgesics for pain, prophylactic antiinfectives
	Corticosteroids are generally contraindicated because they worsen the ultimate outcome; however, a trial dose of steroids may be used if disease progression is unrelenting

General   Plasma exchange to speed recovery of neurological deficit, respiratory monitoring and mechanical ventilation for respiratory paralysis, cardiac monitoring for sinus tachycardia and bradyarrhythmia, communication systems if ventilator is used or with facial paralysis, passive range-of-motion (PROM) exercises, turning to prevent contracture and skin breakdown, rehabilitation to aid neurological recovery, counseling and support of individual and family for long-term adaptation

Hantavirus Infections
(Hantavirus Pulmonary Syndrome [HPS]/ Hemorrhagic Fever with Renal Syndrome [HFRS])

Acute infections transmitted to humans by contact with contaminated saliva or inhaled excreta aerosols of diseased rodents; infection is characterized either by acute renal failure with hemorrhage (HFRS) or by acute noncardiogenic pulmonary edema (HPS).

H

Etiology and Incidence

Hantavirus infections are caused by species of *Hantavirus*, which is a part of the viral family *Bunyaviridae*. They represent one of several zoonotic viruses that can be transmitted from animals to humans. The human diseases associated with Hantaviruses are divided into two distinct clinical and geographical syndromes: (1) HPS is seen in North America and (2) HFRS is found mostly in Asia and Europe or in port cities worldwide. HPS was first reported in 1993 and has been found in more than half of the rodents in the United States. New world rodents (*Sigmodontinae* subfamily) carry the Hantavirus that causes HPS. Old world rodents (*Murinae* subfamily) carry the Hantavirus for HFRS. Infection occurs by being exposed to the rodent droppings, specifically urine and feces. Aerosols from the urine and feces act as the transmission route for infection.

HPS and HFRS occur primarily in adults and are associated with domestic, occupational, or leisure activities that bring humans, usually in rural settings or port cities, in contact with infected rodents. An average of 30 HPS cases is reported each year in the United States and cases have been confirmed in 31 states since 1993. HFRS is an epidemic in many parts of the world, such as China, Korea, Japan, and Russia. Three cases of HFRS have been confirmed in the United States.

Pathophysiology

The pathogenesis is not well delineated in either syndrome. The processes in HPS seem to involve increased permeability of pulmonary capillaries and impaired cardiac contractility. The Hantavirus replicates in the pulmonary epithelium and produces large amounts of highly proteinaceous secretions, which result in pulmonary edema and shock. In HFRS, impaired vascular tone and increased vascular permeability result in generalized damage to the capillaries, widespread vascular dilatation, and hemorrhagic engorgement of organs, such as the kidneys, heart, and anterior pituitary. There seems to be an immunopathological basis for both syndromes since the body launches a specific immune response, producing antibodies and T lymphocytes to fight off the infection.

Risk Factors

Repeated exposure to rodent-infested areas
Any activity that puts the individual in contact with rodent droppings, urine, or nesting materials
Use of infested trail shelters or camp in other rodent habitats
Exposure to crawl spaces under houses or in vacant buildings that may have rodent populations
Houses, yards, or buildings infested with rodents
Dock workers in port cities

Clinical Manifestations

HPS

Incubation Period	1 to 5 weeks from the time of exposure to the onset of symptoms
Prodrome (3 to 5 Days)	Fatigue, fever, muscle aches, headaches, cough, nausea/vomiting, and chills Malaise, diarrhea, shortness of breath, dizziness, abdominal and back pains seen about half the time
Pulmonary Involvement	Coughing; shortness of breath; fast breathing (26 to 30 times/min); ❶ feelings of suffocation rapidly progressing (under 24 hours) to pulmonary edema and hypoxia usually requiring mechanical ventilation; hypotension also present
Diuresis	Diuresis signals recovery with rapid improvement

HFRS
There are five distinct phases but considerable variation is manifested depending on the form and severity of the disease. Phases may overlap or be skipped.

Febrile Phase (5 to 7 Days)	Abrupt onset of fever, chills, lethargy, and weakness; then development of frontal or occipital headache with pain on eye movement, myalgias, backaches, abdominal pain, nausea and/or vomiting, and blurred vision followed by intense thirst and anorexia
Hypotensive Phase (24 to 48 Hours)	About 5th day, hypotension is seen with accompanying shock
Oliguric Phase	Blood pressure (BP) normalizes and intermittently spikes; urine output decreases; nausea and vomiting persist, but other symptoms abate. ◑ In a small percentage (up to 15%) of severely ill individuals, hemorrhagic signs (nosebleeds, bruising, hematuria, bloody sputum, bloody stools, and central nervous system (CNS) bleeds) appear.
Diuretic Phase	Diuresis within 2 weeks of onset signals improvement
Convalescent Phase	Asymptomatic except for frequent urination of very dilute urine

H

Complications

HPS	Disseminated intravenous coagulation (DIC), pulmonary and cardiovascular collapse, and death; fatality rate in United States is 38%.
HFRS	Renal hypertension (HTN), end-stage renal disease, massive hemorrhage, CNS bleeding, coma, and death

Diagnostic Tests

Clinical Evaluation	History of exposure to rodents or rodent-infested areas; presentation of clinical signs
IFA/ELISA	Used in detection of Hantavirus antibodies but difficult to isolate in humans
Laboratory	*HPS:* Fall in serum albumin; rise in hematocrit; WBC count raised with shift to left; atypical lymphocytes; platelet count below 150,000; proteinuria; mild elevation of transaminase, creatine phosphokinase, amylase, and creatinine; prolonged prothrombin time and partial prothrombin time
	HFRS: Unremarkable in initial phase, but thrombocytopenia and leukocytosis seen at end of febrile phase; proteinuria with hemoconcentration about day 5; electrolyte abnormalities during oliguric phase
Radiological	*HPS:* Characteristic radiological evolution is as follows: (1) minimal changes of interstitial pulmonary edema, (2) alveolar edema, and (3) pleural effusions.

Therapeutic Management

Surgery	None
Medications	Opiates/analgesics for pain; sedatives for agitation; broad spectrum antibiotics until diagnosis confirmed; vasopressors to maintain blood pressure; prompt, corrective management of electrolyte, pulmonary, and hemodynamic abnormalities
	Ribavirin therapy for viral reduction in HFRS

General	Supportive in nature; early intensive care management; careful monitoring; strict intake and output (I&O) management; colloids for volume expansion in hypotension; mechanical ventilation, extracorporeal membrane oxygenation in HPS; renal dialysis in HFRS
Prevention/ Promotion	Limiting exposure to rodents and their droppings and nests (e.g., proper storage of materials that might provide food or water to rats; use of traps, rodenticides for rodent control in homes; eliminating entry into homes by sealing holes in eaves, attics, basements; cleaning rodent-infested areas using bleach solution and wearing mask and gloves); vaccines for HFRS strains are in phase II human trials for use in high-risk populations
Education	Educate about rodent control and handling, information available through Centers for Disease Control and Prevention (CDC).

H

Headache

Pain or aching of the head associated with various intracranial or extracranial factors; major categories of headache include tension, cluster, migraine, or traction inflammatory

Etiology and Incidence

Although *tension headaches* are the most common type, their precise cause is not well defined. However, most hypotheses suggest that they are related to muscle tension, minor trauma, increased stress or anxiety, food or environmental allergens, infection or lesions of the oral or nasal cavity, ear infections, or eye strain.

Cluster headaches are idiopathic; however, extracranial vasodilation and the trigeminal nerve are implicated in the pain production. The cause of *migraine headaches* is also unknown but is thought to be related to some neuronal event in the brainstem.

Traction inflammatory headaches can be intracranial or cranial in origin. Intracranial headaches may be caused by increased intracranial pressure stemming from an underlying process, such as a brain tumor, abscess, or hematoma; meningitis; syphilis; tuberculosis; cancer; or subarachnoid hemorrhage. Cranial changes in the skull caused by neoplasms, temporal arteritis, or involvement of the sensory nerves of the scalp with a disease—such as herpes zoster—also can cause headaches.

Headaches are the most common of all pain experiences and are conservatively estimated to have affected at least 75% of the population in the United States. Each year, approximately 30 million Americans seek medical treatment for recurrent headache. Tension headaches are most common and occur in children and adults across age and gender lines, though more women than men report having tension headaches. Migraines affect about 12% of the general U.S. population and women are affected at three times the rate of men. Cluster headaches are 10 times more likely to occur in men, with most happening between ages 30 and 40 with a peak incidence at age 30.

Pathophysiology

Headache pain occurs when afferent pain fibers on the cranial nerves (V, VII, IX, or X) carry sensory stimuli to central nervous system (CNS) tissue. The location and diffusion of the pain are dictated by the cause, the extent of tissue affected, and the cranial nerve or nerves involved. Pain can be highly localized and specific or diffuse and generalized. Involvement of the deep brain structure often causes referred pain.

Clinical Manifestations

Tension	Bilateral, dull, nonpulsatile ache, typically bifrontal or nuchal occipital, transient or chronic lasting an average of 4 to 13 hours
Migraine	Paroxysmal, throbbing, unilateral pain that lasts hours to days; cyclical pattern; possible nausea and vomiting; aversion to light and noise; may be preceded by an aura (shimmering visual manifestation) or prodromal-behavioral alterations ranging from depression to euphoria, or triggering food cravings
Cluster	Deep, agonizing, nonthrobbing pain often beginning during sleep and involving an eye, temple, cheek, and forehead on one side; lasts from 30 minutes to 3 hours, with several headaches occurring each day for several weeks; tearing and redness of affected eye
Traction	Deep, dull, steady ache that is worse in the morning and is aggravated by coughing or straining
Arteritis	Soreness of one or both temples that becomes a chronic, burning, well-localized pain; the affected scalp artery is prominent, tender, incompressible, and pulseless

Complications

Complications are usually associated with an underlying disease process rather than the headache itself. However, headaches associated with temporal arteritis, if left untreated, may cause blindness.

Diagnostic Tests

Diagnosis centers on classification of the head pain and identifying the potential cause. A neurological history and a physical

H

examination, with identification of precipitating or underlying disease, are paramount. CT and MRI are useful in detecting intracranial lesions. Cerebral angiography may help detect vascular abnormality.

Therapeutic Management

Surgery	None
Medications	*Tension:* Nonnarcotic analgesics; antidepressants for chronic headaches
	Migraine: Analgesics, ergotamine preparations, or sumatriptan for acute attacks; beta-blockers or serotonin agonists for prophylaxis in chronic retractable syndromes
	Cluster: Prophylaxis with drugs, such as valproic acid, verapamil, lithium carbonate, methylsergide, or topiramate is more effective than administration of drugs during acute attacks. Sumatriptan is sometimes effective during acute episode.
General	*Tension:* Relaxation, biofeedback, cold or hot compresses, massage, stretching, exercise
	Migraine: Avoidance of triggers such as alcohol, caffeine, tobacco; biofeedback
	Cluster: Inhalation of 100% oxygen at 8 to 10 liters by face mask for 15 minutes
	Traction: Treatment of any identified underlying disease or condition
Prevention/ Promotion	Smoking cessation
	Regular exercise program
	Avoidance of food and environmental triggers (migraines)
	Use of prophylactic medications (cluster headaches)
Education	Education about medications and side effects (e.g., ergotamine poisoning from long-term use); instruction in SC injections if on prophylactic sumatriptan

Hearing Impairment (Deafness)

Acquired or congenital diminished auditory capacity that may be classified as sensorineural, conductive, or central; loss with no organic basis has been called *psychogenic, simulated,* or *functional.* Hearing loss ranges from partial to complete.

Etiology and Incidence

Causes of *sensorineural impairment* include trauma, noise, infection, aging, exposure to certain toxins, and drugs. *Conductive loss* results from disorders of the middle and external ear, such as otitis media, otosclerosis, or perforation of the eardrum. *Central hearing loss* is induced when the brain's auditory pathways are damaged by underlying disorders, such as cerebrovascular accident (CVA) or a brain tumor. *Congenital losses* may result from fetal or neonatal anoxia; delivery trauma; fetal exposure to toxins, rubella, or syphilis; Rh incompatibilities; and bilirubin toxicity. *Psychogenic loss* has no traceable organic basis and is thus thought to be psychological in origin.

Pathophysiology

In *sensorineural* impairment, damage to the cochlea or cranial nerve VIII results in interference with bone conduction of sound waves from the inner ear. *Conductive loss* occurs when injury to the middle or external ear results in interference with air conduction of sound waves to the inner ear. Some individuals have both conductive and sensorineural impairment. *Central* impairments interfere with auditory brainstem pathways. There is no organic pathological condition in *functional* hearing loss.

Clinical Manifestations

The overriding manifestation is a reduced ability to distinguish sound. It is often progressive and may range from a mild loss to total deafness.

Complications

Permanent, nontreatable deafness is the central complication.

Diagnostic Tests

Weber Tuning Fork	Lateralization of sound to deaf ear in conductive loss and to better ear in sensorineural loss
Rinne Tuning Fork	Bone conduction heard longer than or as long as air conduction in conductive loss; air conduction heard longer in sensorineural loss
Schwabach's Test	Examiner hears longer than examinee in sensorineural loss and vice versa for conductive loss.
Audiometry	To distinguish types and identify degree of impairment

Therapeutic Management

Surgery	Stapedectomy for loss caused by otosclerosis; cochlear implants in some cases to treat profound deafness
Medications	None
General	Hearing aids for conductive loss; instruction in sign language, speech, and lip reading for the profoundly deaf; use of specialized assistive devices (e.g., amplified or typed-message telephones, low-frequency or flashing doorbells, closed-caption television decoders, flashing alarm clocks, alarm bed vibrators, flashing smoke detectors); counseling and support groups for adaptation
Prevention/ Promotion	*Conductive:* Prompt treatment of ear infection, trauma to tympanic membrane, immediate removal of foreign bodies or impacted earwax *Sensorineural:* Avoid chronic exposure to loud noises (e.g., music); use of noise suppression devices, such as ear plugs, in noisy occupational settings

Heat Exhaustion

Exposure to high ambient air temperature that leads to excessive body fluid loss and eventual hypovolemic shock and electrolyte imbalance

Etiology and Incidence

Heat exhaustion is caused by exogenous heat gain, increased heat production, and/or impaired heat dissipation in combination with inadequate fluid and electrolyte replenishment. Heat exhaustion is particularly common in hot, humid locales in summer months.

Pathophysiology

Causal agents serve to deplete fluid and electrolytes and disrupt balances, leading to decreased sweat production, dilated blood vessels, and increased cardiac output. This results in further fluid volume reduction and electrolyte depletion. Heat exhaustion then results. If not promptly or adequately treated, heat exhaustion may result in heat stroke (see Heat Stroke).

Risk Factors

Prolonged exposure to hot, humid environment
Loss of body fluids from sweating and failure to drink enough replacement fluids
Extremely young or old age
Chronic disease states such as diabetes, hyperthyroidism, or blood-vessel diseases
Alcoholism or other drug abuse
Recent illness or infection involving fluid loss from vomiting or diarrhea
Heavy or restrictive clothing
Poor acclimation to hot and humid weather
Extreme forms of exercise (marathon running, triathlons) or heavy physical labor

Clinical Manifestations

Dizziness; fatigue; faintness; headache; profuse sweating; pale, clammy skin; rapid, weak pulse; low blood pressure (BP); fast, shallow respirations; muscle cramps; intense thirst; confusion with impaired judgment; malaise; total body weakness are all indicators.

Complications

If not promptly and adequately treated, may result in heat stroke.

Diagnostic Tests

Positive history and clinical evaluation

Therapeutic Management

Surgery	None
Medications	Antipyretics are ineffective
General	Place in a cool, well-ventilated environment and remove clothing to cool body; lie down either flat or head slightly lower than feet; apply cool compresses; use other comfort measures. Provide fluid and electrolyte replacement as tolerated.
Prevention/ Promotion	Adequate fluids when exercising and/or working in heat
	Avoidance of exercise/work in extreme heat/ humidity
	Avoidance of excessive layers of clothing, particularly for infants or the elderly
Education	Educate about importance of adequate hydration and proper precautions when exercising and/or working in hot and/or humid conditions

Heat Stroke ⓘ

Extreme and prolonged hyperthermia of the body in which the core body temperature reaches 103° to 106° F (39.4° to 41.1° C) without the body attempting to cool off by sweating and with altered mentation
(See also Heat Exhaustion)

Etiology and Incidence

This serious and potentially fatal problem occurs when the body becomes overheated, the body's temperature soars, and the body no longer attempts to cool itself through sweating. It is an extension of unchecked and/or untreated heat exhaustion. Incidence of heat stroke in the United States is approximately 20 cases per 100,000.

Pathophysiology

Factors of exogenous heat gain, increased heat production, and/or impaired heat dissipation in combination with inadequate fluid and electrolyte replenishment lead to heat exhaustion, which depletes fluids and electrolytes, dilates blood vessels, and increases cardiac output until the sweat glands stop functioning. When sweating ceases, the core body temperature rises rapidly. The skin becomes hot and dry, and an altered level of consciousness occurs. If not treated, cardiovascular collapse results.

Risk Factors

Prolonged exposure to hot, humid environment
Loss of body fluids from sweating and failure to drink enough replacement fluids to ensure fluid and electrolyte balance
Age extremes
Chronic diseases such as diabetes, hyperthyroidism, blood-vessel diseases
Alcoholism or other drug abuse
Recent illness involving fluid loss from vomiting or diarrhea
Heavy or restrictive clothing
Poor acclimation to hot and humid weather
Prolonged exercise or heavy physical labor

Clinical Manifestations

Usually preceded by heat exhaustion, with an elevated temperature, 103° to 106° F (39.4° to 41.1° C); skin is reddish, flushed, and dry. Early manifestations include elevated blood pressure (BP); bounding, rapid pulse; rapid, irregular respirations; agitation; weakness; dizziness; and nausea and vomiting. Late manifestations are a decreased level of consciousness and coma.

Complications

The most common complication is cardiovascular collapse, leading to coma and death. Mortality rate exceeds 30% in those with severe or prolonged hyperthermia.

Diagnostic Tests

Positive history and clinical evaluation

Therapeutic Management

🕛 Heat stroke is an emergency and must be treated rapidly and aggressively. Transport victim to hospital as soon as possible. First aid before transport to hospital should include rescue breathing or cardiopulmonary resuscitation (CPR) if needed. If the individual is conscious or semiconscious, wrap him or her in cold, wet sheets, or place the individual in cold bath water. *Do not delay transport to initiate these first aid measures.*

Surgery	None
Medications	Sedatives or muscle relaxants as needed to control shivering or muscle twitching; anticonvulsants for seizure activity
General	🕛 Emergency management including airway maintenance with oxygenation and ventilation support if needed; invasive and rapid cooling of the body with constant monitoring; IV fluid and electrolyte replacement
	Cooling methods include tepid water mist; fans; ice packs to the head, groin, neck, and axillae, or invasive cooling such as ice water lavage, cold water peritoneal dialysis, and cardiopulmonary bypass

	Shivering should be avoided. Provide careful body temperature monitoring, cardiovascular and cardiac monitoring, and other supportive therapies as needed.
Prevention/ Promotion	Adequate fluids when exercising and/or working in heat
	Avoidance of exercise/work in extreme heat/ humidity
	Avoidance of excessive layers of clothing, particularly for infants or the elderly
Education	Educate about importance of adequate hydration and proper precautions when exercising and/or working in hot and/or humid conditions.

H

Hemophilia

A hereditary bleeding disorder characterized by impaired coagulability of the blood

Etiology and Incidence

Hemophilia is caused by a deficiency of blood clotting factors that are carried on genes on the X chromosome. Sons of men who are hemophiliacs are normal, whereas daughters are obligatory carriers. Sons of women who are carriers have a 50% chance of being hemophilic, and daughters have a 50% chance of being a carrier. Hemophilia is the most common X-linked genetic disease; it occurs in 1.25 of every 10,000 live male births in the United States.

Pathophysiology

Hemophilia A (absent factor VIII) and hemophilia B (absent factor IX) are the most common types. The absence of the clotting factor interferes with the intrinsic phase of the coagulation process and inhibits the formation of prothrombin activator. This interferes with the rate at which thrombin is formed from prothrombin, slowing clot formation.

Clinical Manifestations

The primary presenting sign is excessive, poorly controlled bleeding. The rate of bleeding depends on the amount of factor activity and the severity of the injury that caused the bleeding. A factor activity level below 1% can cause spontaneous bleeding or severe bleeding from even minor trauma. When the factor activity level is more than 5%, bleeding is usually caused by trauma and is more easily controlled. The bleeding may be superficial, may involve subcutaneous and muscle tissue, or may entail deep bleeding into joints and organ systems.

Complications

Nearly 70% of all hemophiliacs are human immunodeficiency virus (HIV)-seropositive. The virus was transmitted through plasma transfusions from blood banks that had HIV-contaminated blood and blood products during the 1980s before reliable testing. Acquired immunodeficiency syndrome (AIDS) is the leading cause of death in hemophiliacs. The second most common cause of death is intracranial bleeds (usually secondary to trauma), which occur in about 10% of hemophiliacs and are fatal 30% of the time. Other complications of repeat bleeds include joint and musculoskeletal deformities, pericardial tamponade airway compression, and uncontrolled hemorrhage.

Diagnostic Tests

Laboratory tests reveal a normal prothrombin time, a prolonged partial thromboplastin time, and a normal bleeding time (platelet function). Assays are used to determine the factor affected and the level of factor activity. Genetic testing is performed to identify carriers.

Therapeutic Management

Surgery	None; extreme care must be exercised when these individuals need surgery for other conditions
Medications	Desmopressin acetate is used to stimulate factor VIII in mild hemophilia A. Aminocaproic acid is given in cases of persistent bleeding unresponsive to treatment and for inoculation against hepatitis B virus (HBV). *Aspirin and nonsteroidal antiinflammatory drug (NSAID) use and intramuscular injections* should be avoided because they may precipitate bleeding.
General	Replacement of deficient factors with recombinant factor products or plasma is the primary treatment. This may be used as prophylaxis or to stop bleeding episodes. Safety precautions in activities of daily living (ADLs) to prevent injury; dental maintenance to prevent need for dental surgery or tooth pulling; counseling for adaptation to chronic disease. Experimental work is being conducted in gene transfer therapy to replace absent gene.
Education	Education of patient and family about disease process; injury prevention; self-administration of factor replacement products; instruction to wear Medic Alert tag at all times

Hemorrhoids (Piles)

Varicosities of the veins in the rectum (internal) or on it (external) that are often inflamed and thrombosed and have a tendency to bleed

Etiology and Incidence

The exact causal mechanism for hemorrhoid formation is unknown but is hypothesized to be associated with increased pressure, which causes congestion in the hemorrhoidal plexus in the anus. Increased pressure has been attributed to straining on defecation, various occupations that require prolonged standing or sitting, pregnancy, and chronic constipation. Another hypothesis suggests involvement of the vasculature of the hemorrhoidal plexus and its tendency to slide or be displaced with bowel movements in concert with a failure of the internal sphincter to relax. Hemorrhoids occur universally in children and adults and are treated as a normal finding when asymptomatic. It is estimated that 50% of the adult population has hemorrhoids.

Pathophysiology

A hemorrhoid is formed when a portion of the vascular mound of the hemorrhoidal plexus weakens and prolapses after being subjected to increased vascular pressures over time. These projections from the anal lining are subject to ulceration and infection.

Risk Factors

Low-fiber/high-fat diet
Chronic constipation
Pregnancy
Obesity
High-resting anal sphincter pressures
Rectal surgery
Prolonged sitting
Anal intercourse

Clinical Manifestations

Typical symptoms of internal hemorrhoids include painless, bright red bleeding with defecation. External hemorrhoids cause intermittent pain, itching, burning, and bleeding. Strangulation of a hemorrhoid may produce severe pain.

Complications

The most common complication is strangulation of an ulcerated and edematous hemorrhoid. In rare cases, severe bleeding may occur and lead to secondary anemia.

Diagnostic Tests

Hemorrhoids are easily diagnosed by direct rectal examination or anoscopy.

Therapeutic Management

Surgery	Injection sclerotherapy to eliminate bleeding hemorrhoids; rubber band ligation for protruding, nonreducible internal hemorrhoids; photocoagulation (laser, infrared lights), cryodestruction to stop bleeding; hemorrhoidectomy (surgical excision) for severe intractable disease
Medications	Topical anesthetic ointments or corticosteroid cream for pain, stool softeners, analgesics
General	Sitz baths, cold and heat therapy for thrombosis, use of wet wipes instead of toilet paper
Prevention/ Promotion	High-fiber diet, adequate hydration, weight reduction, avoid prolonged sitting, avoid prolonged straining at stool

Hepatitis, Viral

A diffuse inflammation of the cells of the liver that produces liver enlargement and jaundice

Etiology and Incidence

The cause is a variety of hepatotropic viruses. To date, five primary viral types cause hepatitis and are identified as hepatitis A (HAV), hepatitis B (HBV), hepatitis C (HCV), hepatitis D (HDV), and hepatitis E (HEV). Hepatitis F has been tentatively identified but it is unclear whether it is a separate virus. Hepatitis G has been recently recognized but epidemiology is not yet clearly established. HAV is transmitted by contaminated food and water and by the fecal-oral route; HBV and HDV are transmitted by contact with body fluids, HCV by percutaneous exposure to blood, and HEV by contaminated water and the fecal-oral route. NOTE: Hepatitis may also occur as a secondary infection and is associated with viruses from other primary diseases, including cytomegalovirus (CMV), Epstein-Barr, herpes simplex, varicella zoster, coxsackie B, and rubella viruses.

Primary viral hepatitis occurs worldwide. More than 250,000 cases are reported annually in the United States, and the incidence is rising. Hepatitis A is the most common form of acute hepatitis in the United States and is seen most often in children and young adults, but the incidence is rising in those with human immunodeficiency virus (HIV). Hepatitis B affects all age groups; about 10% of all transfusion-related hepatitis is this type. Hepatitis C accounts for about 20% of all cases and for most transfusion-related cases. It is seen across all age groups. Hepatitis C cases are rising rapidly. The Centers for Disease Control and Prevention (CDC) estimate that 4 million Americans are infected and at least 12,000 of these will die annually. The annual number of deaths is expected to increase to 38,000 by the year 2010. Hepatitis D is seen in individuals who are susceptible to HBV or may be HBV carriers, such as hemophiliacs and IV drug users. The disease manifestation is severe in children. Hepatitis E is seen primarily among young adults in developing countries in Africa, Asia, or Central America. It is most severe in pregnant women.

Pathophysiology

The etiologic agent, mode of transmission, and clinical course vary according to the hepatitis type. However, the pathophysiology is the same. The causative agent invades the mononuclear cells in the liver, replicates, and sets up an inflammatory process in the parenchyma and portal ducts, causing hepatic cell necrosis, cellular collapse, and accumulation of necrotic tissue in the lobules and portal ducts. This results in interference with bilirubin excretion. Cellular regeneration and mitosis occur simultaneously with cellular necrosis, and the liver regenerates within 2 to 3 months. Continuation of the inflammatory response sets up a chronic disease process.

H

Risk Factors

HAV, HEV	Poor sanitary conditions, crowding, poor hygiene, recent travel to third-world countries
HBV, HCV, HDV	IV drug use with shared needles; health care workers and other occupational workers who are exposed to blood and body fluids; history of multiple sex partners; anal sex; infants or young children of infected mothers; recipients of blood products (hemophiliacs, recipients of multiple blood transfusions); recipients of hemodialysis

Clinical Manifestations

Incubation	*HAV:* 15 to 50 days
	HBV: 45 to 180 days
	HCV: 14 to 182 days
	HDV: 14 to 70 days
	HEV: 15 to 64 days
Communicability	*HAV:* last half of incubation until 1 week after onset of jaundice
	HBV: during incubation and entire clinical course (carrier state may persist for years)
	HCV: as carrier, 1 week before clinical onset to indefinite period as carrier
	HDV: throughout clinical disease
	HEV: unknown

Preicteric Phase	Malaise, headache, nausea and vomiting, anorexia, myalgia, chills, fever, upper quadrant abdominal pain
	HBV, HDV: hives, itching, erythema, arthritis
Icteric Phase	Appetite returns; malaise continues
	Jaundice with or without itching, dark urine, clay-colored stools

Complications

Occasional relapses and prolonged infection are the most common complications with HAV. Complications for HBV, HCV, and HDV include development of chronic hepatitis, spontaneous relapse, and cirrhosis. Severe fulminant hepatitis with rapid cellular destruction, no regeneration, and accompanying encephalopathy occurs in 1% of hepatitis cases and is usually fatal.

Diagnostic Tests

Serum enzymes (aspartate aminotransferase [ASAT, SGOT], alanine aminotransferase [ALAT, SGPT]) that are 8 to 20 times normal values during the prodromal and clinical phases and lactate dehydrogenase (LDH) that is 1 to 3 times normal often occur. These elevations are the hallmark of the disease. Serum bilirubin is elevated. The differential diagnosis is based on the clinical history and various laboratory tests and may be confirmed by liver biopsy. In HAV, the stool is positive for the virus 2 to 4 weeks after exposure, and the enzyme-linked immunosorbent assay (ELISA) shows a rise in HAV antibodies. Immunoglobulin M (IgM) and hepatitis B surface antigen (HbsAG) are present. In HBV, serum antigen tests detect HBeAg and HBsAg, and serum antibody tests detect a rise in antiHBe. Serum antibody tests are used to detect HCV and HDV. HEV is often diagnosed by exclusion of other causes of hepatitis.

Therapeutic Management

| Surgery | Liver transplant for deteriorating cirrhosis associated with chronic HCV |
| Medications | α-interferon, lamivudine, famciclovir, and/or adefovir for chronic HBV; α-interferon for acute HCV; α-interferon, ribavirin for |

	chronic HVC; antiemetics (chlorpromazine is contraindicated in hepatic disease) for nausea; analgesics for pain (acetaminophen is preferred). *Avoid hepatically metabolized drugs in acute hepatitis.*
General	Bed rest; diet as tolerated, with frequent, small, low-fat, high-carbohydrate meals; adequate fluid intake; appropriate infection precautions dictated by transmission routes; monitoring by liver function tests until normal value is achieved
Prevention/ Promotion	*HAV and HBV:* Immune globulin prophylaxis for exposure; vaccines (Havrix, Recombivax HB, Engerix-B, Twinrix) for prophylaxis in high-risk or exposed individuals. HAV vaccines now routinely recommended for all children in 11 western states, where the rate of HAV is at least 20 cases per 100,000 *HAV, HEV:* Improved hygiene and sanitation *HBV, HCV, HDV:* cease IV drug use or cease needle sharing; meticulous testing of blood; use of condoms during anal sexual contact
Education	Instruction on appropriate infection precautions to prevent spread; demonstration of injection procedures for α-interferon

H

Hernia, External

Protrusion of an internal organ (usually bowel) through an abnormal opening or weakness in the muscle wall

Etiology and Incidence

Causes include congenital malformation, traumatic injury, or muscle weakening caused by factors such as pregnancy, obesity, ascites, abdominal tumors, long-term heavy lifting, surgery, or aging. Herniation may be precipitated by excessive coughing or straining during defecation. Hernias occur in all age groups and are more common in men than women. About 75% of hernias occur in the groin area.

Pathophysiology

External hernias may be classified as inguinal, femoral, umbilical, or incisional. *Inguinal* hernias involve an abdominal wall weakness where the spermatic cord in men or the round ligament in women emerges. The herniation protrudes either through the inguinal ring (indirect) or through the posterior inguinal wall (direct). With a *femoral* hernia, the bowel protrudes through the femoral ring into the femoral canal. *Umbilical* hernias occur when bowel protrudes through the inguinal ring. *Incisional* hernias involve protrusion through an abdominal incision that may have healed improperly.

Clinical Manifestations

The most common sign is a bulge in the inguinal, femoral, or umbilical area, or at the incision site. The bulge may become larger with a shift in position or coughing. Sharp, steady pain in the affected area may also be present. Signs of hernia strangulation include increasing severity of pain and fever, tachycardia, abdominal rigidity, and absence of bowel sounds.

Complications

Incarceration or strangulation may lead to intestinal obstruction and necrosis of bowel tissue.

Diagnostic Tests

The diagnosis is made by the clinical presentation. X-ray studies may be used to confirm a suspected bowel obstruction.

Therapeutic Management

Surgery	Herniorrhaphy to repair the hernia or hernioplasty to reinforce weakened muscle with wire, fascia, or mesh; bowel resection and temporary colostomy if bowel obstruction and necrosis occur
Medications	None
General	Manual reduction of hernia; binder or truss to prevent other herniations if individual is not a candidate for surgery

H

Herniated Disk

Rupture and extrusion of the nucleus pulposus through the external ring of an intervertebral disk, causing back pain; the usual location is the lumbosacral region of the spine.
(See also Back Pain, Low)

Etiology and Incidence

Degenerative changes with or without accompanying trauma can lead to a weakening of the outer ring of the intravertebral disk and act as predisposing factors in the extrusion of the nucleus pulposus. The rupture is associated with severe strain or trauma. Lumbar herniation is most common and generally occurs in adults 20 to 45 years of age. Men are affected more often than women.

Pathophysiology

As the ruptured nucleus pulposus extrudes through the annulus fibrosus, the nucleus moves posteriorly and laterally into the extradural space. This often compresses or irritates the nerve root, causing sciatica and compression of the spinal cord, leading to corresponding muscle weakness and diminished sensation.

Clinical Manifestations

The predominant feature is pain in the lower back radiating down one leg or pain in the neck radiating down one arm, either of which may be sudden or insidious in onset. The pain is exacerbated by activity and jugular compression (caused by laughing, coughing, or straining at stool). Numbness and weakness may also be present in muscles innervated by the affected spinal nerve root.

Complications

Neurological deficits, particularly interference with bowel and bladder functioning, are the most common complications.

Diagnostic Tests

A clinical history, physical examination, and prolapse seen on a CT or MRI scan are used for diagnosis. Electromyography (EMG) may define the particular root involved.

Therapeutic Management

Surgery	Microscopic diskectomy, percutaneous laser diskectomy, diskectomy, laminectomy to remove a bulging disk when lesions are acutely compressing the spinal cord or pain is intractable; spinal fusion used if vertebral processes are unstable
Medications	Analgesics and muscle relaxants to relieve pain
General	Alternating hot and cold compresses, transcutaneous electrical nerve stimulation (TENS) for pain; massage; positioning to avoid strain; strict bed rest on firm surface for an acute episode followed by structured exercise program to strengthen back and abdominal muscles; traction for cervical muscle weakness and sensory loss; back brace with lumbar origin; relaxation techniques
Prevention/ Promotion	Use proper body mechanics, avoid heavy lifting, employ an exercise program that strengthens back, leg, and arm muscles

H

Herpes Simplex Infections
(Fever Blisters, Genital Herpes)

A recurrent viral infection of the skin and mucous membranes characterized by clusters of small, inflamed vesicles filled with clear fluid

Etiology and Incidence

The cause is the herpes simplex virus type 1 (HSV-1) or type 2 (HSV-2). HSV-1 usually affects oral, labial, ocular, or skin tissues and is transmitted primarily by oral secretions. HSV-2 (genital herpes) affects genital structures and is transmitted by contact with genital secretions, primarily through sexual intercourse. Genital herpes is the most common sexually transmitted disease (STD) in the United States, with 500,000 new cases annually. The highest incidence is in men age 15 to 30. The incidence is increasing among women and neonates infected during birth by an infected mother. About 85% of the population have antibodies against HSV-1. The other 15% harbor the virus as carriers and have intermittent outbreaks, often triggered by diminished immune protection, stress, menses, sun exposure, and cold. Almost 25% of the population have antibodies against HSV-2.

Pathophysiology

After initial infection, the virus incubates and then forms the characteristic lesions on mucous membranes and skin. After the lesions resolve, the virus resides in the nerve ganglia and remains dormant until triggered by some stimulus or stressor that reactivates lesion formation. The disease is communicable when the lesions are present, and some transient shedding of the virus occurs even when no lesions are visible.

Risk Factors

Unprotected sexual contact (vaginal, anal, oral) with an infected
    partner in HSV-2
Contact with saliva or oral secretions in HSV-1
Infants of infected mothers in HSV-2

Clinical Manifestations

The classic symptoms are itching followed by the eruption of small, tense, clustered vesicles around the mouth, conjunctivae, or genitalia. These vesicles persist for a few days, then dry and crust over; they disappear in about 21 days. Atrophy and scarring may occur if lesions recur at the same site. Many individuals with HSV are asymptomatic.

Complications

An initial infection of HSV-2 during pregnancy can lead to spontaneous abortion, premature labor, uterine growth retardation, and microcephaly. Blindness may result from ocular infections. Urethral strictures may develop in men, and women are at increased risk for cervical cancer. Herpes infections can be severe in individuals with acquired immunodeficiency syndrome (AIDS), leading to esophagitis, colitis, pneumonia, and neurological syndromes.

Diagnostic Tests

A clinical evaluation and history lead to a tentative diagnosis, which is confirmed by culture of lesions and biopsy results.

Therapeutic Management

Surgery	None
Medications	Analgesics for pain, topical antipruritic lotions, acyclovir, valacyclovir to reduce symptoms in HSV-2 infections, topical and systemic antiinfective drugs for secondary infections; suppressive therapy with acyclovir, famciclovir, or valacyclovir for individuals with more than six recurrences a year
General	Cleansing of lesions with soap and water, lesions kept dry, and mouthwashes for oral lesions; careful monitoring if an infected woman is considering pregnancy; emotional support to assist in coping with diagnosis

| Prevention/
Promotion | Proper hand washing after contact with lesions; use condoms during intercourse when asymptomatic; avoid kissing or oral intercourse with oral lesions; avoid intercourse with active genital disease |
| Education | Instruction about the spread and recurrent nature of the disease; precautions during sexual activity |

Herpes Zoster

(See Shingles [Herpes Zoster])

Hiatal Hernia

Protrusion of the stomach through the esophageal hiatus above the diaphragm

Etiology and Incidence

The cause is unknown but is thought to be related to congenital weakness or abnormalities that often are hereditary or are related to the aging process, obesity, pregnancy, ascites, low-residue diets, and trauma. Hiatal hernias are common and occur in about 30% of the population. They are more common in women and the elderly.

Pathophysiology

Loss of muscle tone around the diaphragmatic opening predisposes a person to hernia development. The two types of hiatal hernia are sliding and rolling. Sliding hernias are more common and occur when the cardioesophageal junction and a fundic portion of the stomach are above the diaphragm, creating a weakened lower esophageal sphincter and gastroesophageal reflux disease (GERD). Rolling hernias involve herniation of the cardia of the stomach above the diaphragm, with possible hemorrhage, obstruction, and strangulation.

Clinical Manifestations

Sliding Type	Asymptomatic or associated GERD and heartburn; possible hemorrhage
Rolling Type	Asymptomatic unless hemorrhage or strangulation occurs, which may cause chest pain and other manifestations imitating myocardial infarction (MI)

Complications

Esophageal laceration, perforation, or rupture with massive hemorrhage and strangulation with gangrene are the most common complications.

Diagnostic Tests

X-ray evaluation or esophagography is used to visualize the hernia. A Bernstein test is performed to distinguish cardiac from esophageal chest pain (a positive test result indicates esophageal pain). Cardiac conditions (e.g., acute MI) must be ruled out if the person has acute symptoms, such as chest pain.

Therapeutic Management

Surgery	Reduction of rolling hernia to prevent strangulation; fundoplication for complete mechanical incompetence of sphincter or persistent, untreatable symptoms
Medications/ General/ Prevention	(See Therapeutic Management section under Gastroesophageal Reflux Disease [GERD])

Hirschsprung's Disease

Congenital abnormality of lower bowel innervation that results in partial or total mechanical obstruction

Etiology and Incidence

Hirschsprung's disease is caused by inadequate motility of the intestine because of the congenital absence of enteric ganglionic neurons in the anus and parts of the lower colon. Rarely the small intestine may also be involved. It occurs in 1 in 5000 live births in the United States and is the most common cause of lower intestinal obstruction in neonates. It occurs four times more frequently in males.

Pathophysiology

The absence of the ganglion neurons translates into a lack of enervation that produces a functional defect that results in an absence of peristaltic movements and allows an accumulation of bowel contents proximal to the affected area, which produces intestinal distention. This can lead to inflammation and ischemia of the large and small bowel with resulting bacterial overgrowth and sepsis (enterocolitis).

Risk Factors

Familial tendencies
Down syndrome
Male gender

Clinical Manifestations

Manifestation patterns vary based on the length of the affected bowel. Neonates may be asymptomatic during the first few months of life.

Complete Obstruction	Delayed passage of meconium, obstipation, massive abdominal distention, refusal to feed, and bilious vomiting
Partial Obstruction	Cycles of constipation and diarrhea with thin ribbon-like stools, abdominal distention, and possible failure to thrive

Enterocolitis	Sudden onset fever, abdominal distention, explosive bloody diarrhea

Complications

Enterocolitis or toxic megacolon is the most serious complication and causes death in about 20% of the cases. Postsurgical complications include stricture, continued diarrhea, and recurring enterocolitis.

Diagnostic Tests

Clinical Evaluation	Clinical signs of obstruction
Barium Enema	Diameter of colon distal to obstruction is narrowed and proximal colon is enlarged
Anorectal Manometry	No sphincter relaxation or a paradoxical rise in pressure with rectal distention
Rectal Suction Biopsy	This is the "gold standard" and shows no evidence of ganglion cells.

Therapeutic Management

Surgery	Temporary ostomy to relieve obstruction; several repairs available including: Soave endorectal pull through; Duhamel procedure to create neorectum; Swenson's procedure to resect aganglionic segment; laparoscopic pull-through procedure; transanal endorectal coloanal anastomosis. Myectomy if only anal segment involved; myectomyotomy if entire intestine involved
Medications	Antiinfectives for infection, enterocolitis; analgesics for pain; antiemetics for nausea/vomiting

General	Saline enemas to prep bowel for surgery; routine preoperative and postoperative care; comfort measures; IV hydration; intake and output (I&O); abdominal measurements; support and reassurance to child and family; colostomy care; wound care
Education	Education about colostomy and instruction in care and cleaning; education about possible continuing soiling incidents after surgery; information on available community resources; genetic counseling for parents

H

Histoplasmosis

An infectious disease caused by inhaling fungal spores and taking several forms, including acute benign respiratory histoplasmosis, progressive disseminated histoplasmosis (PDH), or chronic pulmonary histoplasmosis (CPH)

Etiology and Incidence

The cause is inhalation of the fungal spore *Histoplasma capsulatum*. *H. capsulatum* grows in soils throughout the world. In the United States, the fungus is most prevalent along the Ohio and Mississippi river valleys and along the St. Lawrence and Rio Grande rivers. The fungus grows best in soils that are heavily rich with bat or bird droppings. Disturbances of contaminated materials cause the small *H. capsulatum* spores to become airborne or aerosolized. Once airborne, spores can easily be carried by wind currents over long distances. It is not contagious. Incidence of the acute benign form is unknown but the disease is seen more frequently in males than females (4:1 ratio). CPH is estimated at 1 in 100,000 cases in endemic areas.

Pathophysiology

After inhalation, the spores are deposited in the alveoli, convert to yeast, and set up bronchopneumonia. Once infected, the yeast may be spread from the lungs through the blood and lymphatic system to other body organs, including the liver and spleen. Eventually the body sets up a granulomatous inflammatory response to contain the yeast in discrete granulomas, which contract, fibrose, and calcify over time.

The number of spores inhaled, the individual's age and overall state of health, and the susceptibility to the disease determine who becomes ill and the severity of the illness.

Risk Factors

Living/working in high prevalence areas (e.g., Ohio and Mississippi river valleys; St. Lawrence or Rio Grande rivers)

High risk occupations/hobbies involving contact with contaminated soil or bat or bird droppings (e.g. bridge inspector, construction/demolition worker, farmer/gardener, microbiology lab worker, pest control worker, roofer, spelunker)

Age extremes

Those with weakened immune systems (e.g., cancer, human immunodeficiency virus [HIV])

Clinical Manifestations

Acute Benign Respiratory Form	Usually asymptomatic in immunocompetent individuals, who may have dry or productive cough, malaise, infiltration pneumonia, pleural and/or substernal chest pain, low-grade fever
PDH	*Acute:* High fever; hepatomegaly, lymphadenopathy, splenomegaly
	Chronic: The liver lesions may lead to hepatic calcification; purpura; ulcerated lesions in larynx, mouth, nose, or pharynx
CPH	Pulmonary lesions similar to tuberculosis (TB); purulent sputum; hemoptysis; chronic, low-grade fever; cough; increasing dyspnea; and eventual respiratory distress or progressive emphysema

Complications

Histoplasmosis may lead to secondary infections such as pneumonia, progressive emphysema, septic-type fever, hepatosplenomegaly, severe prostration, and death.

Diagnostic Tests

Blood Test and Culture	Positive serologic test for *H. capsulatum* fungal spore
Radioimmunoassay	Used to determine the level of *H. capsulatum* in the urine, serum, and other body fluids
Chest X-ray	*Acute:* To determine transient parenchymal pulmonary infiltrates
	Chronic: To identify progressive enlarged necrotic areas
Skin Test	A skin test, similar to a TB test, to determine previous infection from *H. capsulatum*

Therapeutic Management

Surgery	None
Medications	Fungicidal and fungistatic antiinfective agents, corticosteroids, antihistamines
General	Supportive, rest, IV fluids
	Monitor for antifungal drug toxicity
Prevention/ Promotion	Institute safety practices and dust control measures to reduce worker exposure to *H. capsulatum*
	National Institute for Occupational Safety and Health (NIOSH) recommends that personnel use respirator protective equipment during some activities, such as removal of an accumulation of bat or bird droppings from enclosed areas, such as an attic, barn, or abandoned building, or when working around areas with a buildup of bat or bird droppings
	Lifelong suppressive therapy (itraconazole or amphotericin B) for individuals with acquired immunodeficiency syndrome (AIDS)
Education	Education about prevention, importance of continuing suppressive therapy with AIDS

Hives

(See Urticaria [Hives, Angioedema])

Hodgkin's Disease

A chronic, progressive cancer of the lymphoid tissue
(See also Cancer)

Etiology and Incidence

The cause of Hodgkin's disease is unknown. Current theory holds that it is a low-grade, graft-versus-host reaction with some type of infectious agent as a cause. The incidence in the United States is low. Each year, about 7600 new cases are diagnosed in the United States and 1300 deaths occur. Hodgkin's disease is the most common cancer in young adults. It occurs most often in two age groups, 15 to 35 and 60 to 80, and it is more common in men and boys.

Pathophysiology

The disease begins with an abnormal proliferation of histiocytes (Reed-Sternberg cells) in one lymph node, replacing the normal cellular structure and causing tissue necrosis and fibrosis. The disease spreads through lymphatic channels to lymph nodes throughout the body and eventually metastasizes to the liver, spleen, bronchi, and vertebrae.

Clinical Manifestations

Most individuals first notice a swelling in the cervical lymph nodes. It may be accompanied by itching, fever, night sweats, and weight loss. Later signs may include cough, dyspnea, chest and bone pain, ascites, and jaundice.

Complications

The prognosis for long-term survival is excellent with treatment. About 95% of individuals with stage I or stage II disease are cured with treatment. Untreated or advanced disease causes multiple organ failure and death.

Diagnostic Tests

The definitive diagnosis is made by lymph node biopsy, which shows the presence of Reed-Sternberg cells.

Therapeutic Management

Surgery	Excision of tumors in advanced disease, therapeutic splenectomy
Medications	Systemic combination chemotherapy used with radiation
General	Radiation is the primary therapy, used alone or in combination with chemotherapy, particularly for stage III and stage IV disease. Colony-stimulating factors (CSFs), autologous peripheral blood stem cell transplants, and bone marrow transplants have also been tried with varying degrees of success.

Human Immunodeficiency Virus (HIV) Infection/ Acquired Immunodeficiency Syndrome (AIDS)

Infection that results in wide range of clinical presentations that can vary from a carrier state to a chronic, secondary immunodeficiency syndrome (AIDS) characterized by progressive deterioration of the immune system and manifested by opportunistic infections and malignancies

(See also Kaposi's Sarcoma and *Pneumocystis carinii* Pneumonia)

H

Etiology and Incidence

The HIV infection is caused by one of two related retroviruses (HIV-1 or HIV-2) that convert viral ribonucleic acid (RNA) into a proviral deoxyribonucleic acid (DNA) copy, which is incorporated into the DNA of the host cell. The proviral copy then is duplicated with normal cellular genes during each cellular division. The cell primarily infected is the CD4 lymphocyte (T cell). HIV is a blood-borne virus and is transmitted through exchange of body fluids from an individual with HIV during sexual contact or through parenteral exposure, or from mother to fetus and/or infant during pregnancy, delivery, or postpartum. Individuals with HIV who are asymptomatic are in a carrier state and may transmit the disease without displaying any of the characteristic signs of AIDS.

HIV-1 infection is a global pandemic, and it is estimated that 1 million to 2 million persons in the United States and 30 million to 40 million persons worldwide have HIV. In the United States, there are more than 40,000 new cases of AIDS diagnosed and more than 14,000 deaths annually. It is the leading cause of death in males age 25 to 44 and the second leading cause of death in females age 25 to 44. All races and ethnic groups are affected. Currently, men far outnumber women as victims of the disease. However, the fastest rise in cases is occurring among minority women. The peak incidence is 30 to 35 years. HIV-2 infection is found predominantly in Africa where the prevalence is about 1% of the population. Infection with HIV-2 is rare in the United States.

Pathophysiology

The current theory holds that as HIV is reproduced, it affects the immune system by infecting the helper T cell lymphocytes, which usually coexist in a 2:1 ratio with suppressor T cells. As the viruses replicate, masquerading as helper cells, the number of real helper cells declines, and the suppressor T cells eventually dominate, leading to immunosuppression and a lowering of the body's prime defense mechanism against intracellular pathogens and the formation of malignant tumors.

Risk Factors

An individual is placed at risk when exposed to body fluids (e.g., blood, semen, vaginal fluid, and breast milk) from an individual with HIV.

High-risk behavior for HIV exposure includes unprotected sexual activity (oral, anal, or vaginal) and IV drug use with shared needles. Unprotected sex with multiple partners or multiple modes of exposure increases the risk. Infants are at risk of acquiring HIV during fetal development, delivery, or breast feeding from a mother with HIV. Occupational transmission to health care workers is possible through needle sticks or other exposure to HIV-infected blood. Transfusion from contaminated blood products is a risk factor that has been mediated by testing of donated blood.

Clinical Manifestations

HIV-1 infection:

Stage I	An acute, retroviral syndrome that develops at the time of initial infection and lasts from 1 to 3 weeks; it may be accompanied by flulike signs and symptoms, such as fever, sore throat, headache, lymphadenopathy, and a rash. HIV antibodies develop during this stage.
Stage II	An asymptomatic state that may persist for years; may display manifestations such as generalized persistent lymphadenopathy, fatigue, headaches, night sweats, and a low-grade fever. Individuals are seropositive at the beginning of this stage. CD4+ counts remain above 500 cells/μl.
Stage III	Chronic infection state is characterized by persistent fever, involuntary weight loss,

	chronic diarrhea, fatigue, night sweats, seborrheic dermatitis, shingles, localized fungal infections, such as thrush, leukoplakia, myopathy, and aseptic meningitis. CD4+ counts drop below 500 cells/μl and viral load increases.
Stage IV	The development of AIDS as manifested by: (1) neurological disease (peripheral neuropathies, paresthesia, myelopathy, and dementia); (2) opportunistic infections (bacterial, viral, fungal, or protozoan) and their accompanying clinical features; (3) secondary neoplasms; (4) other conditions (e.g., endocarditis, interstitial pneumonitis, and immune thrombocytopenic purpura).
	NOTE: The Centers for Disease Control and Prevention (CDC) uses a case surveillance definition for AIDS that lists diseases indicative of a definitive diagnosis of AIDS with or without laboratory evidence and diseases that are presumptive for AIDS with laboratory evidence.
HIV-2 Infection:	Follows the same general course as HIV-1 but develops more slowly, is less infectious, and causes milder immunosuppression

Complications

The complications are numerous and are associated with the various opportunistic infections or neoplasms, and the repetitive nature of the infections. Without treatment, these infections eventually overwhelm the body's compromised immune system, leading to massive infectious invasions in every body system and death.

Diagnostic Tests

| Clinical Evaluation | Any of the above manifestations, history of high-risk behavior |
| Enzyme-linked Immunosorbent Assay (ELISA) | Screening test for HIV antibody (results may be positive for up to 12 months after exposure); if results are positive, then it should be repeated twice on same sample. |

Western Blot/ Immunofluorescent Assay Test	To confirm reactive seropositive results obtained by ELISA
	Reverse transcription polymerase chain reaction (RT-PCR), branched chain deoxyribonucleic acid (bDNA), and nucleic acid sequence-based amplification (NASBA)
	Detects HIV, measures viral load and disease progression, and treatment response to antiretroviral drugs
WBCs/ Lymphocytes	Depressed
T Cell Studies	Reduced reactivity and function of T cells; reduced number of helper T cells, and increased number of suppressor T cells

Therapeutic Management

Treatment descriptions are for HIV-1 infections; protocols for HIV-2 infections have not been established in the United States.

Surgery	Tumor excision of some related neoplasms
Medications	Primary treatment is through various combinations of antiretroviral drug protocols using CD4 lymphocyte counts and viral loads as treatment guides. Drug combinations include nucleosides, such as zidovudine (Retrovir and AZT), didanosine (DDI), zalcitabine (DDC), and lamivudine (3TC); protease inhibitors, such as ritonavir (Norvir), indinavir (Crixivan), and saquinavir (Invirase); or nonnucleoside reverse transcriptase inhibitors, such as nevirapine (Viramune), delavirdine (Rescriptor), and efavirenz (Sustiva).
	Prophylaxis with trimethoprim-sulfamethoxazole tablets is used to prevent *Pneumocystis carinii* pneumonia (PCP) for individuals with CD4 counts 200/mm^3;

rifabutin prophylaxis used for *Mycobacterium avium* infection.

Prophylaxis with zidovudine is used for infants of infected mothers.

Prophylaxis is required for 4 weeks with a 2 to 3 drug cocktail (zidovudine and lamivudine, plus protease or nonnucleoside reverse transcriptase inhibitor) after exposure to HIV through mucous membranes, nonintact skin, or percutaneous injuries.

Drugs specific for various opportunistic infections; chemotherapy for carcinomas is used.

General	Measures to improve overall health (e.g., smoking cessation; balanced nutrition; adequate rest; decreasing stress; avoiding exposure to infectious agents; drug rehabilitation; influenza, pneumococcal, and hepatitis B virus [HBV] vaccines); supportive measures for coping with and adapting to the effects of the disease (e.g., counseling, support groups)
Prevention/ Promotion	Community education in disease transmission, particularly among high-risk groups; emphasis on elimination of high-risk behaviors, such as unprotected sexual activity and sharing needles when engaging in IV drug use; promotion of safe-sex practices, such as use of latex condoms and/or barriers treated with viricidal spermicides; use of universal precautions by health care workers and family members to prevent transmission; prenatal prevention through cesarean section; no breast-feeding activity
	AIDSVAX, an HIV vaccine that is in phase III testing in Thailand
Education	Educate about disease course; early symptom recognition; transmission modes and infection control measures; effects, side effects, and dosing schedules for antiretroviral medications; monitoring treatment with CD4 counts and viral loads.

Hyperparathyroidism

Hyperactivity of one or more of the parathyroid glands, which is manifested as hypercalcemia

Etiology and Incidence

Primary hyperparathyroidism is caused by a parathyroid adenoma, multiple endocrine neoplasia, or a genetic defect. Secondary hyperparathyroidism is caused by underlying disease, such as rickets, renal failure, or osteomalacia; pregnancy; vitamin D or calcium deficiency; or an excessive intake of laxatives. Radiation exposure in the neck region may also be a precipitating factor. The disease most often occurs in adults age 30 to 70. Hyperparathyroidism is diagnosed more often in women than in men (3:2 ratio). It is particularly prevalent in postmenopausal women.

Pathophysiology

In primary hyperparathyroidism, one or more of the parathyroid glands hypertrophies, increasing secretion of parathyroid hormone (PTH) and elevating serum calcium levels. Increased PTH causes an increase in osteoblast formation, which increases bone turnover rate. Cysts and fibrous tissue invade the bone. Increased calcium causes renal calculi, a decrease in neuromuscular excitability, a delay in gastrointestinal (GI) motility, defects in cardiac conduction, and decreased neuronal permeability. In secondary disease the elevated PTH stems from a hypocalcemia-producing abnormality outside the gland that stimulates it to produce more calcium.

Clinical Manifestations

Clinical presentation varies with disease development and the degree of hypercalcemia. Manifestations include the following:

Musculoskeletal	Muscle weakness and wasting, bone pain, backache, pain on weight bearing, pseudogout
Genitourinary	Diluted urine, hematuria, polyuria, nocturia

GI	Constipation, anorexia, nausea, vomiting, ulcers, pancreatitis
Central Nervous System (CNS)	Obtunded senses, confusion, mood swings, and psychosis
Other	Itching, fatigue, band keratopathy of cornea, hypertension (HTN)

Complications

Osteoporosis, pathological fracture, renal failure, cardiac arrhythmias, cardiac failure, CNS coma, and death are complications associated with untreated hyperparathyroidism.

Diagnostic Tests

Increases in total serum calcium, ionized calcium, PTH, uric acid, and chloride are the usual diagnostic findings. A thyroid scan, ultrasound, CT, MRI, or sestamibi imaging may be used to locate parathyroid lesions. X-ray studies reveal bone demineralization. Intact PTH is used to distinguish primary from secondary and malignant disease.

Therapeutic Management

Surgery	Treatment of choice in primary hyperparathyroidism is parathyroidectomy or sestamibi/CT/ultrasound (US)-guided adenectomy to remove adenoma or other abnormal parathyroid tissue.
Medications	Diuretics *(no thiazides, since they can lead to hypercalcemia)* to increase urinary excretion of calcium; phosphate as an antihypercalcemic; bisphosphonates to inhibit osteoporosis and prevent fractures
General	Treatment of the underlying disease in secondary hyperparathyroidism; increased fluid intake to at least 2 liters a day; increased sodium chloride; restriction of dietary intake of calcium; monitoring of serum calcium, BUN, and potassium and magnesium levels; structured exercise

program with weight bearing on long bones; psychiatric evaluation and treatment for mood swings, anxiety, paranoia

Education   Education about diet, exercise, and long-term follow-up

Hypertension (HTN)

An intermittent or sustained elevation in systolic blood pressure (BP) (above 140 mm Hg) or diastolic BP (above 90 mm Hg); systolic pressure of 120 to 139 and/or a diastolic pressure of 80 to 89 is now classified as prehypertension.

Etiology and Incidence

The cause of primary (essential) HTN is unknown. Secondary HTN is related to an underlying disease process, such as renal parenchymal disorders, renal artery disease, endocrine and metabolic disorders, central nervous system (CNS) disorders, and coarctation of the aorta. It is estimated that 60 million to 85 million Americans have HTN, and it is a major factor in cerebrovascular, cardiac, and renal disease.

Pathophysiology

HTN is a disease of the vascular regulatory system in which the mechanisms that usually control arterial pressure within a certain (normal) range are altered. The central nervous and renal pressor systems and extracellular volume are the predominant mechanisms that control arterial pressure. Some combination of factors affects changes in one or more of these systems, ultimately leading to both increased cardiac output and peripheral resistance. This elevates the arterial pressure, reducing cerebral perfusion and the cerebral oxygen supply, increasing the myocardial workload and oxygen consumption, and decreasing the blood flow to and oxygenation of the kidneys.

Risk Factors

Familial history of the disease

Race (African Americans are at higher risk than Caucasians and have increased incidences of mortality and morbidity from related diseases, such as stroke and heart disease.)

Underlying disease such as diabetes mellitus (DM)

Age (BP rises with aging)

Obesity

Sedentary lifestyle

Smoking

Stress

High-fat or high-sodium diet in genetically susceptible
individuals

Elevated serum lipids

Alcohol

Clinical Manifestations

HTN is generally asymptomatic until complications develop. It
is usually discovered on routine evaluation.

Complications

Complications include atherosclerotic disease, left ventricular
failure, cerebrovascular insufficiency with or without stroke,
retinal hemorrhage, and renal failure. When the pathological
process is accelerated, malignant HTN results; the BP becomes
extremely high; nephrosclerosis, encephalopathy, and cardiac
failure rapidly ensue.

Diagnostic Tests

Elevated pressures on at least two occasions from measurements
taken on 3 separate days are needed to diagnose a person as
hypertensive. Secondary causes are then ruled out to make a
determination of primary HTN.

Therapeutic Management

Surgery	None
Medications	Diuretics, alpha- or beta-adrenergic blocking agents, antihypertensives, angiotensin-converting enzyme (ACE) inhibitors, calcium antagonists and/or angiotensin II receptor blockers (ARB) to reduce BP (prescribed according to the stepped-care approach outlined by the 6th Report of the Joint National Committee on Detection, Evaluation, and Treatment of High Blood Pressure)
General	Treatment of underlying disease in secondary HTN; systematic exercise, moderate restriction of dietary sodium, decreased alcohol intake, decreased consumption of

saturated fats, smoking cessation, stress reduction, and weight loss, if indicated; regular monitoring of BP

Prevention/ Promotion
Lifestyle changes (weight loss if overweight, limit alcohol intake, reduce sodium intake, stop smoking, reduce stress, limit saturated fat in diet) in individuals with prehypertension or in high-risk individuals

Routine BP screening every 2 years if BP normal, annually in individuals with prehypertension

Education
Instruction in BP monitoring; education on effects and side effects of medications (including postural hypotension) and the importance of taking medications consistently; instruction to avoid over-the-counter preparations, such as high sodium antacids, appetite suppressants, and cold and sinus medications; ❶ instruction to seek immediate medical attention for edema in hands and feet, sudden weight gain, BP elevations of 20 mm Hg over a 48-hour period, and/or sudden visual changes.

Hyperthyroidism

A syndrome initiated by excessive production of thyroid hormones, which results in multiple system abnormalities ranging from mild to severe

Etiology and Incidence

The cause of hyperthyroidism is an autoimmune disorder of unknown origin with a genetic component. The most common type of hyperthyroidism is Graves' disease, which occurs about 10 times more often in women than in men and is seen in about 2% of the female population in the United States.

Pathophysiology

Thyroid hormones are generally stimulatory, and excess production of these hormones produces a state of hypermetabolism in which the functions of various organ and tissue systems are increased. This is manifested by increased activity of the neuromuscular and sympathetic nervous systems. Compensatory mechanisms are called into play, and cardiac output, peripheral blood flow, body temperature, and respiratory rate increase. Other effects include increased cellular use of glucose and hyperinsulinemia, decreased supply of fats and carbohydrates, increased vitamin metabolism, increased bone mobilization and hypercalcemia, and increased secretion of adrenocorticotropic hormone (ACTH) and melanocyte-stimulating hormone. The organ systems eventually have trouble coping with the increased demand and failure can result.

Clinical Manifestations

The most common signs are goiter; warm, moist skin; tachycardia; palpitations; erythema; sweating; tremor; weakness; restlessness; insomnia; emotional lability; increased food intake; exophthalmos; lid lag; lid retraction; proptosis; tearing; and/or a startled look.

Complications

Cardiac insufficiency, generalized muscle wasting, corneal ulcers, decreased libido, osteoporosis, myasthenia gravis (MG), and impaired fertility are among the complications. The elderly are the most likely to exhibit these complications. ⊕ Thyroid storm is a severe, dramatic form of hyperthyroidism with an abrupt onset and rapid progression. It is a life-threatening emergency requiring immediate treatment to prevent shock, coma, cardiovascular collapse, and death.

Diagnostic Tests

Diagnosis depends on the clinical history and evaluation coupled with elevations in free thyroxine (T_4), free triiodothyronine (T_3), and decreased thyroid-stimulating hormone (TSH) unless pituitary adenoma is the cause of the hyperthyroidism, in which case TSH will be elevated.

Therapeutic Management

Surgery	Thyroidectomy in individuals who cannot receive radioactive iodine, have large goiters, or have toxic adenoma
Medications	Radioactive iodine to destroy thyroid tissue (treatment of choice); thioamides to inhibit hormone synthesis; beta-adrenergic blockers to diminish clinical manifestations; iodines to reduce the size of the thyroid before surgery; corticosteroids for palliation in Graves' disease
General	Monitoring for signs of hypothyroidism, planned rest and exercise cycles, long-term follow-up, counseling for lability
Education	Instruction about medications

Hypertrophic Pyloric Stenosis (HPS)

Hypertrophy of the pylorus muscle resulting in obstruction of the gastric outlet in infants

Etiology and Incidence

Precise etiology is unknown, but there is a genetic association. The incidence is 1 in every 250 live births in the United States. HPS is the most common infantile gastrointestinal (GI) obstruction beyond the first month of life. Males are affected at four times the rate of females, and HPS is diagnosed more frequently in Caucasians than in other races.

Pathophysiology

The circular muscle of the pylorus is enlarged through hypertrophy and hyperplasia, which produce a narrowing of the canal between the stomach and duodenum. Over time, inflammation and edema continue to reduce the size of the canal opening until total occlusion occurs. Vomiting occurs as the outlet narrows, and hydrogen and chloride ions are lost. The kidneys attempt to retain hydrogen ions by substituting potassium, resulting in a hypochloremic and/or hypokalemic acidosis.

Risk Factors

Familial tendencies
Male gender
Caucasian race

Clinical Manifestations

The condition usually develops in the first few weeks of life, and manifestations include emesis that progresses to projectile nonbilous vomiting. The infant displays a ravenous appetite and rapidly consumes an entire feeding and then promptly regurgitates it. Lethargy, dehydration, and electrolyte abnormalities ensue with visible left to right peristaltic waves. Weight loss occurs, but there is no evidence of pain and no "ill" appearance.

Complications

Marasmus and failure to thrive can occur if the condition is not diagnosed and corrected. Prognosis is excellent with treatment.

Diagnostic Tests

Clinical Evaluation	History of emesis, projectile vomiting, and ravenous appetite; peristaltic waves; palpable pylorus aka "classic olive"
Laboratory	Decreased serum chloride, sodium, and potassium levels; increased pH; increased bicarbonate; elevated BUN
Ultrasound	Elongated pyloric channel, thickened pylorus

Therapeutic Management

H

Surgery	Laparoscopic or conventional pyloromyotomy is the definitive treatment
Medications	Analgesics for pain
General	IV fluid and electrolyte replacement and possible gastric lavage and stomach decompression preoperatively; nasogastric (NG) tube and progressive oral fluids and formula postoperatively; positioning of infant with head elevated; comfort and support of infant and parents
Education	Education about nature of defect, instruction about prevention of aspiration with vomiting

Hypoglycemia

A low plasma glucose level; a plasma glucose level less than 50 mg/dl

Etiology and Incidence

Three types of hypoglycemia can be considered as pathological. *Reactive hypoglycemia* occurs 2 to 4 hours after a rich carbohydrate meal. This type of hypoglycemia may be seen in individuals who have had radical gastric surgery where there may be a rapid absorption of carbohydrates, causing an early and very high plasma glucose level. This is followed by an insulin surge that reaches a peak when most of the glucose is absorbed or in individuals with early stage diabetes mellitus (DM) or alimentary hypoglycemia. *Fasting hypoglycemia* may occur when there has been inadequate food and carbohydrate ingestion. This type of hypoglycemia may be found in individuals with insulin-producing islet cell tumors *(insulinomas)*, islet cell hyperplasia *(nesidioblastosis)*, hormonal deficiency, liver disease, pancreatic tumors, insulin autoimmune syndromes, and renal disease. *Induced hypoglycemia* includes exogenous insulin or sulfonylurea used by people with known diabetes, use of insulin by nondiabetics, and individuals with alcohol- or drug-induced hypoglycemia.

Pathophysiology

Regardless of cause, hypoglycemia occurs when the level of glucose in blood glucose drops. Insulin is responsible for maintaining normal blood glucose levels in conjunction with counter-regulatory hormones that oppose the insulin action. Any physiological disruption resulting in an imbalance of insulin and blood glucose may lead to a state of hypoglycemia. A decrease in blood glucose results in increased secretions of epinephrine, glucagon, cortisol, and growth hormones. The release of these counterregulatory hormones results in clinical signs that are seen in hypoglycemia. Hypoglycemia is generally episodic. Symptoms may recur and may last from a few minutes to a few hours. In most cases, the clinical signs of hypoglycemia disappear with the ingestion of food or glucose to increase the plasma glucose level.

Risk Factors

Individuals with history of radical gastric surgery, insulinoma, nonislet cell neoplasms, hormonal deficiency, liver disease, renal disease, and alcohol or drug ingestion.

In diabetics: insulin excess (wrong medication, wrong dose, wrong frequency), decreased food intake, increased activity, use of alcohol, rapid weight loss.

Clinical Manifestations

Symptoms include sweating, anxiety, tremors, tachycardia, palpitations, seizures, fatigue, dizziness, headache, behavioral changes, or visual disturbances, which are relieved by ingestion of carbohydrates.

Complications

The proven presence of hypoglycemia should be used as a sign of another underlying disorder or disease.

Diagnostic Tests

Laboratory Tests	Low plasma glucose level less than 50 mg/dl
Increased Plasma Insulin Level	Presence of insulin antibodies (may be present if the individual has had previous animal product insulin injections; will be absent if human insulin is present)
C-peptide Level (Elevated Fasting in Nesidioblastosis)	72-hour supervised fast
Elevated Insulin	Low plasma glucose level

Therapeutic Management

Surgery	Subtotal pancreatectomy (for nesidioblastosis); insulinoma resection
Medications	Nonlife-threatening hypoglycemia: diazoxide, phenytoin, propranolol
	Life-threatening hypoglycemia: antineoplastic agents, subcutaneous glucagon, IV dextrose
General	Nutritional consultation

	Diet for fasting hypoglycemia (insulinoma or nesidioblastosis): small, frequent meals with rapidly absorbable simple carbohydrates
	Diet for reactive hypoglycemia: small, frequent meals that restrict carbohydrates
Prevention/ Promotion	Balanced diet with distributed carbohydrate intake, adequate rest, consistent exercise, slow weight loss if dieting
Education	Education about signs and symptoms of hypoglycemia, preventive measures through diet

Hypoparathyroidism

Decreased secretion of parathyroid hormone (PTH) by the parathyroid glands, manifested as hypocalcemia

Etiology and Incidence

The cause is usually unintentional damage to or removal of the parathyroid glands during thyroidectomy. There is a rare idiopathic form in which the parathyroids are absent or atrophied, and a genetic form that is part of a polyendocrine syndrome called HAM (hypoparathyroidism, Addison's disease, and moniliasis). The idiopathic form generally occurs in childhood. All forms of hypoparathyroidism are rare.

Pathophysiology

A decrease in the secretion of PTH leads to a reduced resorption of calcium from the renal tubules, decreased absorption of calcium in the gastrointestinal (GI) tract, and decreased resorption of calcium from bone. The serum calcium level falls, increasing neuromuscular excitability and leading to spasms and tetany.

Clinical Manifestations

Hypoparathyroidism is often asymptomatic in the early stages. The most characteristic sign is tetany with paresthesia of the lips, tongue, fingers, and feet; other signs are carpopedal and facial spasms, generalized muscle aches, and fatigue. Encephalopathy, depression, dementia, and papilledema may also be present.

Complications

Acute onset of hypocalcemia leads to laryngospasm, airway obstruction, and cardiac failure. Long-standing disease leads to bone deformities, cataract formation, reduced cardiac contractility, and heart failure. Childhood disease can lead to mental retardation and stunted growth.

Diagnostic Tests

Parathyroid deficiency is characterized by a low serum calcium level, high serum phosphorus level, and normal alkaline phosphatase level. Serum intact PTH is decreased. Chvostek's sign and Trousseau's sign are positive.

Therapeutic Management

Surgery	None
Medications	Calcium supplements; vitamin D to increase calcium absorption in the GI tract
	☻ Tetany necessitates IV infusion of calcium
General	Calcium-rich diet; monitoring of calcium levels three to four times annually
Education	Instruction in long-term nutritional management, drug therapy, and signs and symptoms of calcium deficit and excess

Hypothermia

A systemic lowering of core body temperature below 95.8° F or 35° C, which may be classified as mild, moderate, or severe

(See also Frostbite)

Etiology and Incidence
Hypothermia is caused by prolonged exposure to cold temperatures and occurs when heat produced by the body cannot compensate for the heat lost to the environment. Incidence estimates vary widely, but hypothermia is most common in the very young and the very old, and hypothermia is diagnosed in males more frequently than in females. Death rate is approximately two to four per million in the United States.

Pathophysiology
When the body temperature begins to drop, the hypothalamus sends signals to increase muscle tone and metabolic rate (manifested as shivering) and to shunt blood to vital organs, causing peripheral vasoconstriction. As the body cools, the metabolic rate slows, decreasing CO_2 production and slowing the heart rate. As cooling continues, there is a physiological deceleration of all functions including cardiac dysrhythmias; decreases in neuronal activity and cerebral metabolic activity; depressed respiratory volume; renal diuresis; and decreases in gastrointestinal (GI) motility and hepatic function.

Risk Factors
Age extremes
Environmental conditions (e.g., cold water immersion, exposure to high winds)
Inadequate clothing for weather conditions
Environmental exposure (e.g., homelessness, auto breakdown)
Occupational or recreational pursuits that involve exposure to cold
Infection (e.g., sepsis, meningitis)
Metabolic disorders (e.g., hypoglycemic, hypopituitary, hypothyroid, hypoadrenal)
Extensive skin problems (e.g., psoriasis, burns)

Acute debilitating conditions (e.g., diabetic ketoacidosis, trauma)

Drug intoxication (e.g., sedatives/tranquilizers, narcotics, alcohol)

Mental illness

Central nervous system (CNS) pathology (e.g., head trauma, cerebrovascular accident (CVA), congenital abnormalities, tumors)

Malnutrition, dehydration

Clinical Manifestations

Mild (34° to 35° C/ 93° to 95° F)	Hunger, nausea, lethargy, mild confusion, shivering, dyspnea, clumsiness, apathy or decreased affect, increased pulse and blood pressure (BP), peripheral vasoconstriction
Moderate (30° to 34° C/ 86° to 93° F)	Delirium, slowed pulse, decreased BP, hypoventilation, cyanosis, cardiac arrhythmias, decreased level of consciousness, muscular rigidity, generalized edema, slowed reflexes
Severe (<30° C/ <86° F)	Apnea, coma, absent reflexes, fixed pupils, extremely cold skin, rigidity, respiratory arrest, and ventricular fibrillation

Complications

Complications are multiple, increase as temperature decreases, and include cardiac arrhythmias, pneumonia, pulmonary edema, pancreatitis, GI bleeding, tubular necrosis, intravascular thrombosis, gangrene, compartment syndromes, neurological damage, coma, and death. Mortality rate in those with a co-existing illness exceeds 50%.

Diagnostic Tests

Clinical Evaluation	History of cold exposure; pattern of manifestations delineated above
Arterial Blood Gases	Increased pH and PO_2; decreased PCO_2; initial hypokalemia with hyperkalemia with increasing hypothermia

CBC	Elevated hematocrit (Hct), leukopenia, and thrombocytopenia
ECG	Prolonged PR, QT and QRS segments; depressed ST segments; inverted T waves

Therapeutic Management

Surgery	Cardiopulmonary bypass for extracorporeal blood warming in very severe hypothermia
Medications	Appropriate medications for underlying conditions only if drug effective in reduced temperature conditions
General	Treatment focused on rewarming, managing blood gases, correcting dehydration, treating cardiac arrhythmias, maintaining a patent airway, monitoring intake and output (I&O), and treating underlying conditions
	Mild: Passive external warming (move to warm, dry environment, remove damp clothing, place in warm blankets)
	Moderate: Passive and active external rewarming (body to body contact, fluid- or air-filled warming blankets, radiant heat lamps, warm water immersion); monitor for vasodilatation and hypotension during rewarming process
	Moderate to Severe: Active core rewarming (heated and humidified oxygen, warmed IV fluid, warmed fluids via peritoneal dialysis or gastric or colonic lavage)
Prevention/ Promotion	Avoidance of prolonged exposure to cold; dressing appropriately for cold weather (e.g., layering clothing, covering head, lined boots); carrying supplies in car when driving in cold weather, ice, snow (e.g., extra clothing, coats, blankets, fluids, high-carbohydrate foods, cell phone, hazard markers)
Education	Education about prevention of future hypothermic episodes

H

Hypothyroidism (Myxedema)

A clinical state resulting from a deficiency of thyroid hormone

Etiology and Incidence

The cause of some hypothyroidism is unknown but is thought to be autoimmune in origin. Other hypothyroidism is caused by destruction of thyroid or pituitary tissue by underlying disease, surgery, or radiation treatment. Hypothyroidism is a common disorder that affects all age groups. Women between ages 30 and 60 are most often affected. It also occurs in approximately 1 in every 4500 live births. The incidence is rising in the elderly population.

Pathophysiology

When the supply of thyroid hormone is inadequate, a general depression of most cellular enzyme systems and oxidative processes results, reducing the metabolic activity of the cells. This in turn reduces oxygen consumption, decreases energy production, and lessens body heat. Tissues are infiltrated by mucopolysaccharides, carotene is deposited in epidermal layers, adrenergic stimulation is decreased, protein effusion collects in the pericardial and pleural sacs, and proteinaceous ground substances are deposited in tissue.

Clinical Manifestations

Signs and symptoms are often insidious at onset. They include fatigue and lethargy; mild weight gain; cold, pale, dry, rough hands and feet; reduced attention span with memory impairment, slowed speech, and loss of initiative; swelling in extremities and around the eyes, eyelids, and face; menstrual irregularities; muscle aches and weakness; joint aches and stiffness; clumsiness; hyperstiff reflexes; decreased pulse; decreased blood pressure (BP); agitation; depression; and paranoia.

Complications

⚕ Myxedema coma is a life-threatening complication of hypothyroidism that necessitates immediate treatment. It is preceded by gradual or sudden onset of mental sluggishness, drowsiness, and lethargy. Other complications include ischemic heart disease, congestive heart failure (CHF), pleural and pericardial effusion, deafness, psychosis, and anemia.

Diagnostic Tests

Serum and serum-free triiodothyronine and thyroxine (T_3, T_4) are decreased; serum thyroid-stimulating hormone (TSH) is increased in primary hypothyroidism and decreased or normal in secondary hypothyroidism. Serum lipids and cholesterol levels are increased.

Therapeutic Management

H

Surgery	None
Medications	Oral replacement thyroid hormone; ◑ IV form is used for myxedemic coma; addition of triiodothyronine in some stable patients who continue to have mood or memory problems
General	Lifelong monitoring of TSH level annually ◑ Mechanical ventilation in myxedemic coma
Prevention/ Promotion	Early detection through thyroid screening every 2 to 3 years
Education	Instruction about lifelong thyroid hormone replacement therapy; drug effects and side effects; signs and symptoms of hypothyroidism and hyperthyroidism

Impetigo

A superficial vesiculopustular infection of the skin found primarily on the arms, legs, and face; ulcerative impetigo is called *ecthyma*

Etiology and Incidence

Impetigo is caused by staphylococci or streptococci transmitted by insect bites or directly from person-to-person through skin breaks. A secondary form of impetigo occurs with pediculosis, scabies, and fungal infections. Predisposing factors include poor hygiene, crowding, poor nutritional status, and frequent skin breaks. It is highly contagious in infants and small children, who are the most susceptible.

Pathophysiology

The bacteria colonize and incubate on the skin for as long as several weeks before initiation of the disease process. The lesions begin as small, erythematous macules beneath the stratum corneum that change to vesicles and then pustules, which rupture. In streptococcal impetigo, honey-colored crusts are formed, whereas in staphylococcal impetigo, light brown or clear crusts form. Individuals often have a mixture of both forms.

Risk Factors

Poor hygiene
Crowding
Poor nutrition
Frequent skin breaks

Clinical Manifestations

Intense itching, burning, and regional lymphadenopathy accompany the crusted skin lesions. Scratching often causes satellite lesions.

Complications

Ecthyma is a deeper form of impetigo that affects the dermis and epidermis and forms ulcers that later cause scarring.

Glomerulonephritis is a severe complication that occurs in about 3% of impetigo cases.

Diagnostic Tests

The diagnosis is made by physical examination, Gram's stain, and culture of the lesions.

Therapeutic Management

Surgery	None
Medications	Topical antiinfective drugs on lesions, systemic antiinfective drugs sensitive to causative agent, antipruritics for itching; mupirocin ointment in nares for carriers of *Staphylococcus aureus*
General	Crusts are washed with soap and water, and cool, moist compresses are applied; isolation until lesions have healed; careful personal and family hygiene; protective devices (e.g., mittens, distractions) to reduce scratching; nails kept trimmed; nutritional therapy if needed; treatment of any underlying disease processes

I

Influenza (Flu)

An acute viral respiratory disease with clinical manifestations that often resemble a severe form of the common cold

Etiology and Incidence

Influenza is caused by orthomyxovirus types A, B, and C, which are spread by direct person-to-person contact or by airborne droplet spray. Flu generally occurs in the late fall and early winter and can reach epidemic proportions when a modified form of the virus emerges for which the population has no immunity. All age groups are susceptible, but the prevalence is highest in school-age children. More than 90 million cases are reported annually in the United States. Annual mortality rate exceeds 20,000.

Pathophysiology

After a 48-hour incubation period, the virus penetrates the surface of the upper respiratory tract mucosa, destroying the ciliated epithelium and reducing the viscosity of mucosal secretions. This facilitates the spread of virus-laden exudate to the lower respiratory tract, with resultant necrosis and desquamation of the bronchi and alveoli. The disease is generally self-limiting, with acute symptoms lasting 2 to 7 days and lingering symptoms lasting another week.

Clinical Manifestations

The onset of influenza types A and B is sudden, marked by chills, fever, generalized aches and pains, headache, and photophobia. Respiratory symptoms begin with a scratchy, sore throat; substernal burning, and nonproductive cough. Later cough becomes severe and productive, and weakness, fatigue, and sweating persist. Influenza C produces milder symptoms.

Complications

The most common complication is viral pneumonia or a secondary bacterial pneumonia. Individuals who have a compromised respiratory system and the elderly are most susceptible.

Diagnostic Tests

Tissue culture of nasal secretions or fluorescent antibody staining of secretions is positive for virus.

Therapeutic Management

Surgery	None
Medications	Analgesics for headache, aches, and pains; nasal sprays for congestion *(no aspirin for children because Reye's syndrome may result)*; antitussives for cough; antiviral drugs (amantadine, rimantadine) for early intervention for influenza type A; inhaled antivirals (zanamavir) to treat type A and type B influenza
General	Adequate hydration, rest, careful handling of items in the environment, and proper hand washing to reduce the spread of the virus
Prevention/ Promotion	Flu vaccine should be given annually to adults over 64 and high-risk individuals (e.g., those with compromised immune systems or decreased respiratory function); inhaled live flu vaccine (FluMist) for healthy individuals (5 to 49 years old) with no history of allergy to egg products. Children who are on long-term aspirin therapy should not use FluMist. High-risk individuals should not use FluMist.

Intestinal Obstruction

Intestinal obstruction may be *mechanical* or *functional* and occurs when the contents of the intestines cannot move through the intestinal canal. The obstruction may be partial or complete.

Etiology and Incidence

Bowel obstruction occurs from one of two causes: mechanical blockage or a functional obstruction. The mechanical obstruction is caused by a blockage of the lumen of the bowel by feces, intussusception, adhesions, volvulus (twisting of the bowel), tumor, inflammation, or a foreign body. Functional obstruction, also referred to as *ileus,* occurs where there is a loss of function of the peristalsis of the intestinal tract. Intestinal obstruction accounts for 20% of hospital admissions for acute abdominal conditions in the United States.

Pathophysiology

If there is a blockage or lack of peristalsis within the intestinal tract, an accumulation of fluids and gas builds proximal to the obstruction. The gas, high in nitrogen concentration, and the fluids accumulate and cause the bowel to swell. The edematous bowel secretes more fluids and electrolytes and causes more distention. This continued fluid and gas accumulation causes further compromise. If not treated, the distention may lead to pressure necrosis of the bowel wall. Significant abdominal distention may also cause impaired breathing and can lead to a severe reduction in circulating blood volume resulting in hypovolemic shock.

Risk Factors

Abdominal surgery resulting in adhesions or incarcerated hernia
  or intestinal distention
General anesthesia
Spinal fractures resulting in paresis/paralysis
Use of narcotic drugs or diphenoxylate (Lomotil)
Congenital abnormalities of the intestines
Chronic constipation

Underlying disease (e.g., cholelithiasis, inflammatory bowel disease, diverticular disease)

Ingestion of foreign bodies (e.g., pica, enteric-coated potassium tablets)

Clinical Manifestations

General	History of lack of "normal" bowel movement, early onset of cramping abdominal pain, abdominal distention
Gastrointestinal/ Abdomen	Vomiting, failure to pass gas, blood in stool, localized tenderness, constant abdominal pains, guarding and rebound tenderness
Bowel Sounds	*Mechanical obstruction* peristalsis has a high-pitched, tinkling sound; *paralytic ileus* is absence of bowel sounds or low infrequent sounds

Complications

🅠 If untreated, intestinal obstruction may progress to necrosis and gangrene of the bowel, leading to a life-threatening situation.

Diagnostic Tests

X-ray	*Abdominal series* x-rays indicate large amounts of gas in the bowel; fluid and gas levels may be diagnostic for intestinal obstruction. *Barium enema* stops at the point of obstruction.
Laboratory	Decreased serum electrolytes may indicate electrolyte loss; increased WBC count indicates strangulation of bowel.

Therapeutic Management

Surgery	Surgery exploration with lysis of adhesions, reduction of volvulus, intussusception, or strangulated hernia; enterotomy to remove

foreign bodies, gallstones; resection for obstructing lesions or strangulated bowel; sometimes temporary colostomy/cecostomy may be life saving

Medications Antiinfectives if strangulation and/or sepsis are present; analgesics for pain

General Nasogastric or intestinal suctioning may assist in reducing trapped fluids and gases and to reducing inflammation. Colonoscopy may assist with reduction of volvulus by releasing trapped gas and fluid. Correction of fluid and electrolyte balance with IV fluids and potassium and possible total parenteral nutrition to correct nutritional deficiencies before surgery. Observe strict intake and output (I&O) and bed rest.

Education Preoperative instruction in turning, coughing, deep breathing; instruction postoperatively in care of incision, activity, and diet modifications, and signs and symptoms of possible surgical complications

Irritable Bowel Syndrome (Spastic Colitis)

A noninflammatory motility disorder of the large bowel that alters bowel habits and causes abdominal pain and distention

Etiology and Incidence

The cause of irritable bowel syndrome (IBS) is unknown, but it is associated with diet, drugs, toxins, gastrointestinal (GI) hormones, prostaglandins, and emotional factors. IBS is a common GI disorder that accounts for about half of all presenting GI complaints in the United States. Women are affected more often than men and whites and Jews more often than other ethnic groups. All age groups are affected, although the disease is predominant in those under age 35. Almost half of individuals with IBS also have a psychiatric abnormality, with anxiety disorders being most predominant.

Pathophysiology

The pathophysiology of IBS is still unclear. However, two patterns can be identified: one with painful constipation and diarrhea and the other with painless diarrhea. Hypermotility with high-amplitude pressure waves is present in the sigmoid colon in painful IBS and hypomotility of the sigmoid colon in painless IBS. Myoelectric activity is increased in both patterns, as is contractile activity after meals.

Clinical Manifestations

The primary symptoms are either painless, urgent diarrhea that occurs after meals, or alternating diarrhea and constipation accompanied by abdominal pain, bloating, flatulence, headache, and fatigue.

Complications

IBS is associated with an increased risk of diverticulitis and colon cancer.

Diagnostic Tests

A careful history of bowel habits and emotional stimuli, along with a rectal examination that elicits pain in a tender rectum, is important. Manometric studies are done to evaluate electrical response, as are tests to rule out other bowel diseases.

Therapeutic Management

Surgery	None
Medications	Anticholinergics (dicyclomine) to reduce pain; bulk-forming agents and antidiarrheal drugs to regulate stool; tegaserod for IBS with constipation to increase stool movement; alosetron to treat IBS with diarrhea in women not helped by other therapies; mild tranquilizers or sedatives for those with anxiety; a*void use of laxatives*
General	High-fiber, low-lactose, caffeine-free, low-fat diet; fiber supplements; counseling for emotional effects, relaxation, stress management, acupuncture

Kaposi's Sarcoma (KS)

A malignant vascular tumor of the endothelium that originates in multifocal sites; there are four subtypes: classic, epidemic, endemic, and immunosuppression-related

Etiology and Incidence

The cause is unknown, but a herpes virus (HHV-8/KSHV) has been isolated in tumors of most individuals with KS and is the suspected cause. At one time the incidence of KS was confined to a select population of older men of Jewish or Italian origin (classic type) and to those who were severely immunocompromised (immunosuppression-related). In late 1980, however, an alarming increase in cases occurred among sexually active, homosexual men between ages 25 and 50 (epidemic type). The endemic type is seen on the continent of Africa and affects children and adults. African children are particularly susceptible to a very aggressive form of lymphadenopathic KS.

KS is currently the most common acquired immunodeficiency syndrome (AIDS)-related cancer, occurring in at least 15% of human immunodeficiency virus (HIV)-positive individuals in the United States. KS develops in less than 1% of the general U.S. population. It is endemic in equatorial Africa and accounts for more than 10% of malignancies in Zaire and Uganda. (See also HIV Infection.)

Pathophysiology

Viral transmission appears possible through sexual and nonsexual contact with body fluids. KS lesions begin in the endothelial cells, which originate in the middermis, oral mucosa, lymph nodes, and gastrointestinal (GI) viscera. A vascular or dysplastic endothelial cell is transformed by exposure to the infectious agent. The transformed KS cell then produces an autocrine factor to sustain cell growth and cytokines, which produce cell proliferation and lesions. The lesions spread to the skin, lungs, liver, and bones. Skin lesions are typically reddish brown or purple and are various shapes and sizes.

K

Risk Factors

Homosexual/bisexual men who are HIV+
Other individuals with HIV infections
Immunosuppressed individuals (chemotherapy, transplant)
Elderly males of Jewish or Mediterranean descent
Indigenous populations in equatorial Africa
At-risk individual who has contact with body fluids of an individual infected with HHV-8/KSHV virus

Clinical Manifestations

Individuals can have varying degrees of cutaneous and systemic involvement. The signs are usually multiple skin and oral mucosal lesions that are small, round, and pink, and progress to red or purple. Later symptoms indicate systemic disease and include diarrhea, weight loss, cough, dyspnea, and fever.

Complications

Associated opportunistic infections and the immunosuppression associated with AIDS complicate the course and treatment of KS. Prognosis is much better in endemic and classic types of KS. KS usually regresses in immunosuppression-related types of KS when immune suppression therapy is reduced or stopped.

Diagnostic Tests

The initial diagnosis is made from the presence of the characteristic lesions and a history of HIV infection, immunosuppression, or Jewish or Mediterranean heritage. The definitive diagnosis is made by biopsy of the skin lesions.

Therapeutic Management

Surgery	Excision, electrodesiccation or cryotherapy of skin lesions in classic KS
Medications	Combination chemotherapy for progressive or widespread disease; α-interferon for minimal or slow-progressing disease; interlesional chemotherapy for nodular lesions
General	Watchful waiting with slow progressive classic KS
	Irradiation of skin lesions in non-epidemic types of KS or with large tumor masses; radiation as palliation

Prevention/ Promotion	Routine screening in all HIV-infected individuals for suspicious skin lesions
	Maintain CD4 cell count above 200 in HIV cases
	Cease high-risk sexual behavior in HIV cases
	Modify immunosuppressive therapy in immunosuppression-related KS
Education	Instruction for HIV+ individuals to perform frequent skin and oral mucosa inspections and to report any suspicious lesions

K

Kawasaki Disease (KD)

An acute, self-limited, systemic vasculitis occurring predominantly in children under 5 years of age

Etiology and Incidence

First discovered in Japan, the cause of KD is unknown, but clinical evidence suggests that a microbial agent (e.g., a streptococcal or staphylococcal superantigen) triggers an abnormal immune response. There are approximately 1900 new cases reported each year in the United States, and it is the leading cause of acquired heart disease in children. The incidence in Japan is 10 times that of the United States.

Pathophysiology

The primary area of involvement is the cardiovascular system. The disease begins when a body immune response is triggered, and inflammatory cells (lymphocytes, macrophages, and monocytes) and plasma cells that produce immunoglobulin A (IgA) infiltrate the vascular walls of the arterioles, venules, and capillaries, causing extensive inflammation.

Clinical Manifestations

KD usually progresses in three stages: acute, subacute, and convalescent.

Acute	Begins with a remittent fever (103° to 105° F) and accompanied by extreme irritability, lethargy, and intermittent colicky abdominal pain. The fever typically lasts 7 days to 2 weeks and is unresponsive to antibiotics. After 1 to 2 days, bilateral conjunctivitis occurs. Within 5 days, there is erythema and edema of the hands and feet, a macular rash on the trunk and perineum, strawberry tongue, fissuring of the lips, and reddened pharynx. Cervical lymphadenopathy is present.
Subacute	Ten to 25 days after onset, fever resolves and symptoms diminish. Irritability, anorexia,

and conjunctivitis remain. There is peeling of the hands and feet, arthritis, arthralgia, and thrombocytosis. The greatest risk for coronary artery aneurysm occurs during this stage.

Convalescent	All clinical signs have resolved, but erythrocyte sedimentation rate (ESR) is still abnormal. Stage complete when ESR blood values are normal (about 6 to 8 weeks after onset)

Complications

Complications include coronary arteritis, coronary artery aneurysms, and thrombotic occlusion of an aneurysm leading to a myocardial infarction (MI) and possible death. Prognosis with treatment is excellent, with a mortality rate of less than 0.1%.

K

Diagnostic Tests

Clinical Evaluation	History of fever (5-day duration) is evident with four of five of the following conditions: conjunctivitis, changes in mucosa of oropharynx, edema and erythema of hands and feet, nonvesicular truncal rash, lymphadenopathy
Blood Studies	Elevated WBCs and platelets; elevated ESR; positive C-reactive protein; elevated alanine aminotransferase (ALT) and aspartate aminotransferase (AST)
Chest X-ray	May show pulmonary infiltrates
Echocardiogram	May show depressed left ventricular function; monitor cardiac status during subacute phase

Therapeutic Management

Surgery	Percutaneous transluminal coronary angioplasty, coronary bypass grafting, cardiac transplant for cardiac complications from KD

Medications	IV Immunoglobulin and aspirin to reduce inflammation in acute stage; aspirin therapy until ESR values normal and ECG reveals no coronary abnormalities; anticoagulant and antiplatelet therapy if evidence of coronary thrombosis
	Corticosteroids increase possibility of aneurysm and are contraindicated
General	Supportive care, careful monitoring of cardiac status, careful fluid replacement, intake and output (I&O), comfort measures (lubrication for lips, lotion for skin, cool cloths), quiet soothing environment, parental support in attempting to console irritable child
Education	Parental education about possible cardiac complications; instruction in cardiopulmonary resuscitation (CPR) if cardiac complications are present

Keratitis

Inflammation of the cornea of the eye
(See also Corneal Ulcer)

Etiology and Incidence

Causes of keratitis include dryness, injury, irritations, infections, ischemia, and nutritional deficiencies. This often starts as a superficial inflammation of the epithelium, but if not treated, may invade subepithelial tissue or may go even deeper into the inner layer of the cornea. Prevalence is common and the disease affects all ages and races.

Pathophysiology

The epithelium may become damaged because of injury or irritation resulting in inflammation, pain, blurring of vision, and other visual disturbances. If not treated, the inflammation of the cornea may result in damage to the corneal membrane and loss of membrane integrity. This in turn may lead to infection and/or ulceration of the cornea.

Risk Factors

Overuse or exposure of eye to dryness, trauma, chemical irritation, or use of topical anesthetics
Contact lens wearer with poor lens-cleaning habits

Clinical Manifestations

Eye pain, discharge and/or increased lacrimation, blurred vision, halo vision seen when looking into light, photophobia, and purulent exudate may be noted. Opacity or irregular light reflection may be noted on the corneal surface. The cornea may appear dull and uneven.

Complications

Corneal ulceration, optic atrophy, or loss of sight in affected eye are all possible complications.

Diagnostic Tests

Fluorescein stain applied to cornea of eye to determine a break in epithelium (green color indicates corneal epithelium damage); culture of corneal tissue and/or ulcer scraping to determine infective organism.

Therapeutic Management

Surgery	None unless complications form (see Corneal Ulcer)
Medications	Topical analgesics for pain; mydriatic-cycloplegic agents to dilate pupil and restrict eye movement; antiinfectives or antifungals for infection
General	Pressure dressings on eye and ice compresses for 10 to 15 minutes several times per day may assist with discomfort
Prevention/ Promotion	Avoid finger to eye contact Follow guidelines for contact lens wear; avoid contaminated contact solution; avoid practices such as cleaning or wetting contact lens with saliva
Education	Education about causes and prevention in future

Kidney Cancer (Renal Cancer)

Renal cell and clear cell adenocarcinomas account for 80% of kidney cancer. Other tumor types include transitional cell, squamous cell, and nephroblastoma.

Etiology and Incidence

The cause of kidney cancer is unclear. Environmental factors have been implicated. Hereditary forms have also been identified. Kidney cancer is diagnosed in nearly 32,000 individuals, and about 12,000 die in the United States annually. About 20% of childhood malignancies and 3% of adult malignancies occur in the kidneys. The average age of diagnosis is 55 to 60, and men are affected 1.5 times as often as women.

Pathophysiology

Tumor cells originate in the renal parenchyma and grow into a well-defined tumor, often surrounded by perinephric fat, which slows infiltration of adjacent tissue. Metastasis occurs by venous or lymphatic routes, and the most common metastatic sites are the lungs, bones, liver, and brain.

Risk Factors

Use of tobacco products (implicated in 30% of diagnosed cases)
History of acquired cystic disease, von Hippel-Lindau disease (VHL)
Familial history of hereditary papillary renal carcinoma (HPRC) or hereditary renal carcinoma (HRC)
Chronic irritation from renal calculi
Exposure to petrochemical products, asbestos, cadmium, or radiation
Obesity, particularly in females
Analgesic abuse (phenacetin-containing analgesics)
History of renal dialysis, end-stage renal disease

Clinical Manifestations

Signs and symptoms develop late in the disease; hematuria is the most common presenting sign, followed by flank pain, a palpable abdominal mass, and/or fever of unknown origin.

Complications

The prognosis for metastatic lesions is poor because kidney tumors are resistant to radiation and chemotherapy. Complications include hypertension (HTN) from pedicle compression.

Diagnostic Tests

Abdominal and renal ultrasound, MRI, and abdominal CT scans help detect masses that warrant further diagnostic study. Biopsy by needle aspiration or tissue sample is definitive.

Therapeutic Management

Surgery	Nephrectomy with removal of regional lymph nodes
Medications	Chemotherapy agents are generally not effective; immunotherapy with interleukin-2 has achieved a 15% to 30% response rate; gene therapy trials are showing some promise.
General	None
Prevention/ Promotion	Avoid exogenous carcinogens (petrochemical products, asbestos, cadmium, or radiation) Smoking cessation
Education	Instruction about disease and treatment procedures

Labyrinthitis

Acute onset of transient vertigo, and/or nausea and vomiting from inflammation or infection of the inner ear that involves the cochlear or vestibular portion of the labyrinth

Etiology and Incidence

Causes are multiple and include physiological mismatch of vestibular, visual, and somatosensory systems; lesions in the vestibular pathways; infections (particularly mumps, otitis media); tumors; vasculitis; ototoxic drugs; alcohol intoxication; allergies; ear or mastoid surgery; traumatic brain injury (TBI); and neuronitis. Labyrinthitis is the most common cause of transient vertigo at any age.

Pathophysiology

Cellular infiltration of serous fluid or serofibrinous exudate occurs. If not recognized and treated, soft tissue structures are destroyed. This is what may cause total, permanent hearing loss. Chronic labyrinthitis can develop after an initial bout of labyrinthitis. The internal ear is filled with granulations that begin to change into fibrous tissue and then calcify as new bone in the labyrinth space. When this occurs, complete deafness in the affected ear occurs. In this second type of labyrinthitis, there may be destruction of the soft tissue structures. This in turn may cause permanent hearing loss.

Risk Factors

Nasal or ear surgery
Drug and/or alcohol intoxication
Viral infections
Chronic ear infections
Head trauma

Clinical Manifestations

Vertigo, tinnitus, and sensorineural hearing loss; vertigo or dizziness is manifested when the vestibular structures are involved and causes problems with balance and equilibrium. Tinnitus occurs when the infection is located in the cochlea. Severe cases may also include nystagmus, which is an abnormal rhythmic, jerking movement of the eyes. This accompanies the symptoms of vertigo and occurs during labyrinth dysfunction. Other clinical signs include pain, fever, ataxia, nausea, and vomiting.

Complications

Dehydration and electrolyte imbalance from vomiting; falls secondary to dizziness and vertigo; deafness

Diagnostic Tests

Positional maneuvers of head make vertigo worse; electronystagmography to check nystagmus; CT/MRI for suspected lesions involving cranial nerve (CN) VIII; audiometry to test hearing

Therapeutic Management

Surgery	Myringotomy and/or mastoidectomy for labyrinthitis caused by otitis media
Medications	Antibiotics if the cause is bacterial; antiemetics to treat nausea and vomiting; vestibular suppressants and antivertigo medications to decrease severity of dizziness and vertigo
General	Bed rest in darkened room with decreased head movement during acute attacks; after the episode is over, the individual should have a complete audiology evaluation to determine possibility of hearing loss
Prevention/ Promotion	Institute fall prevention measures and safety precautions

Laryngitis

Acute or chronic inflammation of mucous membranes of larynx

Etiology and Incidence

Acute laryngitis may be the result of a bacterial, viral, or fungal infection that affects the larynx, subglottic area, and epiglottis. Other causes of both acute and chronic laryngitis include membrane irritation and injury from irritants such as smoking, voice overuse, endotracheal intubation, acid reflux, and alcohol ingestion. Other causes of chronic laryngitis include allergies, autoimmune responses, chronic tonsillitis, adenoiditis, tuberculosis (TB), and syphilis. The prevalence is common and peaks during parallel viral epidemics in the fall and winter.

L

Pathophysiology

The inflammation of the mucous membranes in the lining of the larynx and vocal cords may be acute or chronic. Most prevalent is laryngitis associated with voice overuse and/or environmental irritants. When acute laryngitis is found in combination with an upper respiratory infection (URI), a virus is generally the cause. Laryngitis may also occur in conjunction with pneumonia, influenza, tracheitis, and bronchitis.

Risk Factors

Acute	Voice overuse
	Exposure to environmental irritants
	Recent URI
	Immunosuppression
Chronic	History of smoking and alcohol use
	Exposure to environmental irritants
	Allergy, chronic rhinitis, and sinusitis
	Acid reflux

Clinical Manifestations

Acute	Sore throat, change in voice tone, hoarseness that becomes worse throughout the day, aphonia (complete loss of voice), fever, malaise, pain on swallowing, scratchy throat, and dry cough
	In severe cases, stridor and dyspnea present; indirect examination of the larynx shows redness and edema of the vocal cords and swollen lymph nodes
Chronic	Frequent clearing of throat and complaints of a chronic, dry cough
	Change in voice tone; hoarseness worse in the morning and evening and improves during the middle of the day
	Reddened laryngeal mucosa without noted swelling
	Nodules on the cords may be present, especially in individuals with history of smoking; duration of hoarseness often more than 3 weeks

Complications

Laryngeal swelling may cause airway compromise in severe acute cases.

Diagnostic Tests

Acute	Diagnosis apparent on history and physical examination
Chronic	Lateral and anterior-posterior radiographs of the neck; laryngoscopy to rule out other problems

Therapeutic Management

Surgery	Chronic laryngitis with polyps may necessitate surgical polyp removal; vocal cord biopsy of hyperplastic mucosa if cancer or TB suspected
Medications	Analgesics and/or antipyretic agents for discomfort; antibiotics if causative agent is thought to be bacterial
	Steroids may be used in severe cases to decrease laryngeal edema
General	Avoid talking and give the voice rest. Cool or warm steam mist may alleviate discomfort.
Prevention/ Promotion	Modification of predisposing factors such as removal of irritants, correction of faulty voice habits, smoking cessation
Education	Education about predisposing factors

L

Latex Allergy

An immunoglobulin E (IgE)-mediated reaction to proteins retained in finished natural rubber latex products

Etiology and Incidence

Latex is the milky sap of the rubber tree *Hevea brasiliensis*. This natural rubber product contains proteins. Latex allergy is the reaction to certain proteins in the latex rubber. These allergies have emerged in the 1990s as one of the most pervasive problems in health care. It is a serious and growing problem and health care workers are at increasingly greater risk of acquiring latex allergies. It is currently estimated that an allergy caused by repeated exposure to latex protein allergens develops in at least 1 in 10 health care professionals, and as many as 53% of health care workers reported some type of reaction to latex gloves when surveyed. Children with spina bifida and individuals with chronic illnesses that require frequent operations are especially susceptible to sensitization toward latex. There are limited data on the frequency of latex allergy in the general population.

Pathophysiology

The amount of latex exposure necessary to produce sensitization or an allergic reaction is unknown. Increasing exposure to latex proteins increases the risk of allergic symptoms developing. Although products containing latex have only 2% to 3% protein, it is this protein that is thought to be the allergen in type-1 hypersensitive individuals. The precise protein responsible for causing allergic contact dermatitis latex type-1 hypersensitivity has not yet been identified and may be different for individual patients.

Risk Factors

Although all health care professionals are at risk, those at highest risk are surgical workers, emergency care workers, and obstetrics workers.

Children with spina bifida or others with conditions requiring frequent operations

People with congenital urogenital abnormalities requiring indwelling catheters

Employees in the rubber industry

People with a history of other IgE-dependent allergies, such as rhinitis, asthma, or food allergies with a positive skin test

Clinical Manifestations

Clinical signs include local skin redness, dryness, and itching after contact with latex. Inhalation of particles results in respiratory symptoms, such as rhinitis, sneezing, itchy eyes, scratchy throat, or asthma. ❶ More severe manifestations include anaphylaxis with bronchospasm, laryngeal edema, respiratory distress, and/or respiratory failure.

Complications

❶ Complications include anaphylactic shock and respiratory and cardiac arrest leading to death.

Diagnostic Tests

History	Atopic history, hives under rubber or latex gloves, hand dermatitis related to gloves, allergic conjunctivitis after rubbing eye with hand that has been in contact with latex, swelling around mouth after dental procedures or blowing up a balloon, vaginal burning after pelvic examination or contact with condom
Immunological Evaluation	Skin prick, intradermal, and patch-contact skin tests; serological testing (e.g., radioallergosorbent test [RAST] or enzyme-linked immunosorbent assay [ELISA]). The Food and Drug Administration (FDA) has approved a standardized latex reagent for skin testing to be used for research only. This is not yet available for public use.

Therapeutic Management

Surgery	None
Medications	Epinephrine for reaction (may be autoinjector and carried by individual); β-agonist inhaler;

	prednisone; other anaphylactic life-supporting medications
General	Immediate assessment and interventions for acute reaction, including cardiac monitoring and if necessary, respiratory support
Prevention/ Promotion	For latex-sensitive individuals: avoidance of latex products; avoidance of environments with high levels of circulating aeroallergens (e.g., operating rooms, emergency departments, blood banks); wear medical alert bracelet or tag; carry autoinjector for use at first signs of anaphylaxis System-wide phase out of latex product use (particularly latex gloves) in occupational settings, such as hospitals, clinics
Education	Sensitive individuals—education about prophylaxis Health care workers—education about signs and symptoms of latex allergy Occupational settings—education programs that address creation of latex-free or latex-reduced environments

Lead Poisoning

Multisystem abnormalities resulting from excess exposure to lead

Etiology and Incidence

The cause of lead poisoning is the inhalation of lead dust or fumes, absorption of lead through the skin, or ingestion of lead. Lead poisoning is most common in children 1 to 5 years of age with estimated incidence of 17,000 cases per 100,000 persons or 1 in every 50 children in the United States.

Pathophysiology

Lead enters the bloodstream and attaches to proteins that deliver it to various tissues and organs in the body where it builds up deposits. Lead even in small amounts can affect any part of the body particularly the renal, neurological, and hematological systems. Nervous system effects are of particular concern in young children with developing brains. It interferes with mechanisms such as calcium regulation, neurotransmission in the brain, binding of iron to heme, and erythrocyte production in the blood. It leads to fibrosis in the proximal tubules of the kidneys.

Risk Factors

Children under age 6

1960s housing with deteriorating lead paint

Lead or lead-soldered plumbing

Children that teethe on or ingest paint chips, or chew on vinyl mini blinds or playground equipment with lead

Occupational/hobby exposure (e.g., lead smelting, battery manufacture, plumbing, welding, construction, auto mechanic, painting, ceramics, stained glass, or jewelry making)

Eating from ceramics or pottery containing lead; exposure to burning candles with lead wicks

Exposure to or ingestion of soil or dust near lead industries

Clinical Manifestations

Lead poisoning is frequently asymptomatic with mild toxicity. Likely initial manifestations include loss of appetite, abdominal discomfort, constipation, fatigue, irritability, headache, insomnia, and myalgia. Toxicity leads to three major clinical syndromes: cerebral (hyperactivity, behavior problems, learning problems, neurological disability, and/or mental retardation); neuromuscular (peripheral neuritis, paresthesias, poor coordination); and alimentary (anorexia, abdominal cramping, weight loss, intestinal spasm, and rigidity of abdominal wall). Lead exposure in pregnant women can retard fetal development.

Complications

Chronic exposure may lead to renal failure, liver damage, and encephalopathy with blindness, seizures, paralysis, coma, and death.

Diagnostic Tests

Blood	Lead level greater than 10 µg/dl; mild anemia with basophilic stippling

Therapeutic Management

Surgery	None
Medications	Chelation (succimer, edetate calcium disodium) if blood level greater than 45 µg/dl or in refractory cases; EMLA cream before injection of chelation medications
General	Provide adequate amounts of calcium, iron, zinc, Vitamin C, and protein in diet, low fat to reduce lead absorption; recheck blood levels after chelation; case report to local health department for lead levels more than 20 µg/dl; report occupationally related cases to Occupational Safety and Health Administration (OSHA)

Prevention/ Promotion	Elimination of lead sources
	Screening of all children for lead levels starting at 6 months to 1 year of age
	Use of proper safety equipment in high-risk occupational settings (e.g., respirators)
Education	Education about what lead levels mean; family instruction on lead hazards and lead reduction remedies; dietary instruction; preparation for injections if undergoing chelation; information about community resources, such as Alliance to End Childhood Lead Poisoning; importance of long-term monitoring if levels elevated

L

Leukemia
(Acute Lymphocytic Leukemia, Acute Myelogenous
Leukemia, Chronic Lymphocytic Leukemia, Chronic
Myelogenous Leukemia)

An acute or chronic cancer involving the blood-forming
tissue in the bone marrow; may be classified as myeloid or
lymphoid

Etiology and Incidence

The cause of the various leukemias is unclear, although a viral
association is suspected in some types. Exposure to certain
toxins (e.g., benzene and ionizing radiation) has been implicated, as have genetic defects and a genetic predisposition.
There are more than 30,000 new cases and nearly 22,000
deaths annually from all forms of leukemia in the United States.
Leukemias are most prevalent in adult white males. Acute myelogenous leukemia (AML) is the most commonly reported
leukemia and is an adult disease with a median age at onset of
50 years. Acute lymphocytic leukemia (ALL) is most common
in children age 3 to 5 years but is also seen in adults, particularly those over the age of 60. Chronic myelogenous leukemia
(CML) typically occurs between the ages of 20 and 60, with a
peak incidence between 50 and 60 years of age. The median age
of onset for chronic lymphocytic leukemia (CLL) is 60 years.

Pathophysiology

Whatever the etiological agent, a transformation of leukocytes
and leukocyte precursors into malignant cells occurs. Large
numbers of these immature, abnormal cells proliferate rapidly,
accumulating in the bone marrow, replacing the normal cells,
and suppressing normal hematopoiesis. Proliferation also occurs
in the lymph nodes, liver, and spleen. Eventually all body organs
are involved in the leukemic process.

Risk Factors

ALL	Exposure to select viruses (HTLV-1), high-dose radiation, chemical toxins (benzene); previous use of antineoplastic drugs

AML	Certain genetic disorders (Down syndrome, Bloom or Klinefelter's syndrome, Fanconi's anemia); exposure to chemicals (benzene, pesticides), radiation, tobacco smoke; previous use of antineoplastic drugs; diagnosis of CML
CLL	Familial tendency; history of autoimmune disease
CML	Presence of genetic chromosome translocation t (9,22); exposure to ionizing radiation

Clinical Manifestations

Acute forms of the disease are more rapidly progressive than chronic forms, and acute cell forms are less mature and predominantly undifferentiated.

ALL	Fatigue; dyspnea on exertion; anorexia; weight loss; headache; swollen cervical lymph nodes; swollen, painful joints; splenomegaly; about 10% of cases are asymptomatic
AML	Fatigue, dyspnea on exertion, anorexia, weight loss, headache, swollen cervical lymph nodes, recurrent infections unresponsive to standard treatment, easy bruising, epistaxis, gingivitis
CML	Often asymptomatic for a period, followed by insidious onset of nonspecific symptoms (fatigue, dyspnea, anorexia, weight loss, fever, night sweats); lastly, splenomegaly, pallor, bleeding, and marked lymphadenopathy
CLL	Insidious, asymptomatic onset with lymphadenopathy, followed by fatigue, anorexia, weight loss, and dyspnea; anemia, thrombocytopenia, and bacterial, viral, and fungal infections are present in advanced disease

Complications

The prognosis is better among individuals with acute forms of leukemia and for those who experience total remission after the first course of treatment. Children have a better survival rate than adults. Second malignancies are most likely to develop in people with CLL , and people with CML have the shortest survival rates, often dying of a blast crisis. Other complications of leukemia include infection, hemorrhage, organ failure, and recurrence of the disease.

Diagnostic Tests

The leukocyte count is elevated from 15,000 to 500,000/mm^3 or higher; a large number of immature neutrophils are present; bone marrow biopsy shows a massive number of WBCs in the blast phase; and RBCs, Hgb, and Hct are decreased. Cell morphology, cytogenetics, and immunological and histochemical methods are used to stage the leukemia and to identify and classify cell subtypes. CT scan and lumbar puncture can help stage the disease.

Therapeutic Management

Surgery	None
Medications	Chemotherapy combinations (combinations vary by cell types and subtypes) to induce remission, then post remission, consolidation or maintenance chemotherapy in ALL and AML; chlorambucil in symptomatic stage I or II CLL, chemotherapy combinations in stage III CLL cases; interferon, Gleevec in CML; high-dose chemotherapy before bone marrow transplantation, antiinfectives in cases in which neutrophil count is less than 500/μl, or to treat secondary infection; use of Neupogen to reduce and/or prevent infection; erythropoietin to treat anemia

General	Radiation for palliation or as a pretreatment for bone marrow transplantation, transfusions, reverse isolation procedures, support groups, survivor networks
	Bone marrow transplantation is the only curative modality in CML and is used after relapse in acute leukemias
Prevention/ Promotion	Eliminate exposure to agents such as radiation, benzene, fertilizers
	Cease smoking
Education	Education about chemotherapy, effects and side effects of radiation regimens; avoidance of infection; information about available community resources

L

Liver Cancer, Primary

Hepatocellular carcinomas are the most prevalent of the primary liver tumors, although cholangiocarcinomas, angiosarcomas, and hepatoblastomas also are seen.

Etiology and Incidence

Chronic hepatitis B virus (HBV) is a known etiologic agent. Hepatitis C virus (HCV), cirrhosis, and hemochromatosis are also associated with liver cancer development. The incidence of primary liver cancer in the United States is low. Most of these individuals have underlying cirrhosis. In certain areas of Africa and Southeast Asia, however, liver cancer is the leading malignancy and one of the leading causes of death. Most are associated with HBV infections.

Pathophysiology

Most cancer cells originate in the parenchyma and rapidly form a tumor that extends and invades adjacent structures, such as the stomach and diaphragm. Metastasis occurs to the regional nodes, lung, bone, adrenal gland, and brain.

Risk Factors

Ethanol or anabolic steroid abuse
Exposure to vinyl chloride, pesticides, and herbicide
Ingestion of food contaminated with fungal aflatoxins
Chronic HBV or HCV infection
Chronic liver disease

Clinical Manifestations

Abdominal pain, right upper quadrant mass, epigastric fullness, and weight loss are the most common presenting signs and symptoms. Systemic metabolic signs may include hypoglycemia, hypercalcemia, hyperlipidemia, and erythrocytosis.

Complications

The prognosis in liver cancer is grim; the survival rate is only about 5%. Complications include liver failure, gastrointestinal (GI) hemorrhage, and cachexia.

Diagnostic Tests

The alpha-fetoprotein blood value is elevated in 70% of cases; ultrasound (US), MRI, and CT scans can help visualize masses. A biopsy is necessary for definitive diagnosis.

Therapeutic Management

Surgery	Resection of tumor is only a potentially curative modality; percutaneous ethanol injection or cryoablation for local tumor control; liver transplant for small tumors and advanced cirrhosis
Medications	Chemotherapy is experimental and not particularly effective to date
General	Radiation cannot be given in sufficient doses to be effective; radiolabeled antibodies have been used with limited success
Prevention/ Promotion	HBV vaccine for individuals at high risk of contracting HBV
	Cease alcohol, anabolic steroid use
	Reduce exposure to pesticides, herbicides, and vinyl chloride
	Reduce food supply contaminated with fungal aflatoxins
	Screen for tumor marker alpha-fetoprotein (AFP) in individuals with chronic HBV or cirrhosis

L

Lung Cancer

The major histological types of lung cancer are nonsmall cell cancers (squamous cell carcinoma, adenocarcinoma, and large cell undifferentiated carcinoma), which account for 90% of lung cancers, and small cell lung cancers, which make up the remaining 10%.

Etiology and Incidence

Cigarette smoking is implicated in approximately 80% to 90% of all cases of lung cancer. Occupational exposure to asbestos, radon, nickel, chromium, hydrocarbons, and arsenic is linked to 10% to 15% of lung cancers. The role of air pollution and home exposure to radon gas is unclear. Lung cancer is the leading cause of cancer death for both men and women in the United States and kills more than 157,000 persons per year. Nearly 172,000 cases are diagnosed each year; the incidence for men is declining, and the incidence for women has plateaued as more people quit smoking.

Pathophysiology

Squamous cell carcinomas usually begin in the larger bronchi, often causing bronchial obstruction and spreading by direct extension and lymph node metastasis. Adenocarcinomas are peripheral tumors that begin in fibrotic lung tissue and spread through the bloodstream, commonly metastasizing to the brain, liver, and bone. Large cell undifferentiated carcinoma, which may arise in any area of the lung, disseminates early, spreading through the bloodstream. Small cell carcinoma is centrally located and is the fastest growing type of lung cancer, with rapid metastasis to the brain, liver, and bone.

Risk Factors

Smoking

Passive smoking (nonsmokers with chronic exposure to cigarette smoke)

Exposure to asbestos, radon, nickel, chromium, hydrocarbons, and arsenic, particularly in combination with smoking

Exposure to radiation

Clinical Manifestations

A chronic cough, a change in the volume and color of sputum, chronic upper respiratory tract infections (URIs), and aching in the chest are common presenting symptoms. Wheezing, fatigue, and chest tightness may also be present.

Complications

The prognosis is poor. The long-term survival rate in individuals with localized disease is only 35%, and most people have extension and metastasis on diagnosis. Overall the survival rate for all individuals regardless of stage is 13%. Complications include superior vena cava syndrome, paraneoplastic syndromes, and cor pulmonale.

Diagnostic Tests

A history of smoking and a chest x-ray are the principal sources of diagnostic suspicion. A sputum cytology test is positive in about 75% of cases. Retrieval of cells through bronchoscopy or needle or tissue biopsy provides the definitive diagnosis. CT, MRI, or PET scan is used for detection and evaluation of pleural effusion.

Therapeutic Management

Surgery	Resection of tumor and surrounding tissue, lobectomy, or pneumonectomy
Medications	Systemic multidrug combination chemotherapy, biologic response modifiers
General	Radiotherapy before and after surgery and for palliation; dyspnea management (breathing patterns, positioning, oxygen therapy, relaxation), modifications in activities of daily living (ADLs), home health care, hospice
Prevention/ Promotion	Smoking cessation
	Reduce exposure to cigarette smoke, asbestos, radon, nickel, chromium, hydrocarbons, and arsenic
	Public education programs about smoking hazards and environmental irritants

| **Education** | Education about chemotherapy, radiation regimen effects and side effects, dyspnea management; information about available community resources |

Lupus (Systemic Lupus Erythematosus)

A chronic, multisystem, inflammatory connective tissue disorder

Etiology and Incidence

The cause of systemic lupus erythematosus (SLE) is unknown, but it is thought to be an autoimmune disease with interrelated environmental, hormonal, viral, and genetic factors. More than 500,000 individuals in the United States have diagnosed cases of SLE. Seven times as many women as men are affected, and three times as many African Americans, Asian Americans, and Native Americans as Caucasians are affected.

Pathophysiology

After the etiological agent or agents are introduced, the body forms antibodies directed against "self" tissue, cells, and serum proteins. The regulatory components of the immune system are severely compromised by these autoantibodies. The number and activity of suppressor T cells are both diminished, allowing unrestrained proliferation of B cells and resultant hypergammaglobulinemia. Combinations of autoantibodies and autoantigens form, circulate, and are deposited within capillary complexes, renal glomeruli, renal interstitia, serosal membranes, and the choroid plexus, and in the pleural vasculature. The formation of these immune complexes triggers an inflammatory response, leading to chronic destruction of host tissue.

Clinical Manifestations

Signs and symptoms vary with the acuteness of the disease and the distribution of the immune complexes in body tissue. No characteristic clinical pattern exists, but the following manifestations may be seen:

1. *Skin:* malar or discoid rash (butterfly rash) with scaling; plugging of hair follicles; scarring, painless ulcerations of nasal and oral mucosa; photosensitivity-induced rash
2. *Joints:* tenderness, swelling, arthritis-like pain

3. *Lungs:* pleuritis, pleuritic pain, dyspnea, cyanosis
4. *Kidneys:* oliguria, bladder spasms, edema, proteinuria
5. *Neurological effects:* seizure activity, depression, psychoses
6. *Blood:* anemia, thrombocytopenia
7. *Cardiac effects:* pericarditis, murmurs, electrocardiographic changes
8. *General:* fatigue, headache, fever, malaise, nausea, vomiting, anorexia, weight loss, abdominal pain

Complications

SLE is a chronic, relapsing disease often marked by long periods of remission. If acute episodes can be successfully controlled, the long-term prognosis is good. The 10-year survival rate in the United States approaches 95%. Concomitant infections and renal failure are the leading causes of death.

Diagnostic Tests

Antinuclear antibody (ANA) tests are positive in 98% of SLE cases. A positive ANA test should lead to tests for anti-deoxyribonucleic acid (DNA) and anti-SM antibodies. A high titer in these tests is almost specific for SLE.

Therapeutic Management

Surgery	Joint replacement for chronic synovitis, kidney transplant for renal failure
Medications	Nonsteroidal antiinflammatory drugs (NSAIDs) for mild disease, steroids and immunosuppressives for severe disease, antiinfective drugs for secondary infections, antimalarials for skin rash and polyarthritis
General	Plasmapheresis to reduce circulating immune complexes, renal dialysis for renal failure, aggressive management of intercurrent infection, long-term medical monitoring, balanced diet, careful monitoring if pregnant, keeping a disease-related log to trace conditions that trigger flare-ups, early treatment of flare-ups, counseling to adapt to long-term disease

Education   Education about disease exacerbation and triggers; medication effects and side effects; pain management strategies; energy conservation techniques; avoidance of exposure to infection; instruction on regular follow-up care; information about community resources

L

Lyme Disease

A multisystem infectious disease transmitted by a tick bite and characterized by an early skin lesion

Etiology and Incidence

The disease is caused by a spirochete called *Borrelia burgdorferi*. Lyme disease is the most common vector-transmitted disease in the United States. People of all ages are vulnerable, and the highest incidence is among individuals living in and around wooded areas. The peak season for human infection is from May to November. It is endemic in the Northeastern, Midwestern, and Western United States.

Pathophysiology

The spirochete enters the skin at the site of a tick bite. It incubates for 3 to 32 days and then migrates outward to the skin, forming a pinkish-red rash that resembles a bull's-eye target. It may then spread to other skin sites and various organ systems via the lymphatics and bloodstream. An inflammatory cycle is set up, and cardiac, neurological, and joint abnormalities are common developments.

Clinical Manifestations

The disease first manifests itself as a red skin macule or papule at the bite site with accompanying flulike symptoms, such as headache, fever, muscle ache, and fatigue. These are often missed or ignored by the individual. In about 50% of cases, other lesions develop soon after onset.

Complications

After weeks or months, neurological abnormalities such as meningitis, meningoencephalitis, neuritis, and radiculopathies appear in about 15% of cases. Myocardial abnormalities such as atrioventricular block, myopericarditis, and cardiomegaly occur in 8% of cases. Joint inflammation, pain, and arthritis develop in 50% of cases as long as 2 years after transmission.

Diagnostic Tests

A physical examination with characteristic lesions and a positive enzyme-linked immunosorbent assay (ELISA) are indicative of the disease.

Therapeutic Management

Surgery	None
Medications	Antiinfective drugs to combat infection
General	Bed rest, treatment of complications
Prevention/ Promotion	For endemic areas: wear appropriate clothing (long pants tucked in boots) in wooded or grassy areas and use bug repellent with DEET; keep grass mowed; keep woodpiles away from foot-traffic areas and away from house; have pets wear tick and flea repellent and keep them off furniture; remove ticks with tweezers, wash area thoroughly, and apply antiseptic; see physician for single dose of doxycycline within 72 hours of Ixodes tick bite.

L

Lymphoma, Non-Hodgkin's

Neoplasms of the lymphoid tissue

Etiology and Incidence

The cause is unknown, but theories involving immune deficiencies and viral origins are under investigation. More than 53,000 cases are diagnosed and more than 23,000 deaths occur annually in the United States. The peak incidence occurs in preadolescence, with a drop during adolescence and then a steady increase with age in adulthood. Men and Caucasians are at slightly higher risk than women and African Americans. The incidence is on the rise in the United States.

Pathophysiology

Normal cells in the lymph nodes are replaced with immature, rapidly progressive leukocyte cells of either the T cell or B cell type. Rare cases involve histiocytes. Spread is via the lymphatic system to regional and distal sites, including the skin, bone marrow, brain, and gastrointestinal (GI) system.

Risk Factors

Immunodeficiency disorders (acquired or congenital)

Autoimmune disorders (Hashimoto's, Sjögren's, rheumatoid arthritis, lupus)

Infectious agents (Epstein-Barr virus [EBV], HTLV-I, HHV-8, *Helicobacter pylori*, hepatitis C virus [HCV])

Environmental factors (benzene, hair dyes, paint thinners, creosote, lead arsenate, styrene, formaldehyde)

Clinical Manifestations

A wide variety of signs and symptoms is possible, but many individuals have painless lymphadenopathy, typically of the cervical or inguinal nodes. Other symptoms are fatigue, malaise, fever, anemia, weight loss, night sweats, abdominal pain, and skin lesions.

Complications

The prognosis for individuals with low-grade tumors is good with early treatment. Rapidly progressive intermediate- and high-grade tumors have a poor prognosis. Complications include central nervous system disease (CNS), spinal cord compression, and superior vena cava syndrome.

Diagnostic Tests

A definitive diagnosis is made through lymph node biopsy. Bone marrow biopsy, CT scans, bone scan, chest x-ray, and lab studies (CBC, erythrocyte sedimentation rate [ESR], lactate dehydrogenase [LDH], BUN, creatinine, serum calcium, uric acid, liver function tests [LFTs], serum protein electrophoresis) are done for staging.

Therapeutic Management

Determined by stage and histological type

Surgery	Excision of tumors in advanced disease; therapeutic splenectomy
Medications	Systemic combination chemotherapy with radiation; purine analogs, rituximab for salvage therapy
General	Radiation is the primary therapy, used alone or in combination with chemotherapy, particularly for stage III and stage IV cancer; bone marrow or peripheral blood stem cell transplantation is used as a salvage treatment
Education	Education about chemotherapy, radiation regimen effects and side effects; information about available community resources

L

Macular Degeneration

Progressive deterioration of the macula of the retina, which causes loss of central vision; there is an exudative (wet) and an atrophic (dry) form

Etiology and Incidence

No systemic cause has been discovered, but it appears to have a genetic component and has been associated with smoking. *Chlamydia pneumoniae*, a pathogen that causes chronic inflammation, has also been recently associated with macular degeneration. Macular degeneration is the main cause of blindness for individuals over 55 years of age in the United States. The dry form is diagnosed in about 90% of those affected with the disease, however, the wet form accounts for 90% of all severe vision loss. Incidence in both forms increases with age and is more common in Caucasians than in African Americans. At least 5% of the adult population under age 50 and 80% of those over age 75 have some signs of degeneration of the macula.

Pathophysiology

In *exudative* macular degeneration, the formation of new blood vessels behind the retina encroaches on the macula and leaks blood and fluid, causing edema and scar tissue. This causes fairly rapid damage to the macula and relatively quick loss of central vision. In *atrophic* macular degeneration, there is a slow breakdown of the light-sensitive cells in the macula, interfering with the changing of light into nerve signals. Visual loss is gradual, occurring over a period of years. This is thought to be related to some ischemic process. There is no fluid build up, bleeding, or scarring in atrophic degeneration. Exudative degeneration usually involves both eyes, and atrophic degeneration often starts in one eye and may or may not eventually involve the other eye.

Risk Factors

Familial tendencies
Cigarette smoking
Hyperlipidemia
Hypercholesterolemia
Aging

Chlamydia pneumoniae infection
Ultraviolet radiation exposure (sun)

Clinical Manifestations

Atrophic Degeneration	Early manifestations include slightly blurred vision and a need for more light for reading. This progresses to a blurred spot in the center of the visual field that gets larger and darker over time. If only one eye is affected, the individual may not notice any visual changes unless the good eye is closed. Peripheral and color vision remain intact.
Exudative Degeneration	Early manifestations include the tendency for a straight line to appear wavy, vision quickly becomes increasingly distorted with blurring blind spots and rapid loss of central visual field. Peripheral and color vision remain intact.

M

Complications

Blindness in the central visual fields in exudative forms

Diagnostic Tests

Eye Examination	Look for pigmentary, hemorrhagic disturbance, and/or drusen bodies in macula
Visual Field	To evaluate degree of lost visual acuity
Amsler's Grid	Checkerboard lines wavy or missing in exudative form
Fluorescein Angiography	Detect blood vessel leakage in exudative form

Therapeutic Management

Surgery	Laser photocoagulation/photodynamic treatment for abnormal blood vessels
Medications	Role of antioxidants and zinc for slowing disease process is under study

General	Use of low vision devices to augment remaining vision, referral to low vision counseling services
Prevention/ Promotion	Smoking cessation Protection of eyes with sunglasses during sun exposure
Education	Education about low vision devices available to augment vision for various activities of daily living (ADLs) (e.g., large print, talking books, magnifying glasses, kitchen aids, sewing aids, computer aids, telephones, clocks, lighting)

Malaria

An infectious disease transmitted by a mosquito bite and characterized by fever, sweats, and chills

Etiology and Incidence

Malaria is caused by four species of protozoan parasites: *Plasmodium vivax, P. falciparum, P. malariae,* and *P. ovale.* Infection occurs through the bite of an infected mosquito or by contact with blood products from an infected individual. It is estimated that there are more than 400 million cases of malaria worldwide each year; 1 million persons die of the disease annually in Africa alone. Most endemic areas are in the tropics, and underdeveloped countries are particularly hard hit. Approximately 1500 cases are reported in the United States annually, and most involve travel to endemic regions.

M

Pathophysiology

A mosquito carrier bites a human host and injects the sporozoites, which reside and multiply in the parenchymal cells of the liver. After a maturation period averaging 2 to 4 weeks, merozoites are released and invade the erythrocytes. The infected erythrocytes rupture and release merozoites, pyrogens, and toxins, which cause hemolysis, sluggish blood flow in the capillaries, and adherence of infected erythrocytes to venous walls, obstructing blood flow, increasing the permeability of the capillaries, and causing tissue extravasation, particularly in the brain and gastrointestinal (GI) system.

Clinical Manifestations

The incubation period is followed by a 2- to 3-day prodromal period marked by low-grade fever, malaise, headache, joint aches, and chills similar to the flu and often misdiagnosed and treated as such. A paroxysmal pattern is then established, beginning with a shaking chill and followed by fever and sweats. After the fever and sweats (usually lasting 1 to 8 hours) the person feels well until the next chill begins. One cycle ranges from 20 to 72 hours, depending on the parasite involved.

Complications

Chronic malaria with accompanying parasitemia may occur in partially immune individuals in hyperendemic areas. It is characterized by recurring symptoms resembling a mild, short attack of acute malaria. Blackwater fever is a rare complication characterized by severe hemolytic anemia and renal failure. Uremia and renal failure are common complications. Cerebral malaria causes seizure, psychosis, and coma. Pulmonary edema and splenic rupture are also seen. Untreated malaria caused by *P. falciparum* has a 20% death rate.

Diagnostic Tests

A physical examination revealing the paroxysmal pattern and an enlarged spleen plus a history of exposure to an endemic area within the year are notable. A thick and thin blood smear that isolates the parasite provides the definitive diagnosis.

Therapeutic Management

Surgery	None
Medications	Antimalarial drugs for acute attacks and as prophylaxis if traveling to endemic areas; new deoxyribonucleic acid (DNA)–based vaccines are in development
General	Infusion and monitoring of glucose
Prevention/ Promotion	Use of antimalarial drugs when traveling to endemic area; selection of the correct drug for chemoprophylaxis depends on medical and allergic history, the endemic area, and the length of the trip. Other individual prophylaxis when in endemic areas includes use of insect repellent with DEET, wearing light-colored long-sleeved clothing, long-legged pants tucked into boots, use of mosquito netting for bed, and avoidance of outdoors between dusk and dawn. Hygiene products (e.g., shampoo, deodorants, and cosmetics) should be unscented. Avoid perfumes, colognes, and aftershaves.

Community prophylaxis includes control of mosquito breeding grounds and protection of the blood supply.

Education   Education about importance of taking full course of prophylactic medication beginning a week before travel, every week during travel, and continuing 1 month after travel

Measles

(See Rubella and Rubeola)

M

Ménière's Disease

A chronic disease of the inner ear characterized by recurrent vertigo, tinnitus, and hearing loss

Etiology and Incidence

The cause of Ménière's disease is unknown, although auto-immune or viral causes have been proposed. Adults of both genders between 30 and 60 years of age are usually affected, and most cases are unilateral, although 15% to 30% become bilateral 2 to 5 years after a unilateral onset.

Pathophysiology

The pathogenesis of Ménière's disease is poorly understood but is thought to center on overproduction or decreased absorption of endolymph, which causes a degeneration of the neural end organ of the labyrinth and cochlea and rupture of the labyrinth. The rupture allows endolymph into the perilymphatic space, causing a temporary paralysis of sensory structures.

Clinical Manifestations

The hallmark manifestations are an attack of prostrating vertigo with nausea and vomiting, worsening tinnitus, and sensory hearing loss with a feeling of fullness or pressure in the affected ear. The attack may last from a few hours to a day, and then it gradually subsides. Between acute attacks the person has progressive hearing loss and a persistent background humming and has an intolerance to loud noises.

Complications

Progressive hearing loss is the primary complication.

Diagnostic Tests

A history of the characteristic symptoms and a positive caloric test are indicative of Ménière's disease.

Therapeutic Management

Surgery	For persistent incapacitating episodes (10% of all cases): decompression of the endolymphatic sac; labyrinthectomy or vestibular neurectomy to destroy end organs and neural connections to relieve vertigo and stabilize hearing loss
Medications	Vestibular suppressants or anticholinergics for symptomatic relief of vertigo; antiemetics and sedatives to prevent vomiting and promote rest during acute attack; diuretics, antihistamines, and vasodilators during remission
General	Bed rest with safety precautions, avoidance of sudden head movements during acute attack; low-sodium diet to reduce fluid retention is helpful in some cases

M

Meningitis, Bacterial ●

An infection and inflammation of the meninges of the brain and spinal cord resulting in altered neurological function

Etiology and Incidence

Bacterial meningitis can be caused by any number of bacteria, but 80% of cases are caused by one of three strains: *Neisseria meningitidis, Haemophilus influenzae,* and *Streptococcus pneumoniae.* The disease occurs worldwide and is both endemic and epidemic. Approximately 17,500 cases are reported in the United States annually. Spread is through droplet contact, and the disease can be transmitted as long as the respiratory tract contains the causative bacteria. Children under age 5 are at greatest risk. *Neisseria* meningitis is now the most common form of meningitis.

Pathophysiology

The bacteria invade the respiratory passages and are disseminated by the bloodstream to the cerebrospinal fluid (CSF) space and the meninges of the brain and spinal cord. A growing exudate damages cranial nerves, obliterates CSF pathways, and induces vasculitis and thrombophlebitis. The exudate also generates metabolites and cytokines, which damage cell membranes, disrupt the blood-brain barrier, and cause cerebral edema and ischemic brain damage.

Clinical Manifestations

A prodromal respiratory illness may precede symptoms of fever, severe headache, stiff neck, and vomiting. Changes in consciousness then occur, beginning with irritability, drowsiness, and confusion, followed by stupor and coma. Seizures are common.

Complications

Complications include cranial nerve dysfunctions, hydrocephalus, blindness, deafness, arthritis, myocarditis, pericarditis, and cognitive deficit. ● When left untreated, mortality rates approach 100%.

Diagnostic Tests

Cultures of CSF, respiratory secretions, and blood are positive for the causative agent. CSF pressure greater than 100 to 200 mmHg, CSF glucose less than 40 mg/dl, and CSF protein greater than 50 mg/dl are indicators of meningeal infection.

Therapeutic Management

Surgery	None
Medications	Immediate IV infusion of antiinfective drugs if meningitis suspected, continuing antiinfectives specific for the causative agent after culture results, analgesics for muscle pain and headache, aspirin/acetaminophen for fever, antiseizure drugs for seizure activity, corticosteroids for adults with mental status changes, early course of dexamethasone in children to prevent hearing loss
General	Adequate hydration and balancing of electrolytes, monitoring and control of intracranial pressure (ICP), hemodynamic monitoring, ventilatory support if necessary, seizure precautions, secretion precautions to prevent spread, comfort measures for photophobia, rehabilitation measures for neurological sequelae
Prevention/ Promotion	Vaccine for prevention in at-risk populations Monitoring of contacts with infected individuals Prophylactic antiinfective drugs for those in close contact with an infected individual

M

Meningitis, Viral

Acute aseptic inflammation of the meninges of the brain and spinal cord

Etiology and Incidence

Viral meningitis is usually caused by an enterovirus though many other viruses (e.g., arboviruses, adenoviruses, human immunodeficiency virus (HIV), herpes viruses, and measles and/or mumps) can also cause viral meningitis. It is more common and milder than bacterial meningitis and usually occurs in late summer or early fall in children or adults under 30 years of age. There are approximately 11 cases per 100,000 persons annually in the United States, and 70% of those occur in children under age 5.

Pathophysiology

The virus enters the central nervous system (CNS) after it replicates itself in another location, such as the gastrointestinal (GI) tract for the enterovirus; the respiratory tract for the measles, mumps, and flu viruses; or the subcutaneous tissue for arboviruses. Thus, fecal-oral contamination, inhalation, and direct inoculation by an animal or insect bite are the major routes of infection. Herpes and HIV viruses may be sexually transmitted. Viruses usually enter the CNS via the bloodstream by crossing the blood-brain barrier. Following CNS entry, the virus spreads by infecting other cells. The immune response of the CNS to viral infection is not fully understood, but inflammation is mediated predominantly by T cell and B cell lymphocytes sensitized by the infecting agent. The sensitized lymphocytes are activated by cytokines, and an inflammatory response develops in an attempt to clear the virus.

Clinical Manifestations

The manifestations may vary from individual to individual. Common symptoms include fever, severe headache, stiff neck, drowsiness, mild confusion, nausea, vomiting, diarrhea, and photophobia.

Complications

Although serious, viral meningitis rarely causes disability or death. Encephalitis rarely develops.

Diagnostic Tests

Done to rule out bacterial meningitis; CSF pressure greater than 200 to 250 mmHg, normal or slightly decreased CSF glucose, normal or slightly elevated CSF protein, mononuclear pleocytosis, and CSF cultures negative for bacteria. Blood, respiratory, and/or stool cultures may show viral organism.

Therapeutic Management

Surgery	None
Medications	Analgesics for fever and pain; intravenous acyclovir for herpes simplex infection
General	Supportive care with bed rest and fluid balance
Prevention/ Promotion	Good hand washing technique

M

Migraine

(See Headache)

Mononucleosis

An acute viral infectious disease characterized by fatigue, fever, pharyngitis, and lymphadenopathy

Etiology and Incidence

Mononucleosis is caused by the Epstein-Barr virus (EBV) and transmitted via prolonged contact with infected saliva or through blood transfusion. After the primary infection, the virus remains in the host for life and is periodically shed in nasal secretions. At any given time, 15% to 20% of the adult population are active carriers. Mononucleosis is common in the United States, Canada, and Europe, particularly among adolescents and young adults.

Pathophysiology

EBV invades the host and incubates for 4 to 6 weeks. It then replicates in the nasopharynx and moves to the lymphatic system, where it infects B lymphocytes and stimulates the secretion of an antigen. T lymphocytes proliferate in response to the antigen, producing a generalized lymph node hyperplasia.

Clinical Manifestations

The hallmark signs are profound fatigue; a fever that peaks in the late afternoon at 101° F to 105° F (38.3° C to 40.6° C); severely painful and exudative pharyngitis; and symmetric lymphadenopathy. Splenomegaly is usually present in the second or third week. Mild hepatomegaly may also be present. A maculopapular rash, palatal petechiae, and periorbital edema are less common signs. Fatigue and general malaise may persist for months after infection clears.

Complications

The prognosis is excellent; complications are rare but include splenic rupture, anemia, Guillain-Barré syndrome (GBS), meningitis, and encephalitis.

Diagnostic Tests

The presence of clinical manifestations plus a differential WBC count showing lymphocytes and monocytes more than 50%; a heterophil agglutination antibody test with an antibody titer greater than 1:40; and an EBV-immunoglobulin M (IgM) test with antibodies more than 1:80 are all suggestive of mononucleosis. Liver function tests (aspartate aminotransferase [AST], alanine aminotransferase [ALT], and bilirubin) elevated if the liver is involved.

Therapeutic Management

Surgery	Removal of the spleen in cases of rupture
Medications	Nonaspirin analgesics and antipyretics; steroids for treating impending airway obstruction, severe thrombocytopenia or hemolytic anemia
General	Supportive care with bed rest during the acute phase, saline throat gargles, adequate hydration; avoidance of heavy lifting and contact sports for 2 months after recovery to prevent injury to spleen
Prevention/ Promotion	Prevention is impossible as more than 95% of the adult population are carriers of the EB virus and intermittently shed the virus in their saliva

M

Mood Disorders
(Bipolar, Cyclothymia, Depression, Dysthymia)

A group of common, typically recurring psychiatric ill-nesses (including depressive, dysthymic, bipolar, and cyclo-thymic disorders) characterized by dysregulation of emotion and psychomotor dysfunction with disturbances to sleep, appetite, and sexual function.
(See also Depression, Major)

Etiology and Incidence

The exact cause of mood disorders is unknown though theories point to a multicausal origin involving neurobiological, psycho-logical, genetic, and personality factors in combination with life events. Mood disorders are the most commonly reported of the psychiatric disorders, and mood disturbances necessitating clinical attention affect more than 20% of women and 12% of men in the United States at some point during their lifetimes.

Pathophysiology

The disruption in neurophysiological processes is unclear, but certain areas in the brain become abnormal during depressive or manic episodes. Neurotransmitters such as norepinephrine in the brain are depleted, and the synthesis, transport, and action of serotonin are impaired. MRI and PET scans of the brain have shown increased blood flow to some areas of the brain during depression. The prefrontal cortex and the limbic system also display physiological disruptions. Triggers may be multiple.

Risk Factors

Familial tendencies
Female gender
Substance use/abuse (alcohol, marijuana, digitalis, thiazide diuretics, reserpine, propranolol, anabolic steroids, oral con-traceptives, disulfiram, sulfonamides)
Stressful life events/prolonged stress/lack of social support
Chronic illness (hypothyroid or hyperthyroid, mononucleosis, diabetes mellitus [DM], Cushing's, pernicious anemia, pan-creatitis, hepatitis, human immunodeficiency virus [HIV], multiple sclerosis [MS])

Introverted or anxious temperament for depression; extroverted or achievement-oriented temperament in bipolar disorders

Prior episodes of depression and/or mania

Clinical Manifestations

Depression	Mood is depressed, irritable or anxious, slumped posture, poor eye contact, inability to cry, disinterest and withdrawal from usual activities, decreased ability to concentrate, sleep problems, helplessness, hopelessness, recurrent thoughts of suicide and death, and a pervasive feeling that the world is meaningless. Delusions indicate psychosis.
Dysthymia	A long-standing, fluctuating, low-grade depression, which begins in childhood or adolescence; individuals are habitually gloomy, humorless, lethargic, hypercritical, self-derogatory, and preoccupied with inadequacy and failure. They display low energy, decreased concentration, and difficulty in making decisions.
Bipolar	Patterns of depression (see above) alternating with patterns of mania or hypomania; manic manifestations include pressured, loud, and rapid speech; no need for sleep; elevated, expanded, or irritable mood; impulsivity; grandiosity; belligerence; tearfulness; agitation; easy distractibility; and engagement in risky behavior. Functioning is greatly impaired and delusions and/or hallucinations may be present.
Cyclothymia	Chronic mood swings of at least 2 years with multiple periods of hypomania, depression, and anhedonia. Symptoms are not severe enough to meet criteria for bipolar disorder. The person may display chaotic life patterns characterized by unstable relationships and uneven performances at work or school.

M

Complications

Suicide is the most serious complication in individuals with mood disorders and is the cause of death in 15% to 25% of untreated patients. Overdoses with lithium or heterocyclic antidepressants can be life threatening.

Diagnosis

Diagnosis is based on the clinical picture of symptoms and past history. Assessment should be made for suicide potential.

Therapeutic Management

Surgery	None
Medications	Antidepressants for depression and dysthymia; monoamine oxidase inhibitors (MAOIs) if other antidepressants fail; haloperidol for extreme mania; mood stabilizer (lithium) or anticonvulsants (carbamazepine, valproate) for bipolar disorders; mood stabilizers (divalproex) for cyclothymia; antipsychotics for delusions
General	Hospitalization for severe acute episodes, psychosis, severe functional deficits or high suicide potential; intermittent supportive psychotherapy for acute episodes of depression or periods of inertia in dysthymia; group/family therapy for bipolar disorders; enlisting aid of significant other to increase drug compliance in bipolar disorders; phototherapy for seasonal affective disorder; vocational counseling for dysthymia and cyclothymia; electroconvulsive therapy for severe depression or uncontrolled mania; transcranial magnetic stimulation and vagal nerve stimulation are being investigated for depression
Education	Education about disorder and cyclic nature; effects and side effects of medications and importance of not stopping antidepressants or mood stabilizers abruptly

Multiple Myeloma

A progressive, hematological neoplastic disease of the plasma cells

Etiology and Incidence

The etiological factors are not clearly understood, but chromosomal abnormalities, genetic factors, viruses, and chronic antigen stimulation have been implicated as probable contributors. Multiple myeloma is a relatively rare disease that occurs primarily in those over age 40 and peaks around age 60. Men and women are equally affected, but the disease rate for blacks is more than two times that of whites. More than 14,500 cases are diagnosed in the United States each year, with 10,900 deaths.

Pathophysiology

Multiple myeloma involves an abnormal growth and proliferation of plasma cells and the development of single or multiple plasma cell tumors in the bone marrow. This leads to mass destruction of bone marrow and bone throughout the body. Plasma cells also produce an M protein immunoglobulin that coats the RBCs and inhibits the production of effective antibodies; this can lead to anemia. Metastasis is via the lymph nodes to the liver, kidneys, and spleen.

Risk Factors

Occupational exposure to petroleum products (benzene), asbestos, pesticides, herbicides, or radiation
Familial tendencies

Clinical Manifestations

Early symptoms are nonspecific and include fatigue, weakness, anorexia, and weight loss. These are followed by complaints of bone pain, particularly in the back and thorax, and frequent bacterial infections, particularly pneumonia and anemia. Later manifestations include thrombocytopenia and leukopenia; urinary changes; changes in cognitive, sensory, and motor functions; pathological fractures and vertebral collapse; spinal cord compression; and paraplegia.

Complications

The disease is progressive and currently has no cure. Life expectancy is tied to the extent of disease at time of diagnosis; the median survival rate is 10 years in those with no lytic bone lesions and a serum myeloma protein concentration less than 3 g/dl. Complications include infection, hyperuricemia, hypercalcemia, pyelonephritis, renal failure, and gastrointestinal (GI) bleeding.

Diagnostic Tests

The diagnosis is made based on one or more of the following criteria: plasma cell infiltration above 10% in bone marrow, a monoclonal spike on serum electrophoresis, presence of Bence Jones protein in blood, radiographic visualization of osteoporosis and osteolytic lesions, soft-tissue plasma cell tumors.

Therapeutic Management

Surgery	Laminectomy and fusion for spinal cord compression
Medications	Chemotherapy is the primary treatment, antiinfective drugs for bacterial infections, allopurinol for hyperuricemia, corticosteroids or zoledronic acid for hypercalcemia, epoetin alfa for anemia, analgesics for pain, bisphosphonates to prevent skeletal complications
General	Radiation in chemotherapy-resistant disease and for palliation of bone pain; bone marrow/stem cell transplantation has been used with limited success; ambulation maintained as long as possible; physical therapy to maintain function; fracture

	precautions; adequate hydration to prevent dehydration associated with proteinuria; transfusions for anemia; monitoring for bleeding episodes; precautions against exposure to infections; emotional support for adaptation to chronic, terminal disease
Prevention/ Promotion Education	Eliminate exposure to agents such as asbestos, radiation, benzene, fertilizers, and herbicides
	Education about chemotherapy, radiation, medication regimen effects and side effects; prevention of infection; information about available community resources

M

Multiple Sclerosis (MS)

A chronic, progressive central nervous system (CNS) disease with a disseminating demyelination of the nerve fibers of the brain and spinal cord, characterized by exacerbation and remission of varied multiple neurological symptoms

Etiology and Incidence

The exact cause of MS is unknown, but an immunological abnormality, allergic response, or slow-acting virus is suspected. MS is the most prevalent demyelinating disease and the third leading cause of disability in young and middle adulthood. More than 10,000 cases are diagnosed in the United States each year. MS is five times more prevalent in temperate climates, such as those in the northern United States and Canada, than in tropic climates. The geographic area is linked to the location for the individual's first 15 years of life. Age of onset is typically from 20 to 40 years of age, and Caucasians and females are at greatest risk.

Pathophysiology

Some factor or factors in a genetically susceptible individual trigger an activation of T cells that migrate to the CNS and produce an antigen-antibody response. Multifocal plaques of demyelination form and are distributed throughout the white matter of the CNS. This produces destruction of oligodendroglia and formation of a perivascular inflammation. As myelin breakdown continues, lipid byproducts undergo phagocytosis, and the myelin sheath is destroyed. This leads to decreased velocity and blocked nerve conduction and interferes with impulse transmissions. Eventually the axons are stripped bare. Lesions grow and coalesce into larger lesions, and older lesions form scar tissue. The scars stop the inflammation of the lesion, leading to remission early in the disease process. However, as the disease progresses, symptoms become permanent.

Risk Factors

Growing up in temperate climate
Viral infections
Familial tendency
Altered human leukocyte antigen (HLA) patterns

Clinical Manifestations

Signs and symptoms depend on the size, age, activity, and location of the lesions. Remissions may last months or years early in the disease. Later remission intervals are shorter, and eventually permanent, progressive disability occurs.

Early	The onset is generally insidious, and symptoms are transient, beginning with paresthesia in extremities, trunk, or face; clumsiness and muscle weakness; transient visual disturbances and optic pain; ataxia; bladder incontinence; and vertigo.
Midcourse	Emotional lability, apathy, and shortened attention span; seizures; diplopia; dysarthria; static tremor; spasticity, gait disturbances; transient bowel incontinence
Late	Dementia, scanning speech, nystagmus, intention tremor, hemiplegia, generalized muscular weakness and atrophy, inability to stand and walk, loss of bowel and bladder control

M

Complications

Some individuals have frequent attacks, leading to rapid incapacitation with an unremitting, progressive course that ends in death within 1 to 2 years. Others are prone to complications related to progressive disease and disuse syndrome, such as pressure sores, contractures, pathological fractures, pneumonia, renal infection, and septicemia. Death usually is caused by complications rather than the primary disease.

Diagnostic Tests

Clinical Evaluation	Clinical features present
T1 MRI of Brain	Shows lesions of recent or active disease
T2 MRI of Brain	Shows presence of lesions but not age of development
Magnetic Resonance Spectroscopy (MRS)	Shows biochemistry alterations in brain
Evoked Potential Studies	Show slowed nerve conduction
Lumbar Puncture	Shows elevated immunoglobulin G (IgG), increased WBCs, elevated proteins, identification of oligoclonal bands

Therapeutic Management

Surgery	Rhizotomy for unresponsive spasms; contracture releases for joint immobility; thalamotomy or deep brain stimulation for unmanageable tremor
Medications	Corticosteroids for acute attacks; immunomodulators (interferon, glatiramer acetate) to reduce relapse frequency; immunosuppressive drugs (methotrexate, cyclophosphamide, cladribine) for progressive disease; baclofen or tizanidine for spasticity; clonazepam for tremor; amantadine or pemoline for fatigue; carbamazepine, tricyclic antidepressants or nonsteroidal antiinflammatory drugs (NSAIDs) for pain; antidepressants for depression; oxybutynin or propantheline for urinary urgency
General	Balance of rest and activity; long-term rehabilitation (occupational, physical, and speech therapy) to maintain activities of daily living (ADLs), adapt to progressive loss of function, prevent disuse syndrome, and promote bowel and bladder control; assistive

devices (canes, walkers, bracing, casting, wheelchairs); counseling and psychological support of individual and family; respite home care; ventilatory assistance and communication devices in end-stage disease; care in feeding if dysphagia is present; evaluation for cognitive dysfunction

Education	Education about relapsing-remitting nature of disease, effects and side effects of medications; planning of long-term strategies for diet, exercise, rest, bowel regulation, communication, ADL aids; information about resources, such as National Multiple Sclerosis Society

M

Mumps (Parotitis)

An acute, contagious viral disease, characterized by unilateral or bilateral edema and enlargement of the salivary glands

Etiology and Incidence

The causative agent is the paramyxovirus, and the disease is spread by droplet or direct contact with infected saliva. It is most communicable immediately before and during the glandular swelling. There were more than 200,000 cases annually in the United States in 1967, the year the vaccine was introduced. In 2001, 231 cases were reported.

Pathophysiology

After a 2- to 3-week incubation period, the virus invades one or more salivary glands, causing tissue edema and infiltration of lymphocytes. Cells in the glandular ducts degenerate and produce necrotic debris, which plugs the ducts.

Clinical Manifestations

Onset begins with fever, headache, and malaise about 24 hours before swelling of the gland or glands (usually the parotid glands), either unilaterally or bilaterally. Pain is noted on chewing and swallowing. The glands remain swollen about 72 hours before receding.

Complications

Occasionally, particularly in adults, other glands in the testes, ovaries, breasts, and thyroid are involved, and the disease course is often more severe. Complications include meningoencephalitis, pericarditis, deafness, arthritis, nephritis, and in rare cases, sterility in men.

Diagnostic Tests

Characteristic swelling
Positive cell cultures from saliva or urine

Therapeutic Management

Surgery	None
Medications	Analgesics and antipyretics for pain and fever
General	Bed rest, hydration, isolation during communicability, compresses on swelling, support of scrotum with orchitis
Prevention/ Promotion	MMR (measles, mumps, rubella) vaccine given at age 1 with second dose at ages 4 to 6
	Adult immunization to healthy adults born after 1957 with no demonstrated immunity

M

Muscular Dystrophy

A group of inherited, progressive, degenerative muscle disorders characterized by an insidious loss of muscle strength in a variety of muscle groups; Duchenne's muscular dystrophy (DMD) is the most common of the disorders.

Etiology and Incidence

DMD and Becker's muscular dystrophy (BMD), a clinical variant of DMD, are X-linked recessive disorders involving the gene that encodes dystrophin. Males are exclusively affected, and the incidence in the United States is 1 in every 3500 live male births. These disorders typically manifest in boys ages 3 to 7. Females are carriers. Other dystrophies (Landouzy-Dejerine dystrophy [LDMD], Leyden-Möbius dystrophy [LMMD], Erb's dystrophy, and mitochondrial and congenital myopathies) are also inherited, but the specific genetic link is less clear. These disorders are seen in children and adults, affect males and females, and are milder.

Pathophysiology

Dystrophin, a protein product in skeletal muscle, is absent in individuals with DMD and reduced in those with BMD. The resulting pathogenesis is not clear, but lack of dystrophin is thought to impair fast-muscle fiber function and to induce a number of biochemical anomalies, including intracellular accumulation of calcium. A number of systemic sequelae have also been noted. Serotonin in the platelets is reduced, and non-muscle cells have reduced adhesiveness and generalized membrane abnormalities. Abnormalities of the central nervous system (CNS) are noted, as is reduced gastrointestinal (GI) motility. Platelet function and the vascularity of endothelial cells are abnormal.

Clinical Manifestations

DMD	Delays in gross motor development; difficulty walking, running, climbing stairs, and riding a tricycle appears at about age 3 to 5; progressive weakness with waddling gait,

	lordosis, difficulty rising from a sitting or supine position; calf muscle hypertrophy; scoliosis; contractures and joint deformities; inability to ambulate by about age 12; mild mental retardation; respiratory and accessory muscles involved in end-stage with cardiomegaly
BMD	Onset occurs at age 5 to 25; symptoms are similar to but milder than DMD Ambulation is lost about 20 years after onset. Contractures, scoliosis, and ventilatory failure are rare, and the life span usually is normal.
LDMD	Onset from age 7 to 20; weakness of facial and shoulder girdle muscles; difficulty whistling, closing eyes, and raising arms; footdrop develops late; life span is normal
LMMD/ Erb's	Adult onset with weakness of pelvic girdle (LMMD) and shoulder girdle (Erb's)

M

Complications

The major complications of DMD are disuse atrophy, contractures, and cardiopulmonary problems, resulting in respiratory infections. Death is usually a result of complications rather than the primary disease.

Diagnostic Tests

DMD and BMD are diagnosed through clinical evaluation and the characteristic manifestations; electromyography (EMG) shows rapidly recruited myopathic motor units without spontaneous activity; muscle biopsy shows necrosis and varied muscle fiber size; dystrophin immunoblotting is done in which dystrophin is absent (DMD) or abnormal (BMD). Other types are distinguished primarily on clinical grounds.

Therapeutic Management

Surgery	Contracture release, spinal instrumentation to correct scoliosis, tracheostomy in end-stage DMD

Medications	Random clinical trials are being conducted with steroids; antiinfective drugs for bacterial infections in end-stage DMD
General	Long-term rehabilitation (occupational and physical therapy) to maintain activities of daily living (ADLs) and help adapt to progressive loss of function, prevent disuse syndrome, and promote bowel and bladder control; assistive devices (canes, walkers, bracing, casting, wheelchairs); counseling and psychological support of individual and family; respite home care; ventilatory assistance and communication devices in end-stage DMD; family genetic counseling, identification of carriers
Education	Education about long-term activities to maintain function and prevent disuse syndromes (e.g., stretching and range of motion (ROM) exercises, weight bearing, balance of rest and activity)

Myasthenia Gravis (MG)

A progressive neuromuscular disease of the lower motor neurons characterized by muscle weakness and fatigue

Etiology and Incidence

The cause of MG is unknown, although evidence points to a systemic autoimmune disorder. More than 80% of individuals with MG also have thymic abnormalities, but the link is unclear. The incidence is 2 to 5 per 1 million individuals in the United States annually. The age of onset is either 20 to 30 years (primarily in women) or 50 to 60 years (primarily in men).

Pathophysiology

An antigen attack on the acetylcholine receptor of the postsynaptic neuromuscular junction results in dysfunction of the receptor, which fails to act on the acetylcholine. Because of this, nerve impulses do not pass on to the skeletal muscle at the myoneural junction.

Clinical Manifestations

The most common manifestations are ptosis, diplopia, and muscle fatigue after exercise. Dysarthria, dysphagia, ocular palsy, head bobbing, and facial and proximal limb weaknesses are also reported. Symptoms are milder on awakening and become worse as the day progresses. Rest temporarily improves symptoms. Respiratory involvement leads to breathlessness and reduced tidal volume and vital capacity. Manifestations can be remitting, static, or progressive. Factors such as stress, menses, heat, and illness can exacerbate symptoms.

Complications

Myasthenic crisis is an acute exacerbation of symptoms; it usually involves respiratory distress and can lead to respiratory failure or aspiration and cardiopulmonary arrest.

Diagnostic Tests

A characteristic pattern of fatigue and weakness on exertion that improves with rest and a positive Tensilon test are indicators. A CT scan may indicate the presence of thymoma; electromyography (EMG) may show muscle fiber contraction with progressive decremental response.

Therapeutic Management

Surgery	Thymectomy for treatment of thymoma and remission of adult-onset MG
Medications	Anticholinesterases and corticosteroids to counteract muscle weakness and fatigue; immunosuppressants with autoimmune pathogenesis; influenza shots to prevent respiratory infection
General	Plasmapheresis to treat weakness and fatigue, ventilatory support in respiratory crisis, physical therapy to prevent disuse problems, and occupational therapy to aid in activities of daily living (ADLs), balance of exercise and rest; counseling for long-term adaptation to disease
Prevention/ Promotion	Prevent exacerbations by avoiding temperature extremes, prompt treatment of infection and stress reduction; avoid medications (e.g., aminoglycoside antibiotics, class I antiarrhythmics, penicillamine, tetracyclines) known to exacerbate MG
Education	Instruction about cholinergic crisis caused by excessive anticholinesterase medication, information about the importance of preventing respiratory infection or recognizing and treating symptoms early; information about resources such as Myasthenia Gravis Society

Myocardial Infarction (MI) (Heart Attack)

Ischemic necrosis of the myocardium resulting from inadequate coronary artery blood flow

Etiology and Incidence

More than 90% of all MIs are caused by obstruction of a plaque-lined coronary artery by an acute thrombus. MI also may be caused by arterial embolization from valvular stenosis or endocarditis and by arterial spasm after cocaine ingestion. Each year, nearly 1 million persons in the United States have an MI; one in three dies, and more than half of these deaths occur within 1 hour of onset (see also Coronary Artery Disease and Angina Pectoris).

Pathophysiology

Occlusion of a coronary artery causes a persistent cellular ischemia that interferes with myocardial tissue metabolism, causing rapid, permanent cell damage and necrosis. The extent of necrosis is dictated by the size of the infarct, the vessel occluded, and the length of time that it remains occluded. Damage initially occurs to the left ventricle but often extends to other cardiac chambers. Infarcts may be classified by the thickness of the myocardial tissue involved. Transmural infarcts (Q wave) involve the full thickness of the myocardium from the epicardium to endocardium and cause abnormal Q waves on the ECG. Nontransmural infarcts (non-Q wave) do not extend through the ventricular wall and cause ST segment or T wave ECG abnormalities.

Risk Factors

Familial history of heart disease
History of hypertension (HTN), diabetes mellitus (DM)
Smoking
Sedentary lifestyle
Obesity
Elevated cholesterol and triglycerides
Stress

Clinical Manifestations

Most individuals have prodromal symptoms such as fatigue, shortness of breath, and crescendo angina days or weeks before the acute attack. The first symptom of the attack is usually a deep, substernal, visceral pain that may be described as aching, squeezing, or crushing, or as a heavy weight on the chest. The pain may radiate to the back, neck, jaw, teeth, or left arm, and it is not relieved by rest, nitroglycerin, or antacids. Other signs and symptoms include anxiety; restlessness; sweating; nausea; vomiting; cold, clammy skin; low-grade fever and dyspnea. Females may have a different set of symptoms than males. Their symptoms are often vague, diffuse, and less pronounced in nature, and ECG changes may be less visible. Common symptoms in women include nausea, vomiting, fatigue, dizziness, shortness of breath, and neck and shoulder pain.

Complications

Complications include arrhythmia, cardiogenic shock, heart failure, pulmonary edema, cerebral or pulmonary emboli, myocardial rupture, pericarditis, postmyocardial infarction syndrome, and sudden death. Forty-four percent of women and 27% of men die within the first year of an MI.

Diagnostic Tests

Clinical History	Manifestations, risk factors, and health history
12-lead ECG	Wave elevations in the ST-T segment on two or more contiguous leads; T wave inversion, and/or deep Q waves (ECG changes may be less visible in women)
Serum Cardiac Markers	Serial measurements (on presentation and 8 hours later) show increases of troponins and creatine kinase (CK)
Albumin Cobalt Binding Test	Changes seen in MI
Echocardiogram	To detect contraction abnormalities of ventricles

Therapeutic Management

Surgery	Primary angioplasty within 6 hours with adjunctive glycoprotein IIb/IIIa is the current treatment of choice; coronary stents are used to decrease ischemia and improve long-term patency.
Medications	Thrombolytic drugs given within 6 hours of onset to interrupt MI evolution, if angioplasty not available; glycoprotein receptor inhibitors, aspirin, and heparin to reduce ischemia in non-Q wave MI; glycoprotein receptor inhibitors also used with angioplasty to reduce closure postangiography; beta-adrenergic blockers to reduce reinfarction and infarct size; angiotensin-converting enzyme (ACE) inhibitors to reduce ventricular enlargement; vasodilators and narcotic analgesics for pain, antihyperlipidemics to lower cholesterol and triglyceride levels; stool softeners to prevent straining at stool; sedatives and tranquilizers to increase rest
General	Cardiovascular monitoring; oxygen therapy; bed rest; decreased environmental stimuli; monitoring for and treatment of depression, particularly about the third day; quitting smoking; restriction of caffeine and cholesterol; antiembolism hose; rehabilitation with stepped exercise program, sexual counseling; regular medical follow-up
Prevention/ Promotion	Smoking cessation
	Weight reduction if necessary
	Regular exercise program
	Stress reduction modalities (e.g., deep breathing, meditation, biofeedback)
	Cholesterol, lipid level reduction
	Alcohol in moderation
	Control of HTN, DM
	Low-dose aspirin therapy in those at risk for coronary artery disease (CAD)

M

| **Education** | Education about decreasing risk factors, cardiac conditioning, exercise, diet, medications' effects and side effects, importance of long-term follow-up |

Neuroblastoma

A solid malignant tumor that begins along the sympathetic ganglion chain or in the adrenal medulla in infants and children

Etiology and Incidence

The cause of neuroblastoma is unknown, but genetic abnormalities are strongly suspected. The incidence is 10 cases per 1 million in children less than 15 years of age in the United States. It is the most common tumor in children less than a year old and accounts for 8% of all solid tumors in childhood. In 80% of the cases, children are under age 8 at time of diagnosis.

Pathophysiology

Neuroblastoma cells arise from primitive adrenergic neuroblasts in embryonic neural crest tissue. Malignant transformation is thought to result from inappropriate cell response to signals for morphological differentiation. Neuroblastoma can spontaneously regress or mature into benign ganglioneuromas. Common metastatic sites include the liver, bone, bone marrow, skin, and lymph nodes. It may also metastasize to the brain.

Risk Factors

Familial tendencies
Maternal phenytoin treatment
Fetal alcohol syndrome, EMG syndrome
Pancreatic islet cell dysplasia, Hirschsprung's disease

Clinical Manifestations

Signs and symptoms depend on site of origin and stage of disease. More than half of diagnosed cases are not discovered until they have metastasized.

Localized Tumors
Often asymptomatic

Abdomen	Large, firm, irregular, nontender, abdominal mass that may cross the midline
Pelvis	Disturbances in bowel or bladder function

| Thorax | Dry persistent cough, respiratory distress, dysphagia |
| Neck | Cervical lymphadenopathy, ptosis, miosis, heterochromia of iris, enophthalmos |

Metastasis

Bone Marrow	Pancytopenia, anemia, fever, weight loss, fatigue, bleeding, infection
Liver	Rapid liver enlargement, jaundice, abdominal distention, respiratory distress
Bone	Bone pain, bone masses; bone lesions in orbit of eye cause proptosis and ecchymoses of eyelids (raccoon eyes).
Intracranial	Meningeal signs, separation of cranial sutures, lytic skull lesions
Spinal Cord	⬤ Paresis, paralysis, incontinence of bowel and bladder
Adrenal	Flushing, hypertension, sweating, tachycardia
Skin	Bluish nodules that flush then blanch when palpated
General	Pallor, weakness, irritability, anorexia, weight loss from widespread metastasis

Complications

Overall survival rate is 64%. Infants have a better outcome than children over the age of 1. Those with localized tumors with no lymph node involvement have a greater than 99% survival rate.

Diagnostic Tests

Clinical Evaluation	Symptom patterns and detection of tumor masses require follow-up.
Tissue Biopsy	Definitive diagnosis
Bone Marrow	Detect monoclonal antibodies in spinal metastasis aspirate
24-hour Urine	Urinary excretion of catecholamines with adrenal or sympathetic tumors
CT Scans/MRI	To detect tumor formation in suspected areas

| Bone Scans | To detect bony lesions |
| MIBG Scintigraphy | Assess extent of primary tumor and metastasis |

Therapeutic Management

Surgery	Partial or total surgical resection of primary tumor depending on tumor location
Medications	Single agent or combination systemic chemotherapy as adjunct to surgery or in metastatic disease
General	Radiation in extensive disease, palliation, or in emergencies (e.g., tumor producing respiratory distress or spinal cord compression); radiation as conditioning regimen with bone marrow transplant; psychological support to family to aid in coping with diagnosis and outcomes
Education	Family and patient education about treatment modalities and their effects

N

Obesity

Excess body fat as defined by a body mass index (BMI) of = 30kg/m^2. Overweight is defined as a BMI of 25 to 29.9kg/m^2.

Etiology and Incidence

The ultimate cause of obesity is an unequal balance between energy consumption and energy expenditure. However, there are multiple genetic, environmental, and regulatory factors that affect consumption, storage, and expenditure. It is the most common nutritional problem in the United States and there are more than 97 million adults who are overweight or obese.

Pathophysiology

The regulation of body weight is a complex homeostatic mechanism that balances intake and expenditure. The hypothalamus serves as the central coordinating area for all these activities. There are a number of hormones and neurotransmitters that stimulate appetite or produce satiety. Some theories suggest that obese people may have impaired feedback signals about satiety or faulty feedback receptor centers that produce hyperphagia. Thermogenesis is the process that controls energy expenditure. Other theories suggest that the thermogenic process is impaired or super efficient in the obese.

Risk Factors

Familial tendency
Lower socioeconomic status
Increased food intake
Sedentary lifestyle
Increased number of fat cells
Brain trauma (tumor, injury)
Drugs (steroids, some antidepressants, benzodiazepines, lithium, and antipsychotics)
Endocrine factors (pancreatic neoplasm, Cushing's disease, hypothyroid)
Eating patterns (binge eating, night eating syndrome)
Pregnancy

Clinical Manifestations

Weight greater than norms for height

Complications

Morbidity and mortality is increased in the obese. Complications include predisposition to diabetes mellitus (DM), hypertension (HTN), hyperlipidemia, coronary artery disease (CAD), cerebrovascular disease, osteoarthritis, sleep apnea, and certain cancers.

Diagnostic Tests

Overweight is determined by a BMI of 25 to $29.9 \, \text{kg/m}^2$ and obesity is a BMI = $30 \, \text{kg/m}^2$. Body fat distribution can be assessed by waist to hip ratios, with a ratio of greater than 1.0 for men and greater than 0.8 for women signaling increased risk from obesity.

Therapeutic Management

Surgery	Gastroplasty, gastric partitioning, gastric bypass for severe obesity; lipectomy
Medications	Drugs that suppress appetite (sibutramine) or limit nutrient absorption (orlistat)
General	Diet therapy, nutrition consult, exercise program, lifestyle and behavioral modifications, counseling, support networks
Prevention/ Promotion	Maintenance of loss through long-term lifestyle changes that include balanced diet and regular exercise
Education	Instruction in diet and exercise, medication effects and side effects; long-term nature of the problem

O

Oral and Oropharyngeal Cancer

Oropharyngeal cancer is classified anatomically rather than by cell type and includes cancers of the oral cavity, pharynx, and salivary glands. The oral cavity includes the lips, oral mucosa, gums, most of the tongue, and teeth. The oropharynx begins anteriorly where the oral cavity stops. It includes the base of the tongue, soft palate, uvula, tonsils, and pharyngeal walls.

Etiology and Incidence

The cause of oropharyngeal cancers is unknown, but the aerodigestive tract is exposed to a wide range of carcinogens, including tobacco products and alcohol. More than 27,500 cases occur annually and approximately 7,200 persons die each year in the United States. Men have oropharyngeal cancer twice as often as women and African Americans are more susceptible than Caucasians. Most oropharyngeal cancers occur in men over age 50.

Pathophysiology

Most oropharyngeal cancers are squamous cell cancers arising on the floor of the mouth, the ventrolateral aspect of the tongue, and the soft palate complex.

Risk Factors

Chronic exposure to tobacco including cigarettes, pipes, cigars, and smokeless tobacco (chewing tobacco, snuff)
Poor oral hygiene
Prolonged heavy use of alcohol
Poorly fitting dentures that cause chronic lesions and/or ulcers
Chronic exposure to ultraviolet (UV) radiation from the sun

Clinical Manifestations

Early	Dysphagia; local pain; pain on swallowing; leukoplakia (white patch that does not rub off); reddened areas; mouth or throat ulcers that do not heal; hoarseness; localized pain

| Later | Difficulty swallowing, excessive secretions, airway disturbance, enlarged lymph nodes |

Complications

The 5-year survival rate for oral and oropharyngeal tumors is 56%. Those with oral cancers have a better chance of survival than those with oropharyngeal cancers. Complications include disfigurement; loss of hard or soft palate; nerve damage that may lead to impaired eating, chewing, or swallowing; paralysis; and difficulty with communication.

Diagnostic Tests

| Biopsy | Scraping of leukoplakia and/or biopsy of a lesion for histopathological confirmation is diagnostic |
| X-ray and/or CT Scan | To determine evidence of muscle, bone, or lymphatic involvement |

Therapeutic Management

Surgery	The decision for surgery is determined on disease staging, location, and functional deficit or anticipated outcome for the disease. Surgery may range from simple tumor removal to radical resection of the cancer; tracheostomy with radical neck dissection; gastrostomy to aid in feeding
Medications	Chemotherapy may be used to shrink tumors before surgery or radiation therapy in advanced disease.
General	Radiation therapy may be used as treatment for early disease or as treatment when the functional deficit by surgery may be great or as an operative adjunct; good oral hygiene; communication devices; speech therapy; counseling and support
Prevention/ Promotion	Cessation of tobacco use
	Limit sun exposure, use sun protection on lips

	Limit alcohol intake
	Maintain good dental hygiene
Education	Instruction in oral hygiene; importance of dental and medical follow-up; instruction on management of gastrostomy/tracheostomy tubes at home

Organic Mental Syndromes

(See Delirium/Dementia)

Osteomyelitis

An infection of the bone and bone marrow

Etiology and Incidence

Osteomyelitis is caused by a pathogen that is introduced directly through an open fracture, penetrating trauma, or surgical procedure or indirectly from another infection that spreads through the bloodstream or from adjacent tissues. The most common pathogens are *Staphylococcus aureus, Streptococcus pneumoniae, Escherichia coli, Pseudomonas aeruginosa,* and *Haemophilus influenzae.* The incidence is highest in childhood and early adolescence, and the disorder occurs more often in boys. Those undergoing hemodialysis, drug abusers, and individuals with diabetes, sickle cell anemia, tuberculosis (TB), decubitus ulcers, and peripheral arterial insufficiency are also at risk.

Pathophysiology

The long bones are most often involved. The invading pathogen travels to the metaphysis, located between the shaft and the epiphysis. The pathogen grows and multiplies in the metaphysis, producing pus, which eventually interferes with the blood supply in the bone, causing necrosis. An inflammatory response is set up, and macrophages are produced to combat the pathogens; necrosis continues, and the enlarging mass spreads through the bone cortex to contiguous tissue. New bone trabeculae are formed in an effort to keep the infection localized. The infection can spread to the bone marrow and to the skin through sinus tracts. Periodic drainage occurs until all dead bone is destroyed or excised. In adults the spine is often affected.

Clinical Manifestations

Pain, tenderness, edema, and warmth at the site are the most common manifestations. Bone pain on use or on palpation may be evident, as well as systemic symptoms such as fever, chills, sweats, malaise, weakness, headache, and nausea. Later signs include drainage from sinus tracts to the skin and fractures.

Complications

Osteomyelitis can lead to chronic infection, joint and skeletal deformities, and (in children) disturbed bone growth and limb shortening.

Diagnostic Tests

Clinical Evaluation	A history of antecedent infection or open trauma in the preceding 2 to 4 weeks
Blood Tests	An elevated WBC count and erythrocyte sedimentation rate
Radionucleotide Scan	Positive
MRI/CT Scan	Identify extent of infection
	Bone/wound cultures frequently positive for the pathogen
	Bone/soft tissue biopsy positive for pathogen
Serum Cultures	Positive for blood-borne pathogens
X-ray Examination	May reveal bone destruction but only after 2 weeks or longer

Therapeutic Management

Surgery	Surgical excision (saucerization) of infected and dead bone, sterilization of the abscess, bone grafts to affected site, amputation in some cases related to underlying diabetes
Medications	Antiinfective drugs specific for pathogen
General	Splints to reduce joint pain; external fixation or casting for weakened bones to prevent fractures; initially bed rest, followed by progressive ambulation; dressing changes for draining wounds; hyperbaric oxygen therapy to increase circulating WBCs

Osteoporosis

A generalized, progressive reduction of bone mass as bone resorption outstrips bone formation, causing skeletal weakness and fractures

Etiology and Incidence

The causes of primary osteoporosis are unknown but are presumed to be multifactorial. Secondary osteoporosis may be caused by endocrine disorders, such as hypogonadism, hyperthyroidism, hyperparathyroidism, and diabetes mellitus (DM); prolonged use of substances (corticosteroids, barbiturates, or heparin); underlying disease (renal or liver disease, malabsorption syndrome, chronic obstructive pulmonary disease (COPD), rheumatoid arthritis, or sarcoidosis); and prolonged weightlessness or immobility. Postmenopausal women are the most susceptible to primary osteoporosis; an estimated 50% of postmenopausal women will have osteoporosis develop and 33% will have an osteoporotic fracture in their lifetime.

Pathophysiology

O

As bone resorption outstrips bone formation, bone tissue mass progressively declines but the bone is morphologically normal. Cortical thickness also declines, as do the number and size of trabeculae with normal osteoid seams.

Risk Factors

Menopause or other loss of ovarian function
Race and gender (white women are most susceptible; Asian women are also more vulnerable)
Nulliparity
Familial history of osteoporosis
History of underlying skeletal disease
Chronic malnutrition, long-term lack of calcium intake
Diet high in red meat and/or sugar
Underweight, particularly coupled with intense exercise (women with anorexia are susceptible)
Smoking
Heavy intake of alcohol
Sedentary lifestyle, immobility

Clinical Manifestations

Individuals are typically asymptomatic early in the disease. The first symptom is usually a dull, aching, constant pain in the bones, particularly the back and chest. The pain may radiate down the leg, and muscle spasms may be present. As the spinal column mass diminishes, dorsal kyphosis and cervical lordosis increase, leading to multiple compression fractures of the spine and a reduction in height. Other fractures occur with minimal or no trauma.

Complications

Immobility from increased fractures and deformity from spinal crushing are common complications.

Diagnostic Tests

Clinical Evaluation	Reveal risk factors or secondary causes; bone pain
BMD Tests	Reveal loss of bone mineral density— BMD greater than 2.5 standard deviations above young adult reference mean
X-rays	Show decreased radiodensity after 25% to 40% loss of bone calcium

Therapeutic Management

Surgery	Open reduction internal fixation of fractures of femur
Medications	Calcium and vitamin D supplements; calcitonin, bisphosphonates (etidronate, alendronate, pamidronate) or selective estrogen receptor modulators (raloxifene) to prevent bone resorption; nonsteroidal antiinflammatory drugs (NSAIDs) for pain; use of estrogen-progestin supplements *is controversial*

General	Consistent exercise regimen, including moderate, weight-bearing hyperextension and resistance exercises to slow calcium loss and strengthen musculature; heat and massage for muscle spasm; orthopedic supports for back and neck to prevent stress fractures; cane to aid in walking; high-protein diet; monitoring of calcium levels
Prevention/ Promotion	Bone density surveys every 1 to 3 years after age 49 for early detection
	Calcium and vitamin D supplements
	Regular weight-bearing exercise program
	Balanced diet
	Adequate fluoride ingestion
	Smoking cessation
	Moderate alcohol intake
Education	Instruction in fall and fracture prevention; medication effects and side effects

0

Otitis Externa

Inflammation and/or infection of the external canal or the auricle of the external ear, which may be categorized as acute localized, acute diffuse (swimmer's ear), chronic, eczematous, fungal, and necrotizing (malignant)

Etiology and Incidence

Causes are multiple and include infection from bacteria, fungi, viruses; trauma from foreign objects in the external ear canal; contact dermatitis or neurodermatitis, eczema, or seborrhea; medication side effects and allergies. This common external ear problem is seen more often in adults than in children. The condition is seen most often during hot, humid weather.

Pathophysiology

The etiological agent, often in the presence of moisture, causes a pruritic reaction that becomes erythematous with increasing swelling and occlusion of the external ear canal.

Risk Factors

Underlying immune compromise, diabetes mellitus (DM), or diabetes insipidus
Underlying skin disorder (e.g., seborrhea, psoriasis, eczema)
Poor external ear hygiene and improper drying after bathing
Swimming in dirty or polluted water
Known exposure to allergic substances (e.g., nickel or chromium, or chemicals in hair sprays; cosmetics; hearing aids and earrings)
Improper use of Q-tips for cleaning
Medications such as the sulfonamides and neomycin
Aging adults
Hot humid weather

Clinical Manifestations

The two most common symptoms are otalgia (e.g., itching and/or ear pain exacerbated by motion) and otorrhea (discharge from the canal). The external ear canal appears red and swollen. Additional manifestations are unique to the category of disease:

Acute Localized	Pustules, furuncles, or blisters in canal, auricle, and/or concha
Acute Diffuse	Occlusion of canal, hearing loss, serous secretions, dull infected tympanic membrane (TM)
Chronic	Dry atrophic canal with no cerumen, thickening of canal walls
Eczematous	Pustules, crusts, and scales in canal and pinna
Fungal	Fungal growth in a variety of colors
Necrotizing	Ulceration, tissue granulation, tissue necrosis, facial nerve palsy

Complications

If untreated or inadequately treated, otitis can lead to necrotizing otitis media and infection of nearby bone or central nervous system (CNS) structures.

Diagnostic Tests

No test, other than direct clinical evaluation, is necessary. Culture may be done to determine infective organism.

Therapeutic Management

Surgery	Incision and drainage for superficial pointing furunculosis
Medications	Topical antiinfective agents for infection; opiates, analgesics for pain; antipruritics/antihistamines for itching; topical corticosteroids to reduce inflammation; prolonged course of IV antibiotics for necrotizing otitis
General	Thorough cleansing and/or debridement of ear canal; ear wick for occluded canal; local heat for furuncles
Prevention/ Promotion	Proper cleaning and drying of external ear and ear canal after bathing, swimming
	Avoidance of known allergic substances
	Avoidance of swimming in dirty water
	Treatment of underlying diseases and dermatologic conditions
Education	Education about preventive actions

Otitis Media

Inflammation of the middle ear

Etiology and Incidence

Acute otitis media is usually the result of a bacterial or viral infection of the upper respiratory tract. When acute otitis goes unresolved, it leads to an effusion of the middle ear, called *secretory otitis media*. Otitis media is one of the most prevalent diseases of early childhood. The highest incidence is in children 6 months to 2 years of age with a gradual decline with age and a second rise in incidence at age 5 to 6. It is rarely seen after age 7. It is typically seen in the winter and early spring.

Pathophysiology

Microorganisms migrate from the nasopharynx via the eustachian tube to the lining of the middle ear, where an inflammatory reaction is set up with edema and hyperemia, retraction of the tympanic membrane, and serous exudation. If a bacterial superinfection develops, the exudate becomes pus-filled, causing the tympanic membrane to bulge.

Risk Factors

Familial tendencies
Congenital craniofacial abnormalities (cleft palate)
Native American and Eskimo populations
Passive exposure to tobacco smoke
Blocked eustachian tubes
Day care attendance

Clinical Manifestations

The first manifestation is a severe, resistant earache marked by an erythematous tympanic membrane. Fever, nausea, vomiting, and diarrhea may be present. Hearing loss and fullness in the ears are common.

Complications

Perforation of the eardrum, acute mastoiditis, petrositis, labyrinthitis, facial paralysis, epidural abscess, meningitis, brain abscess, sinus thrombosis, hydrocephalus, and subdural empyema are all possible complications.

Diagnostic Tests

Diagnosis is made by clinical evaluation and confirmed with tympanometry. If pus is present, it may be cultured for the causative organism.

Therapeutic Management

Surgery	Myringotomy to drain pus or fluid from the middle ear if the tympanic membrane is bulging; tympanotomy ventilating tubes to create artificial eustachian tube in exudative otitis media
Medications	Antiinfective drugs to combat pathogens and infection recommended only if child has had more than three infections in a year, or there is a positive respiratory culture, or the child is at high risk for bacterial infection (e.g., immunosuppression, cystic fibrosis (CF), sickle cell disease, attendance at day care, living with smoker); analgesics and antipyretics for pain and fever, antihistamines in allergic individuals to improve eustachian tube function, bronchodilators for adults
General	Autoinflation techniques taught to children to prevent surgical placement of tubes; hearing evaluation; ear kept clean and dry after surgery with use of precautions when bathing to prevent getting water in the ear; humidifier, hydration, heat/cold application to ear to reduce pain
Prevention/ Promotion	Avoidance of tobacco smoke Holding infant upright while feeding Avoidance of known allergens Pneumococcal vaccinations for children age 2 to 6
Education	Instruction on taking antibiotics; precautions with PE tubes

Ovarian Cancer

Seventy-five percent of ovarian carcinomas are epithelial in origin; these include serous cystadenocarcinoma and mucinous, endometrioid, and clear cell tumors. Germ cell tumors make up fewer than 5% of all cancerous ovarian tumors, but in women under 20 years of age, they account for 65% of diagnosed ovarian cancers.

Etiology and Incidence

The cause has not been established, but an increasing incidence among nulliparous women suggests that uninterrupted ovulation and abnormal endocrine activity are predisposing factors. Ovarian cancer accounts for nearly 4% of all cancers among women. There are more than 25,000 cases diagnosed annually and the death rate is more than 14,000. Ovarian cancer is most common in Western industrialized nations among older white women of Northern European descent. Peak incidence is from age 60 to 65.

Pathophysiology

Ovarian cancer begins in the various tissues of the ovary and then spreads by direct extension and lymphatics to the regional nodes in the pelvis and paraaortic region and to the abdominal and pelvic peritoneum. Metastasis is commonly to the liver and lungs.

Risk Factors

Nulliparity (risk is decreased by 5-year or greater history of use of oral contraceptives)
Infertility
Delayed menopause
Family history of the disease (presence of *BCRA* gene mutations)
History of breast or uterine cancer
High-fat, low fiber, vitamin A–deficient diet
Occupational exposure to asbestos and talc

Clinical Manifestations

Symptoms of early disease are often absent or mild and associated with other common problems. They include such things as vague abdominal discomfort, dyspepsia, bloating, flatulence, and digestive disturbances. Later stage signs and symptoms include ascites, abdominal and pelvic pain, abdominal and pelvic masses, persistent gastrointestinal (GI) symptoms, urinary complaints, and menstrual irregularities.

Complications

The prognosis is good with diagnosis at an early stage, with a 5-year survival rate of 95%. However, because early ovarian cancer is typically asymptomatic, the chances of prompt diagnosis are slim. Five-year survival rates with regional disease are 81% and with distant disease are 31%. Complications include intestinal obstruction, ascites, and cachexia.

Diagnostic Tests

An enlarged ovary on manual examination is often the first diagnostic sign. A transvaginal ultrasound may be used to confirm the presence of a tumor. A definitive diagnosis is made by biopsy through laparoscopy or laparotomy. Serum tumor markers include CA-125, alpha-fetoprotein, beta-human chorionic gonadotropin, and lactate dehydrogenase (LDH).

Therapeutic Management

Surgery	Salpingo-oophorectomy with or without hysterectomy is the primary treatment.
Medications	Systemic chemotherapy as adjuvant to surgery; replacement estrogen therapy and calcium supplements after removal of both ovaries
General	Radiation therapy as adjuvant to surgery
Prevention/	Annual bimanual pelvic exams
Promotion	Annual serum CA-125 and transvaginal ultrasound in high risk women
Education	Education about effects, side effects of chemotherapy and radiation; information about resources and support services for cancer survivors

Ovarian Cysts

Fluid- or semifluid-filled sacs on the ovary that may be classified as functional, inflammatory, endometrial, inclusion, and parovarian

Etiology and Incidence

Etiology is largely unknown but may be associated with hormonal changes, infection, and endometriosis. While an ovarian cyst may occur at any time, they most often form from puberty to menopause. Most ovarian cysts are small and disappear within a few months. Only a few cysts require surgical removal. Infrequently, ovarian cysts may be related to a malignancy. These are most prevalent in perimenopausal and post-menopausal women.

Pathophysiology

Functional cysts related to the process of ovulation often appear and disappear spontaneously within a couple of months from development. *Inflammatory cysts* may form after an acute infection, such as a sexually transmitted disease (STD). *Endometrial cysts* probably occur secondary to endometriosis. The cysts may vary in size from very small to 3 to 4 inches in diameter. *Germinal inclusion cysts* of the ovary result from infolding of the surface epithelium after ovulation. *Parovarian cysts* are found in young females and are clear-filled cystic structures within the broad ligament arising from the paroophoron and epoophoron, which are both mesonephric remnants.

Risk Factors

Pelvic infection or STD
Cigarette smoking increases risk twofold for functional cysts
Menstruating women
Endometriosis

Clinical Manifestations

Most ovarian cysts are asymptomatic. Abdominal discomfort and bloating, dull ache, local pain and tenderness, pressure on bladder or bowel, hypermenorrhea may be present.

Complications

Rupture of cyst may lead to peritonitis; torsion may cause severe pain and tissue necrosis.

Diagnostic Tests

Pelvic and Rectal Examination	To determine location and size of cyst
Ultrasonography	To confirm presence and size of cyst and to distinguish functional cysts from neoplasms
Laparoscopy	Used infrequently to determine presence of endometriosis and to examine cyst

Therapeutic Management

Surgery	If necessary (e.g., large cysts, cysts that do not resolve, torsion or rupture, cysts with worrisome ultrasound features), laparoscopy, cystectomy or laparotomy to drain and/or remove cyst and to rule out malignancy
Medications	Analgesics for discomfort, antiinfectives for rupture
General	Pelvic examinations to monitor cyst size and position
	Watchful waiting for reabsorption of cysts less than 10 cm in diameter
	Exercise and positioning to decrease discomfort
	Emotional support during diagnostic process
Prevention/ Promotion	Oral contraceptives for suppression
Education	Information about cysts versus ovarian cancer
	Preoperative and postoperative instructions
	Information on available patient resources from organizations such as American Acadamy of Family Physicians (AAFP) and American College of Obstetricians and Gynecologists (ACOG)

O

Paget's Disease (Osteitis Deformans)

Chronic inflammatory disease of the bones that results in thickening, softening, and eventual bowing

Etiology and Incidence

The cause is unknown, although a familial pattern has been noted and a viral link is suspected. Paget's disease occurs worldwide but is more common in Europe, Australia, and New Zealand. Paget's disease has been diagnosed in about 2.5 million persons in the United States. Men are more likely to be affected, as are individuals over age 40.

Pathophysiology

The disease begins with an initial phase of excessive bone resorption followed by a reactive phase of excessive and abnormal bone formation. The result is large, multinucleated osteoblasts; thickened lamellae and trabeculae; and fibrotic tissue, which produces enlarged, weakened, and heavily calcified bone.

Risk Factors

Familial tendencies

Clinical Manifestations

Early disease is asymptomatic, with an insidious onset of aching, deep pain, stiffness, fatigue, headaches, and decreased hearing. Later signs include bowing and other bone deformities, such as an increasing skull size. Fractures occur with minor trauma.

Complications

Complications include vertebral collapse and resulting paralysis; blindness, deafness, or vertigo from impingement on cranial nerves; vascular collapse from increased cardiac demands; gout; renal calculi, osteosarcoma, and fibrosarcoma.

Diagnostic Tests

The diagnosis is often incidental to examinations done for other reasons.

X-rays	Show increased bone density, abnormal architecture, cortical thickening, bowing, and bony overgrowth
Serum Alkaline Phosphatase	Level markedly elevated in advanced disease
Radionuclide Bone Scans	Increased nuclide uptake at bone lesion sites

Therapeutic Management

Surgery	Hip and knee replacement; spinal decompression; fracture reduction
Medications	Nonsteroidal antiinflammatory drugs (NSAIDs) for pain; chemotherapy to suppress bone cell activity before surgery or to prevent complications in poor surgical candidates; bisphosphonates or calcitonin to inhibit bone resorption and manage disease; calcium and vitamin D supplements
General	Orthoses (cane, quad cane, walker) for gait correction; firm mattress, corset, or brace for back pain; balance of exercise and rest; balanced diet; reduce heavy lifting and twisting body motions; physical therapy and exercise program to increase strength; referral to support groups
Prevention/ Promotion	Fall and fracture precautions
Education	Education about disease, medication effects and side effects; instruction about fall precautions, correct use of gait orthosis, proper body mechanics

P

Pancreatic Cancer

Tumors arise from exocrine glands (95%) and endocrine glands (5%) in the pancreas. Ductal adenocarcinomas constitute 90% of all pancreatic tumors. Other histological types include squamous cell and giant cell carcinomas, sarcomas, plasmacytomas, and lymphomas.

Etiology and Incidence

Cigarette smoking is strongly linked to the development of cancer of the pancreas though the precise cause is unknown. Nearly 31,000 cases of pancreatic cancer are diagnosed each year in the United States, and more than 30,000 persons die annually. The peak incidence is in the seventh and eighth decades of life.

Pathophysiology

Most tumors begin in the head of the exocrine gland, obstruct the bile duct, and extend to the duodenum, intestines, and spine. Spread occurs to the regional lymph nodes, and common metastatic sites include the liver and lungs.

Risk Factors

Smoking
Diet rich in animal fat
Alcohol abuse
Occupational exposure to solvents and petrochemicals
History of chronic pancreatitis, diabetes mellitus (DM), gallstones

Clinical Manifestations

Symptoms occur late in the disease and include anorexia; weight loss; flatulence; bloating; constipation; upper abdominal pain, which radiates to the back and abates in a fetal position; jaundice; and thrombophlebitis.

Complications

The prognosis is extremely poor, with a 4%, 5-year survival rate. Complications include DM and alterations in mental status.

Diagnostic Tests

Ultrasound, CT scans, and endoscopic retrograde pancreatography are used to locate masses and to assist in staging of the tumor. The definitive diagnosis is made by needle or tissue biopsy.

Therapeutic Management

Surgery	Pancreatectomy or Whipple procedure; bypass of obstructions for palliation
Medications	Chemotherapy has not been effective to date, although several combination drugs are under study; insulin after removal or resection of pancreas; analgesics for pain
General	Radiation limits tumor progression and provides pain relief but does little for the survival rate. Use of hospice care and/or support groups is beneficial.
Prevention/ Promotion	Smoking cessation
	Moderate alcohol intake
	Decrease animal fat in diet
	Limit occupational exposure to solvents and petrochemicals
Education	Education about disease and treatment options; instruction on eliminating alcohol, smoking, caffeine, fat restrictions; instruction about DM if pancreas removed or resected; information about support groups

P

Pancreatitis

Acute or chronic inflammation of the pancreas

Etiology and Incidence

The most common causes of acute pancreatitis are heavy alcohol consumption and biliary tract disease. Other causes include infections (e.g., mumps, hepatitis); drugs (thiazides, steroids, azathioprine, pentamidine); vasculitis; and surgery on pancreas, stomach, or biliary tract. The most common cause of chronic pancreatitis is alcoholism. Other causes are hyperparathyroidism, stenosis of the pancreatic duct, and carcinoma. The incidence varies with location and is high where the incidence of alcoholism is high. In tropical countries, such as India, Indonesia, and Nigeria, a form of idiopathic pancreatitis occurs in children and young adults. There are more than 80,000 cases of acute pancreatitis diagnosed annually in the United States.

Pathophysiology

Acute pancreatitis is a result of autodigestion in which normally excreted pancreatic enzymes digest pancreatic tissue. Bile and phospholipase A combine to cause severe tissue necrosis. Elastase dissolves elastic fibers in the blood vessels and causes hemorrhage. Release of kinins causes vasodilation, vascular permeability, and pulmonary edema. Hypercalcemia and transient hyperglycemia develop. Chronic pancreatitis results from repeated acute episodes or from a slow sclerosing process, resulting in fibrosis and obstruction of the pancreatic ducts.

Risk Factors

Alcohol abuse
Biliary tract disease
Infections (mumps, hepatitis)
Abdominal trauma/surgery
Underlying disease (duodenal ulcer, cystic fibrosis (CF), hyperparathyroidism, renal failure)
Drug side effects (e.g., steroids, sulfonamides, nonsteroidal antiinflammatory drugs (NSAIDs), thiazides, tetracycline, angiotensin-converting enzyme (ACE) inhibitors)

Occupational exposure to chemicals (e.g., methanol, cobalt, zinc, creosol, lead, organophosphates, naphthalenes)
Severe malnutrition

Clinical Manifestations

Acute	Severe abdominal pain radiating to the back; fever, sweating, rapid pulse, shallow respirations, and decreased breath sounds; decreased blood pressure (BP); blunted sensorium
Chronic	Intermittent or chronic dull, boring abdominal pain relieved somewhat by sitting and leaning forward; weight loss, steatorrhea, diarrhea, nausea, vomiting

Complications

Adult respiratory distress syndrome (ARDS); disseminated intravascular coagulation (DIC); cardiac, renal, or pulmonary failure; infected necrosis of the pancreas and pancreatic pseudo-cyst, leading to hemorrhage and rupture of the pancreas, are all possible complications that often lead to death.

Diagnostic Tests

Acute	Elevated amylase 2 to 12 hours after onset, dropping to normal within 72 hours; elevated lipase, WBCs, glucose, and serum bilirubin levels; CT scan to determine extent and severity
Chronic	Pancreatic calcification, enlarged ducts, or abnormal size and consistency of pancreas on CT scan or ultrasound; endoscopic retrograde cholangiopancreatography to evaluate presence of dilated ducts, strictures, pseudocysts, and intraductal stones; secretin test with normal volume and low bicarbonate

P

Therapeutic Management

Surgery	*Acute:* Débridement of tissue in necrotizing pancreatitis, drainage of pancreatic pseudocyst or abscesses, removal of stones obstructing the common bile duct
	Chronic: Pancreaticojejunostomy, pancreatectomy, Whipple procedure, autotransplantation for severe intractable pain and complications
Medications	*Acute:* Narcotic analgesics for pain, antacids by nasogastric tube, histamine receptor antagonists for gastrointestinal (GI) bleeding, antiinfective drugs for abscesses, adrenergics for hypotension
	Chronic: Analgesics for pain, pancreatic enzyme supplements to treat steatorrhea; antacids, histamine receptor antagonists to improve effects of enzyme supplements; insulin or oral hypoglycemic therapy if indicated; glucocorticoids in sclerosing pancreatitis to induce remission
General	*Acute:* Endoscopic sphincterotomy for biliary pancreatitis; hemodynamic monitoring; central venous pressure (CVP) catheter; nasogastric tube; peritoneal lavage; correction of electrolyte imbalances; total parenteral nutrition; discontinue alcohol or drug use; nothing by mouth (NPO) to rest GI tract and diminish pancreatic activity, then low-fat, high-carbohydrate diet
	Chronic: Enteral nutritional support if indicated; discontinue use of alcohol with alcohol rehabilitation program
Prevention/ Promotion	Moderate alcohol intake
	Balanced diet low in animal fat
	Reduce occupational exposure to known etiological chemical agents
	Watch for side effects with medications known to cause pancreatitis

Education   *Acute:* Instruction on diet modifications (no
             alcohol or caffeine, restricted fats, increase
             in carbohydrates); avoidance of rapid weight
             loss; education about manifestations of
             recurrence

             Chronic: Instruction on dietary control (no
             alcohol or caffeine, frequent low-volume
             meals, restrict fat); education about
             pancreatic enzyme supplements and antacid
             use; education about diabetes mellitus (DM)
             and its control

P

Parkinson's Disease

A slowly progressive, degenerative neurological disorder, characterized by slow, impoverished movement; muscle rigidity; resting tremor; and postural instability. It occurs in primary and secondary forms.

Etiology and Incidence

The exact cause of Parkinson's is not known although one form of primary Parkinson's has been linked to a genetic defect on the parkin gene for the alpha-synuclein protein. Individuals with this form of Parkinson's comprise less than 10% of known cases, and onset is generally early (before age 50). Secondary Parkinson's has been linked to a number of factors including drugs (phenothiazides and butyrophenones); toxins (carbon monoxide, carbon disulfide, manganese, and MPTP [a byproduct of heroin synthesis]); cerebrovascular disease; hypoparathyroidism or hyperparathyroidism; and encephalitis. Parkinsonism is the fourth most common neurodegenerative disease of the elderly. It affects about 3% of those over age 65 in the United States, and an estimated 40,000 to 50,000 new cases are diagnosed each year. Men and women are equally affected. The mean age of onset is 57, and peak onset is in the seventh decade.

Pathophysiology

Some agent or event triggers a degeneration and loss of pigmented neurons in the substantia nigra, locus ceruleus, and other brainstem dopaminergic cell groups. The loss of these neurons leads to a depletion in neurotransmitter dopamine and interferes with the motor production of the basal ganglia. Interneuronal inclusion bodies (Lewy bodies) are left in surviving pigmented neurons and serve as biological markers of the disease. Clinical manifestations emerge only after 75% to 80% of the dopamine innervation has been destroyed.

Risk Factors

Presence of parkin gene mutation in familial Parkinson's

Exposure to toxins (MPTP, carbon monoxide, carbon disulfide, manganese)

Drug side effects (phenothiazides, butyrophenones, neuroleptics, select antiemetics, nonselective monoamine oxidase (MAO) inhibitors, reserpine)

Underlying disease (cerebrovascular, hypoparathyroidism or hyperparathyroidism, encephalitis)

Clinical Manifestations

Early	Infrequent blinking; lack of facial expression; deliberateness of speech; impaired postural reflexes, particularly in the arm; resting pill-rolling tremor of one hand that is absent during sleep
Midcourse	Progressive rigidity, slowness, and poverty of movement, and difficulty initiating movement; muscle aches and fatigue; masklike, open-mouthed facial expression; stooped posture; gait begins slow and shuffling and quickens to a run with a forward lean; hypophonic speech with stuttering dysarthria; drooling; dysphagia; forgetfulness; resting tremors of lips, jaw, tongue, and limbs; depression
Late	Severe postural instability, urinary retention, orthostatic hypotension, paranoia with visual hallucinations, delirium, dementia

Complications

Injury from falls is a common threat. Other complications include aspiration pneumonia, drug reactions, and disuse syndrome.

Diagnostic Tests

The diagnosis is based primarily on the pattern of clinical manifestations and must be distinguished from individuals with essential tremor in which the tremor is action related and without facial or gait involvement.

Therapeutic Management

Surgery	Stereotactic thalamotomy, bilateral posteroventral pallidotomy, deep brain stimulation to alleviate tremors and rigidity in drug-resistant individuals; human embryonic dopamine neuron transplants in younger patients with severe symptoms
Medications	Antiparkinsonian agents—such as levodopa, carbidopa/levodopa (Sinemet), or dopamine receptor agonists (ropinirole, pergolide, bromocriptine), or amantadine to reduce bradykinesia, tremor, and rigidity; antihistamines (diphenhydramine, orphenadrine) and anticholinergics (trihexyphenidyl, benztropine mesylate) to extend the effects of levodopa and inhibit drooling; antidepressants for depression.
General	Treatment of underlying cause in secondary Parkinson's; long-term physical therapy to maintain muscle tone, function, and range of motion (ROM), gait and transfer training; occupational therapy to maintain activities of daily living (ADLs) and teach safety skills; speech therapy to evaluate and improve swallowing abilities, reduce dysarthria, and strengthen facial muscles; warm baths and massage to relax muscles; consistent weight-bearing exercise program; assistive devices (canes, walkers, wheelchairs, electric lift chairs, grab bars, raised toilet seats, bath seats, eating, and hygiene devices); counseling for depression and long-term adaptation; measures to prevent skin breakdown, urinary tract infections (UTIs), falls, and corneal abrasions; deep breathing to maintain vital capacity; balanced, low-protein diet; bowel and bladder programs; home care assistance; respite care for caregiver

Prevention/ Promotion	Avoidance of medications that induce or worsen disease (phenothiazides, butyrophenones, neuroleptics, select antiemetics, nonselective MAO inhibitors, reserpine); use of anticholinergics with neuroleptics to prevent Parkinson's
	Reduce exposure to toxins (MPTP, carbon monoxide, carbon disulfide, manganese)
Education	Education about chronic progressive nature of disease; instruction on prevention of falls, corneal abrasions, UTIs; information about availability and use of assistive devices; instruction about diet, exercise, deep breathing, bowel and bladder routines; information about available support resources, such as National Parkinson Foundation and respite care services

P

Pediculosis (Lice)

Infestation by lice of the head, body, or pubic areas

Etiology and Incidence

Two species of lice cause pediculosis. *Pediculus humanus* affects the head and body, and *Phthirus pubis* infects the pubic area, eyebrows, eyelashes, and axillae. In pediculosis capitis (head lice), the lice on the scalp are transmitted by personal contact and through objects such as combs and brushes. In pediculosis corporis (body lice), the lice live in unclean underclothing and periodically feed on the skin. In pediculosis pubis (pubic lice), the lice live at the base of curly hairs, chiefly in the genital region, and are transmitted primarily by sexual contact or very close personal contact. The presence of *Phthirus pubis* in the eyebrows or eyelashes of young children generally indicates sexual abuse. Body lice infestation is widespread in areas with crowded, unsanitary living conditions. There are somewhere between 6 million and 12 million cases of head lice annually and infestation is common in day care centers, schools, and other places with large numbers of children who share personal items.

Pathophysiology

The lice bite the skin and inject saliva during feeding, causing severe pruritus. Scratching causes excoriation and secondary infection. Each day, female lice lay eggs (nits), which cement themselves to the base of the hair shaft in the head or pubic area. These eggs hatch in 8 days.

Clinical Manifestations

Itching, excoriation, and secondary infection of bite lesions are common signs. Grayish-white nits may also be observed at the base of hair shafts, as can the lice themselves.

Complications

Furunculosis is an occasional complication. The lice also serve as vectors for organisms that cause typhus, trench fever, and relapsing fever.

Diagnostic Tests

A physical examination revealing nits or lice. The examination may be enhanced using fluorescent light and microscopic examination of hair shafts.

Therapeutic Management

Surgery	None
Medications	Antiinfective shampoos, creams, lotions, and ophthalmic solutions to kill lice and nits; must be used again about 8 to 10 days after initial treatment to kill remaining hatching nits
General	Nit combs to comb out nits from hair shafts; elimination of body lice from clothing and bedding by washing, boiling, and steaming; elimination of lice from combs and brushes by boiling; vacuuming of carpets and upholstered furniture; cutting fingernails short and using gloves to prevent damage by scratching; notification of recent (within last month) sexual partners about pubic lice; follow-up with social services for children with infestation of *Phthirus pubis*
Prevention/ Promotion	Institute sanitary conditions to prevent body lice; encourage children not to share combs, brushes, caps, scarves, and other articles of clothing to prevent head lice; encourage school and community prevention and early detection programs for head lice
Education	Education about importance of follow-up to initial drug treatment; instruction on elimination of lice and nits; education that head lice do not indicate poor hygiene

P

Pelvic Inflammatory Disease (PID)

Infection of the fallopian tubes, which may extend to the ovaries, pelvic peritoneum, or uterine connective tissue

Etiology and Incidence

PID is caused by a pathogen, the most common of which is *Chlamydia trachomatis*. The pathogen is usually transmitted during intercourse but may also be introduced during abortion and childbirth. Women with intrauterine devices (IUDs) are at greater risk, as are sexually active women with multiple partners. Adolescent and young adult women are most often affected. As many as 1 million women are suspected of being infected annually.

Pathophysiology

The infection typically begins intravaginally and spreads upward through the entire genital tract to the fallopian tubes. The infection, which may be unilateral or bilateral, produces a profuse exudate in the tubes that leads to agglutination of the mucosal folds, adhesions, and tubal occlusion. Peritonitis from spreading exudate is common, and the ovaries may also be invaded.

Risk Factors

Unprotected sex
Multiple sex partners
Sexual contact with urethritis or gonorrhea
Previous history of PID
Frequent vaginal douching
Infection after abortion, childbirth, insertion of IUD, uterine
    biopsy, or pelvic surgery
History of immunological or renal disorders

Clinical Manifestations

PID may be either acute or chronic.

Acute	Onset typically occurs after onset of menses
	Progressive lower abdominal pain with guarding and rebound tenderness, fever, copious purulent cervical discharge, nausea

and vomiting, malaise; urinary urgency and frequency, vaginal itching and maceration

Chronic   Chronic pain, menstrual irregularities, recurrence and exacerbation of acute symptoms

Complications

Common complications include generalized peritonitis, sterility, and ectopic pregnancy.

Diagnostic Tests

Clinical manifestations, coupled with elevated WBCs and erythrocyte sedimentation rate plus a positive culture of secretions, are diagnostic. On pelvic examination, moving of the cervix causes severe pain and rebound tenderness that is present in abdomen. Transvaginal ultrasound may show thickened fluid-filled fallopian tubes or adnexal mass. MRI for evidence of pelvic abnormalities; laparoscopy may be used as a differential diagnostic tool.

Therapeutic Management

Surgery	Laparoscopy to drain antibiotic-resistant abscesses; salpingolysis to remove adhesions; salpingostomy to reopen blocked fallopian tube; salpingo-oophorectomy for ruptured tube or ectopic pregnancy; in vitro fertilization for sterility
Medications	Antiinfective drugs, usually in combinations to control and alleviate infection
General	Bed rest in semi-Fowler's position, adequate hydration, removal of IUDs, tracking and treatment of sexual partners, sexual abstinence, and avoidance of tampons and douching during treatment
Prevention/ Promotion	Safe sexual practices; avoidance of multiple sexual encounters
	Early recognition and treatment of vaginal and/or cervical infection
Education	Instruction about sexually transmitted diseases (STDs) and safer sexual practices

P

Peptic Ulcer Disease (Gastric or Duodenal Ulcers)

A circumscribed excavation of the gastric or duodenal mucosal wall that penetrates the muscularis mucosae and exposes it to acid and pepsin

Etiology and Incidence

Infection by *Helicobacter pylori* bacteria is the major etiological factor in ulcer formation. Use of nonsteroidal antiinflammatory agents (NSAIDs) has been implicated. There continue to be a minority of individuals that have no apparent demonstrable cause. About 80% of all peptic ulcers are duodenal in origin, and the remaining 20% are gastric. Gastric ulcers strike men and women equally, with the peak incidence occurring between ages 55 and 65. Duodenal ulcers occur in men two to three times as often as in women, and the incidence increases with age. There are an estimated 500,000 new cases and close to 4 million recurrences of peptic ulcers annually in the United States.

Pathophysiology

Peptic ulceration occurs when *H. pylori*, NSAIDs, or other causative factors—in concert with certain predisposing factors—upset the balance between ulcer-promoting factors, (e.g., secretion of acid and pepsin) and epithelial defense mechanisms (e.g., mucus and bicarbonate production and replacement of damaged mucosal cells). This sets up an inflammatory process with resultant ulceration, thrombosis, fibrosis, and scarring of the muscularis mucosa layer of the stomach or duodenum.

Risk Factors

H. pylori infection
Use of NSAIDs, acetaminophen, other antiinflammatory drugs
Smoking
Familial history
Stress
Age 50 or older

Underlying disease processes, such as pancreatitis, gastritis, alcoholic cirrhosis, and hepatic disorders

Clinical Manifestations

Manifestations vary with location, and ulcers are often asymptomatic or associated with vague symptoms. Only about 50% of individuals have a characteristic pattern of symptoms. The characteristic pain is described as burning, gnawing, or aching and is located in a well-circumscribed epigastric area. In duodenal ulcers the pain usually appears midmorning, is relieved by food, and then reappears 2 to 3 hours after eating. It also wakens the individual 2 to 3 hours after falling asleep. It occurs daily for 1 week or longer and may then disappear without treatment. With a gastric ulcer, the pain usually occurs after eating food, is located in the left midgastric area, and often radiates to the back. Epigastric pain occurs with an empty stomach. Pain in both instances is typically relieved by antacids or milk. ◑ Sudden sharp unremitting stomach pain, black tarry stools, coffee-ground emesis or bloody vomitus, and/or rigid abdomen are indicators of probable perforation and hemorrhage and necessitate emergency care.

Complications

Complications include ◑ hemorrhage and perforation of the stomach or duodenum, with resulting peritonitis and obstruction of the pylorus or gastric outlet.

Diagnostic Tests

Endoscopy/ Biopsy	To establish presence of ulcer, obtain specimens for *H. pylori* testing, and determine whether malignancy is present
Upper GI Series	May show ulcers overlooked on endoscopy
Gastric Analysis	Increased output with duodenal ulcer; decreased or normal output with gastric ulcer
Carbon-13 Urea Breath Test	Low levels of 13C in exhaled breath indicative of *H. pylori* infection

P

Therapeutic Management

Surgery	Surgery is rarely performed; options include ulcer removal with antrectomy or hemigastrectomy in intractable cases, or for gastric ulcers with complications; fundic vagotomy with chronic duodenal ulcer disease
Medications	Proton pump inhibitors or bismuth compounds in combination with antiinfective drugs or triple combination antibiotics for eradication of *H. pylori* bacteria
	Histamine receptor antagonists to block gastric acid output; antacids to reduce pain; cytoprotectives (sucralfate) to form a protective coating in the base of the ulcer; proton pump inhibitors (omeprazole, pantoprazole) to inhibit gastric secretion
	Prostaglandins in clinical trials for treatment associated with NSAID use
General	Acute in hospital treatment: Rest, nothing by mouth (NPO), nasogastric (NG) tube, fluid replacement, blood if necessary for 24 to 48 hours; progressive, individual diet
	Avoidance of NSAIDs and cigarettes and any other food or fluid substances that aggravate pain; stress reduction therapy; repeat endoscopy after 4 to 6 weeks of treatment to affirm healing for those with gastric ulcer
Prevention/ Promotion	Avoidance of NSAIDs and cigarettes and any other food or fluid substances that may trigger or aggravate recurrence
	Misoprostol or proton pump inhibitor prophylaxis for individuals on long-term NSAID therapy
	Screening for gastric cancer and/or Zollinger-Ellison syndrome (ZES) in those with recurrent disease

	Maintenance drug (proton pump inhibitor, histamine receptor antagonists, cytoprotectives, antacids) therapy for those with recurrent ulcer
Education	Education about possible recurrence, importance of completing all drug therapy; importance of follow-up to determine treatment effectiveness

Pericarditis

A chronic or acute inflammation of the parietal and visceral layers of the pericardium and outer myocardium

Etiology and Incidence

Pericarditis is most commonly idiopathic in origin but may result from viral, bacterial, fungal, or parasitic pathogens from infectious diseases (acquired immunodeficiency syndrome [AIDS], tuberculosis [TB], influenza, histoplasmosis); underlying connective tissue disorders (systemic lupus erythematosus [SLE], rheumatoid arthritis, rheumatic fever, scleroderma, periarteritis); neoplastic disease (breast cancer, lymphoma, bronchogenic cancer); metabolic disease (renal failure, myxedema); postmyocardial infarction; trauma to the chest cavity; chest surgery or hemodialysis; drugs (procainamide or phenytoin); and irradiation. Pericarditis occurs in 2% to 6% of the population in the United States. All age groups, races, and both genders are vulnerable. Pericarditis is the most common manifestation in those with AIDS.

Pathophysiology

Inflammation of the pericardium occurs by irritation or by direct extension of another disease state. The normally clear fluid in the pericardial sac is filled with an exudate of fibrin, WBCs, and endothelial cells, which coat the parietal and visceral layers of the pericardium. Friction occurs between the layers, setting up an inflammatory process in the surrounding tissue. This process may remain localized or become widespread. Pericarditis may be fibrinous or may create a pleural effusion that is serous, sanguineous, hemorrhagic, or purulent. Chronic pericarditis leads to pericardial thickening, adhesions, and scarring, which may in time calcify, rendering the pericardium useless. This impedes the diastolic filling of the heart, reduces stroke volume, and decreases cardiac output.

Risk Factors

Any individual with one of the listed causative agents under the etiology section is at risk.

Clinical Manifestations

Acute	Retrosternal or precordial chest pain radiating to the neck and back; pleuritic pain that increases on inspiration and in a horizontal position; shallow, rapid breathing; dyspnea; dysphagia; restlessness; anxiety; fever, chills, and weakness
Chronic	Asymptomatic unless constriction is present, then symptoms appear with exertional dyspnea; paroxysmal nocturnal dyspnea; fatigue; peripheral edema; orthopnea; cough

Complications

Rapidly forming effusion interferes with cardiovascular dynamics and leads to ◑ cardiac tamponade, shock, and cardiovascular collapse if not treated immediately. Chronic disease leads to cardiac and liver failure.

Diagnostic Tests

Acute

Clinical Evaluation	History of pain; precordial friction rub
Blood	Elevated WBCs, erythrocyte sedimentation rate
Culture	Blood/urine cultures to identify organism if infectious process is involved
ECG	Early: ST-T segment elevation, PR interval depression, QRS voltage decrease
Serial Chest X-rays	Enlarging cardiac silhouette
Echocardiogram	Detect pericardial effusion

Chronic

Clinical Evaluation	Pericardial knock on auscultation
Chest X-ray	Calcifications; enlarged cardiac silhouette

P

ECG	Widened P wave in leads I, II, and V6; deep Q waves; flattened or inverted T waves
MRI	Thickened pericardium
Echocardiogram	Presence of pericardial effusion

Therapeutic Management

Surgery	Pericardiocentesis to remove fluid, pus, or blood from pericardium in acute effusive disease or tamponade; pericardiectomy to remove visceral and parietal pericardium in chronic constrictive disease
Medications	Antiinfective drugs to treat underlying infection; antiinflammatory drugs for effusion, fever, and pain; analgesics for pain; diuretics for chronic congestion *Anticoagulants contraindicated because they can cause intrapericardial bleeding and contribute to tamponade*
General	Treatment of underlying disease *Acute:* Cardiac monitoring for complications, bed rest, adequate hydration, comfort measures *Chronic:* Restricted activity, instruction about surgery
Prevention/ Promotion	Use of thrombolytic agents postmyocardial infarction
Education	Education about early manifestations of cardiac tamponade, constrictive pericarditis

Peripheral Arterial Disease (PAD)

Occlusion of the arterial blood supply to the lower extremities by atherosclerotic plaques

Etiology and Incidence

The most common cause is underlying atherosclerosis. PAD affects approximately 8 to 10 million persons in the United States.

Pathophysiology

The pathological processes involved in atherosclerosis are detailed under coronary artery disease (CAD). In PAD, an artery (aortoiliac, femoral, popliteal, or tibial) in a lower extremity is narrowed and occluded after a long-term buildup of plaque in the vessel, leading to insidious development of tissue ischemia.

Risk Factors

Cigarette smoking
History of hypertension (HTN) or diabetes mellitus (DM)
Hyperlipidemia
Elevated levels of homocysteine and fibrinogen in blood

Clinical Manifestations

The classic symptom is intermittent claudication progressing to pain at rest; decreased pulses; pallor after elevation; dry, scaly skin with sparse hair and nail growth on affected extremity; numbness and tingling; slow healing of wounds

Complications

Necrosis and gangrene, with resultant limb loss, are the most common complications.

Diagnostic Tests

Clinical evaluation, Doppler ultrasound to locate the obstruction, and angiography or magnetic resonance angiography to the define extent of disease are used for diagnosis.

Therapeutic Management

Surgery	Thromboendarterectomy or resection with or without graft to remove obstruction and make vessel patent; amputation for uncontrolled infection, necrosis, or gangrene
Medications	Antiplatelet agents (aspirin, ticlopidine, clopidogrel) for chronic disease; cilostazol for intermittent claudication; antiinfective drugs for infection; antihyperlipidemics
General	Percutaneous transluminal angioplasty to remove obstruction and placement of stents to keep artery open; progressive exercise program to develop collateral circulation; aggressive management of DM and HTN; avoidance of all tobacco products and any other known vasoconstrictors; hyperlipidemia control; careful protection of affected limb from injury and infection (inspection, cleaning, lubrication); careful monitoring of wounds, cuts and ulcers on feet or legs to prevent infection and gangrene
Prevention/ Promotion	Cessation of smoking Good management of DM and HTN Reduction or avoidance of hyperlipidemia through diet, exercise, and/or medication
Education	Education about importance of smoking cessation and careful control of blood pressure (BP) and DM; instruction about foot and skin care and skin inspections

Peripheral Vascular Disorders

A complex of vascular diseases affecting the extremities and involving the arteries, veins, and lymphatics

(See specific diseases, such as Peripheral Arterial Disease, Raynaud's Phenomenon, Thrombosis, Venous [Phlebo-thrombosis, Thrombophlebitis], and Varicose Veins)

Peritonitis

Local or general inflammation of the abdominal peritoneum

Etiology and Incidence

Peritonitis is caused by the contamination of the peritoneal cavity by bacteria or chemicals. The condition may be either primary or secondary. Primary peritonitis is a rare condition caused by acute or subacute bacterial infection of the peritoneum not associated with any underlying bowel disorder. ☻ Secondary peritonitis is the result of contamination of the peritoneum from perforation of the gastrointestinal (GI) tract. Secondary peritonitis generally occurs secondary to a perforation or rupture of one of the organs of digestion. A life-threatening irritation and/or infection of the peritoneum results. Perforated peptic ulcer, ruptured appendix, trauma, ischemic bowel disease, intestinal obstruction, pancreatitis, and perforated colon are common causes of generalized peritonitis. Secondary peritonitis is common in a number of etiological conditions.

P

Pathophysiology

The peritoneum is a semipermeable saclike closure within the abdominal cavity, enclosing the abdominal viscera and mesentery. The peritoneum also lines the abdominal wall, the undersurface of the diaphragm, and the pelvic floor. If there is a rupture of the intestinal wall, the peritoneum attempts to wall off the contamination, and a large number of polymorphonuclear leukocytes pour into the area and, through phagocytosis, remove bacteria and foreign matter. The body's generalized health and systemic tissue perfusion often determine how the body fights off the potential infection. Often the contamination body insult is significant, and the body is unable to cope. Vascular dilation, hyperemia, and fluid shifts occur. The rate of fluid shift is proportional to the degree of peritoneal insult and the success of the body's peritoneal defense mechanism.

Risk Factors

Underlying disease (e.g., peptic ulcer, ischemic bowel disease, pancreatitis, cirrhosis)
Ruptured appendix
Intestinal obstruction and/or decreased tissue perfusion
Abdominal trauma, either blunt or penetrating
Recent abdominal surgery
Elderly state
Corticosteroids
Peritoneal dialysis

Clinical Manifestations

History	Sudden onset of severe abdominal pain that worsens with movement or coughing; nausea and vomiting
Clinical Evaluation Bowel Sounds Systemic	Guarding and report of generalized and rebound tenderness during abdominal palpation; abdominal distention; decreased or absent bowel sounds; rapid, weak, thready pulse; decreased blood pressure (BP); tachypnea; decreased urinary output; fever; appears ill

Complications

Complications are more likely in the elderly, those with poor tissue perfusion, and those with abdominal cavity contamination. Complications include hypovolemia, septicemia, septic shock, acute renal failure (ARF), acute respiratory difficulties, and liver failure and abscess formations. ◑ Untreated peritonitis leads to death.

Diagnostic Tests

Laboratory Tests	CBC with differential shows increased leukocytes; hemoconcentration; metabolic acidosis; respiratory alkalosis

X-rays	Abdominal x-ray to determine gas and fluid collection in large and small bowel; free gas in the abdominal cavity; bowel walls may appear thick
Peritoneal Aspiration	To determine organism; aspirate appears cloudy, blood-tinged, may contain fecal material

Therapeutic Management

Surgery	Indicated to treat the primary cause of the peritonitis and to prevent further peritoneal infection
Medications	Antibiotics to treat multiple bacterial flora contaminating the peritoneal cavity; analgesics to control pain
General	Immediate hospitalization; nasogastric suctioning for decompression; aggressive intervention with IV fluids, electrolytes, and colloid solutions to correct hypovolemia; cardiopulmonary monitoring with assist if necessary; nothing by mouth (NPO) until bowel sounds return; total parenteral nutrition (TPN) if indicated; blood transfusions if necessary to correct anemia; oxygen; bed rest
Prevention/ Promotion	Antibiotic prophylaxis when undergoing abdominal surgery
Education	Routine preoperative and postoperative instruction

P

Personality Disorders

A group of clustered disorders that are characterized by long-standing, rigid, and pervasive maladaptive personality traits that result in emotional distress and impaired interpersonal and/or vocational function. *Cluster A* is the odd and/or eccentric and includes paranoid, schizoid, and schizotypal personalities. *Cluster B* is the dramatic and/or errant and includes borderline, antisocial, narcissistic, and histrionic personalities. *Cluster C* is the anxious and/or inhibited and includes obsessive-compulsive, avoidant, and dependent personalities.

Etiology and Incidence

There is no clearly defined cause for these personality disorders, but research supports multifactorial origins with the interaction of genetic, neurobiological, early developmental, and sociocultural factors. Ten percent to 13% of the population in the United States is thought to have personality disorders, with dependent, borderline, and schizotypal disorders being the most prevalent. Prevalence rate is considerably higher in the clinical psychiatric population and ranges from 20% to 40% in outpatient populations and 30% to 60% in inpatient populations. Many individuals have more than one personality disorder. These disorders are usually manifested in early adulthood and persist throughout life.

Pathophysiology

There appear to be structural deficits and impaired neurophysiological pathways of the brain with multiple triggers that precipitate manifestations of the disorders, but precise mechanisms are not known.

Risk Factors

Familial tendencies
Childhood abuse and/or neglect
Involuntary social isolation

Clinical Manifestations

Cluster A

General mistrust and misinterpretation of actions of others; odd beliefs and tendency toward social isolation

Paranoid	Cold, distant, distrustful, suspicious, controlling, jealous, projection of malevolent motives onto others, unwillingness to forgive, short-tempered
Schizoid	Introverted, withdrawn, solitary, emotionally cold, detached, self-absorbed, lacking in strong emotions
Schizotypal	Manifestations of schizoid plus magical thinking, clairvoyance, preoccupation with the paranormal, inappropriate affect, and anxiety in social settings

Cluster B

Generally labile, unpredictable, impulsive, and unlikeable

Antisocial	Callous disregard for rights/feelings of others, exploitation of others for personal gain/satisfaction; lack of guilt, cold, manipulative, blaming, lack of empathy, irritable, hostile, impulsive, irresponsible, low frustration tolerance, dishonest, deceitful, frequent involvement in illegal activities/substance abuse
Borderline	Unstable mood, behavior, and self-image; impulsivity (binging, spending sprees, reckless behavior) self-mutilative/suicidal ideations; negative affect; fears of abandonment; intense stormy relationships; others classified as good/bad dichotomy
Histrionic	Conspicuous attention seeking; dramatic; conscious of appearance; exaggerated, superficial emotions; sexually seductive; superficial, transient relations
Narcissistic	Grandiose; feelings of superiority; need to be admired; sensitive to criticism; preoccupation with fantasies about success or beauty; lack of empathy; impatience

P

Cluster C
Generally anxious, timid, perfectionistic, and conflict avoidant

Avoidant	Hypersensitive to criticism, disapproval, or rejection; fear of starting anything new; avoids social interaction; withholds thoughts and/or feelings; openly distressed at self-imposed isolation and inability to relate
Dependent	Surrender self-responsibility; submissive; clingy; inability to make independent decisions; difficulty following through; inability to express negative emotions
Obsessive-Compulsive	Conscientious, orderly, reliable; rigid, inflexible; preoccupation with perfection, organization, and control; reluctance to delegate; pack-rat tendencies; difficulties in decision making; difficulty completing tasks; highly rule-conscious and unforgiving of own mistakes

Complications

There is a high likelihood that the individual will have a comorbid psychiatric illness. Disorders are strongly resistant to treatment.

Diagnostic Tests

Diagnosis is based on observing repetitive patterns of perception or behavior. The general diagnostic criteria listed by DSM IV are: an enduring pattern in two or more areas (cognitive, affective, impulse control, and/or interpersonal relationship) of inner experience/behavior that deviates from cultural expectations. Pattern is stable, long standing, inflexible, and pervasive across broad range of situations and causes distress and/or impairs function. The pattern can be traced back to adolescence or early adulthood and is not better accounted for as a consequence of some other mental disorder/physical condition or chemical substance.

Therapeutic Management

Surgery	None
Medications	Psychotropic drugs are generally not effective except for managing concomitant axis I psychiatric disorders or select symptoms. Targeted symptoms, such as perceptual distortions or brief psychotic symptoms, are treated with low-dose neuroleptics or antipsychotics. Severe affective dyscontrol can be treated with carbamazepine or high-dose beta-blockers. Anger, anxiety, and impulsivity are treated with selective serotonin reuptake inhibitors (SSRIs).
General	Individual and group therapies with emphasis on problem exploration and solutions; family therapy focusing on family dynamics; occupational therapy to increase daily functioning; vocational counseling to improve job skills; art and/or music therapy to improve expression; movement therapy to promote relaxation; recreational therapy to strengthen social skills; hospitalization for severe dysfunction and/or high risk for harmful behavior (self-mutilation, suicide); provision of limit setting and structure, protection from self-harm, behavioral contracting, milieu therapy
Education	Education about disorder; effects and side effects of medications; instruction in using activities (diary keeping, relaxation exercises) to modify impulsive behavior

P

Pertussis (Whooping Cough)

An acute, highly communicable bacterial infection of the mucous membranes of the bronchus characterized by a spasmodic cough

Etiology and Incidence

Whooping cough is caused by *Bordetella pertussis,* a nonmotile, gram-negative coccobacillus. It is usually transmitted through aspiration of droplet spray produced by an infected individual during paroxysms. Pertussis is endemic throughout the world and becomes epidemic in 2- to 4-year cycles. It occurs in all age groups, but infants and toddlers are the most susceptible. The incidence had been greatly reduced in the United States since the 1940s, when a pertussis vaccine was introduced, but an upsurge in reported cases began in the late 1980s and continues currently. There are approximately 5000 new cases a year in the United States.

Pathophysiology

When inhaled, *B. pertussis* attaches itself to the cilia of the respiratory epithelial cells and incubates for about 7 to 10 days before producing symptoms. The pertussis toxin is absorbed from the respiratory tract into the lymph system, causing a lymphocytosis. The pathogenesis of the paroxysmal cough is unknown.

Clinical Manifestations

Pertussis has three stages, each lasting about 2 weeks. The individual is contagious from the onset of the first symptom until the end of the second stage, or until the patient is treated with antibiotics.

Catarrhal   Drippy nose, sneezing, tearing, and low-grade fever; listlessness; hacking nocturnal cough

Paroxysmal   Exhausting paroxysms of prolonged coughing two to three times an hour that often end with an inspiratory whooping sound or choking and vomiting accompanied by

	production of copious, viscid, tenacious mucus with cyanosis and apnea
Convalescent	Diminished coughing and production of mucus

Complications

Complications most commonly occur in infants and very young children; they include bronchopneumonia, asphyxiation, convulsions, and cerebral hemorrhage, with resultant spastic paralysis and mental retardation.

Diagnostic Tests

The diagnosis is often missed in the catarrhal phase, since the disease mimics influenza or bronchitis at this point. Lymphocytosis in an afebrile individual is suggestive and should lead to culture of nasal secretions. A definitive diagnosis is made by a positive culture of nasal secretions in the catarrhal or early paroxysmal stage. Direct fluorescent antibody staining of secretions may also isolate the pathogen but is less sensitive than a culture.

Therapeutic Management

P

Surgery	Tracheostomy if necessary
Medications	Antiinfective drugs to treat bronchopneumonia or otitis media, erythromycin in incubation or catarrhal stage to arrest pathogen, prevention through immunization, prophylactic treatment of contacts with antiinfective drugs
General	Hospitalization of infants with IV fluids, oxygen, possible ventilatory support, and suctioning; close monitoring of fluids, electrolytes, and nutritional needs; respiratory isolation during catarrhal and paroxysmal stages; home treatment for older children and adults with bed rest; minimal stimulation; small, frequent feedings;

	adequate hydration; humidifier; well-ventilated and restful environment (free of dust, smoke, sudden temperature changes), and respiratory isolation
Prevention/ Promotion	Pertussis vaccination per schedule
Education	Education about isolation procedures, hand washing techniques, home care

Pharyngitis (Sore Throat)

An acute or chronic inflammation of the pharynx, including the pharyngeal walls, tonsils, uvula, and palate

Etiology and Incidence

Pharyngitis is caused by viral agents, such as respiratory syncytial virus (RSV), influenza A and B, Epstein Barr virus (EBV), adenovirus, herpes simplex; bacterial agents, such as *Streptococcus pyogenes*, *Neisseria gonorrhoeae* or *Arcanobacterium haemolyticum*, or by *Mycoplasma pneumoniae or Chlamydia pneumoniae*. A sore throat is most often the result of viral pharyngitis. Pharyngitis is the most common of all throat disorders. Of all sore throats, about 10% of adults and 30% of children have streptococcal pharyngitis. Even fewer individuals providing a history of oral-genital sexual activity will have gonococcal pharyngitis.

Pathophysiology

It is often preceded by a common cold and is characterized by a mild sore throat, difficulty and pain in swallowing, and a low-grade fever.

Risk Factors

Upper respiratory infection (URI)
Children are more likely to acquire streptococcal infections
Winter months
Unprotected oral-genital sex with infected partner

Clinical Manifestations

Viral	Runny nose, conjunctivitis, cough, red and swollen pharynx, no tonsillar or pharyngeal exudate
Streptococcal	High fever, headache, fatigue, malaise, tonsillar exudate, anterior cervical adenopathy
Gonococcal	History of oral-genital sexual activity, pharyngeal exudate, cervical lymphadenopathy
Herpes Simplex	Vesicles

P

Complications

Pharyngeal abscess or ulcerations are common complications. Rare complications from streptococcal pharyngitis include scarlet fever, rheumatic fever, or acute glomerulonephritis.

Diagnostic Tests

Clinical evaluation with presenting signs and symptoms; rapid strep screen and throat culture may be used to diagnose streptococcal or gonococcal pharyngitis.

Therapeutic Management

Surgery	None
Medications	Antiinfective agents if bacterial organism is identified; analgesics for comfort; antipyretics for fever
General	Rest, humidified air, warm saline throat gargles, adequate fluid intake

Phlebitis

(See Thrombosis, Venous [Phlebothrombosis, Thrombophlebitis])

Pleurisy

An inflammation of the visceral and parietal pleurae that envelop the lungs

Etiology and Incidence

Pleurisy arises from a pleural injury, which may be caused by an underlying lung disease (e.g., pneumonia, asbestosis, or infarction); an infectious agent, neoplastic cells, or irritants that invade the pleural space (e.g., amebic empyema, tuberculosis [TB], pleural effusion, systemic lupus erythematosus [SLE], pleural carcinomatosis, rheumatoid disease); or pleural trauma (e.g., rib fracture).

Pathophysiology

The pleura becomes edematous and congested, cellular infiltration ensues, and fibrinous exudate forms on the pleural surface as plasma proteins leak from damaged vessels. This causes the visceral and parietal pleural surfaces to rub together rather than slide over each other during respiration. The pleura becomes increasingly inflamed and stretched, causing pain on each breath.

Clinical Manifestations

The primary symptom is sudden onset of pain in the chest or abdominal wall that may vary from vague to an intense stabbing sensation. The pain is aggravated by breathing and coughing. Respirations are rapid and shallow, with guarding and decreased motion on the affected side.

Complications

Permanent adhesions that restrict lung expansion may develop.

Diagnostic Tests

Auscultation reveals a friction rub, along with the characteristic presentation of pain. A chest x-ray may show pleural effusion.

Therapeutic Management

Surgery	None
Medications	Narcotic analgesic to relieve pain during deep-breathing and coughing exercises, analgesics and antipyretics
General	Treatment of underlying disease, positioning and splinting of chest, coughing and deep breathing to prevent atelectasis and infection
Education	Instruction in turn cough and deep breathing; splinting of chest, positioning

Pneumocystis carinii Pneumonia (PCP)

A fungally induced pneumonia most commonly seen as an opportunistic infection secondary to acquired immunodeficiency syndrome (AIDS)

(See also Pneumonia, Bacterial/Nonbacterial and Acquired Immunodeficiency Syndrome [AIDS])

Etiology and Incidence

Pneumocystis carinii, the cause of this type of pneumonia (PCP), is a fungus. PCP, or pneumocystosis, was relatively rare—seen in only a handful of severely immunosuppressed patients—until the advent of AIDS. PCP is now seen in about 80% of individuals with AIDS and is the initial AIDS-defining condition in more than 60% of human immunodeficiency virus (HIV)-positive individuals. More than 50% of all AIDS deaths are attributable to PCP infections.

Pathophysiology

The fungus lies dormant in the person's lung until the body's defenses are compromised. At that time a usually benign resident becomes an aggressive pathogen. The organisms proliferate in the alveolar spaces, facilitated by diminished cell-mediated and humoral host defenses. The organisms attach to alveolar epithelial cells, impairing replication and inducing degeneration and increased membrane permeability. This causes formation of exudate in the alveolar space, reduces surfactant levels, and results in intrapulmonary shunting of blood, decreased lung compliance, and hypoxemia.

Risk Factors

HIV infection
CD4 lymphocyte counts less than $100/mm^3$
Immunosuppression

Clinical Manifestations

Fever, fatigue, dyspnea, and a dry, nonproductive cough that evolves over several days or weeks are the first symptoms. Increasing shortness of breath usually prompts the individual to seek treatment. The onset tends to be more acute in individuals who do not have AIDS.

Complications

Pulmonary insufficiency, pulmonary failure, and death can occur. The overall mortality rate with treatment is about 20%.

Diagnostic Tests

The definitive diagnosis is established through a histopathological examination, preferably of induced sputum. A bronchoscopy with lavage or lung biopsy may be done if sputum cultures are negative. A chest x-ray may show fluffy infiltrates. A gallium scan may show increased lung uptake even if the x-ray is normal.

Therapeutic Management

Surgery	Tracheostomy if necessary; thoracotomy for pneumothorax
Medications	Antiinfective drugs to combat the pathogen (trimethoprim-sulfamethoxazole [TMP/SMX] or pentamidine); adjunctive corticosteroid therapy; lifetime prophylaxis with TMP/SMX or aerosol pentamidine for patients who are intolerant of other forms of prophylaxis
General	Oxygen therapy, adequate hydration, adequate ventilation or ventilatory support, adequate nutrition, strict medical asepsis, and universal precautions
Prevention/ Promotion	Prophylaxis with TMP/SMX for individuals with a CD4 cell count below $250/mm^3$ or less than 20% of total lymphocyte count Smoking cessation
Education	Education of HIV-positive individuals about early signs and symptoms of PCP and importance of regular long-term follow-up; importance of adequate rest, regular exercise, balanced diet

Pneumonia, Bacterial/Nonbacterial

An acute infection and inflammation of the bronchioles, alveolar spaces, and interstitial tissue of the lung parenchyma

Etiology and Incidence

Pneumonia is caused by bacteria, viruses, fungi, or parasites. Each year in the United States, pneumonia is diagnosed in more than 4 million persons, and more than 62,000 of those individuals die, making pneumonia the seventh leading cause of death in the United States. In developing countries pneumonia is either the first or second leading cause of death. The most common types, which are bacterial, are *Pneumococcus, Staphylococcus, Streptococcus, Klebsiella,* and *Haemophilus* pneumonia.

Pathophysiology

Organisms reach the lung through aspiration, aerosolization, or hematogenous spread. This usually occurs through droplet inhalation or by aspiration of fluids in the oropharynx. Pneumonia results if a series of host defense mechanisms fails to keep the respiratory tree free of infection. Upper airway mechanisms such as nasal filtration may be bypassed, the normal flora altered, immunoglobulin A (IgA) secretion impaired, or the glottis depressed. Lower airway mechanisms such as coughing, cilia mucus, and mucociliary transport may be altered or impaired. Macrophages or cell-mediated immunity may be impaired, and immunoglobulins, complement, or surfactant may be deficient in the alveoli.

The pathophysiology varies by etiological agent. Bacterial pneumonia is marked by an intraalveolar suppurative exudate with consolidation. Mycoplasmal and viral pneumonias produce interstitial inflammation with infiltrate in the alveolar walls; there is no accompanying exudate or consolidation. Pneumococcal and streptococcal pneumonia have four distinct stages: (1) *congestion,* characterized by serous exudate, vascular engorgement, and rapid proliferation of the pathogen; (2) *red hepatization,* when RBCs, fibrin, and polymorphonuclear cells fill the alveoli; (3) *gray hepatization,* when leukocytes and fibrin pack the alveoli; and (4) *resolution,* marked by lysis and resorption of exudate by macrophages.

Viral pneumonia begins with an inflammatory response in the bronchi, which damages the ciliated epithelium. The lungs become congested and may be hemorrhagic. Intracellular viral inclusions form with many viruses. In aspiration pneumonia, the bacteria are aspirated with food or liquid. If the pH of the aspirated substance is below 2.5, atelectasis, pulmonary edema, and hemorrhage occur, followed by tissue necrosis and the formation of exudate.

Risk Factors

History of viral respiratory infection

Alcoholism

Smoking

Age extremes (very young and very old at greater risk)

History of debility, dysphagia, altered consciousness

Use of therapies that depress the immune system

Underlying disease states, such as diabetes mellitus (DM), heart failure, chronic obstructive pulmonary disease (COPD), asthma, or immunosuppressive disorders

Hospitalized individuals, particularly those postoperative from chest or abdominal surgery

Clinical Manifestations

Bacterial	Abrupt onset with shaking chills, cough, dyspnea, sputum production (often rust or salmon colored), pleurisy; nausea, vomiting, malaise, and myalgia also may be present
Viral	Headache, fever, myalgia, cough with mucopurulent sputum
Mycoplasmal	Malaise, sore throat, dry cough with rapid progression to productive cough with mucoid, purulent, and blood-streaked sputum
Fungal	(See *Pneumocystis carinii* Pneumonia)
Aspiration	Dyspnea, cyanosis, hypotension, tachycardia

Complications

Septic shock, lung abscess, respiratory failure, bacteremia, endocarditis, pericarditis, and meningitis are possible complications.

Diagnostic Tests

Sputum Examination	Must be obtained from lower respiratory tract; positive for pathogen
WBC Count	Leukocytosis; neutrophilia in mycoplasmal or viral infection
Radiology	Consolidation in bacterial infection, bronchopneumonic type of infiltrate in viral infection, clear in early mycoplasmal infection, atelectasis in aspiration pneumonia
Pulmonary Function	Decreased lung volumes and compliance, increased airway resistance

Therapeutic Management

Surgery	Thoracentesis with chest tube if empyema or collapse occurs; tracheostomy if necessary for patent airway
Medications	Antiinfective drugs (broad spectrum or specific to pathogen), analgesics for pain
General	Rest, humidification with nebulizer to loosen secretions, oxygen if PaO_2 is below 60 mm Hg, coughing and deep-breathing exercises, adequate hydration to liquefy secretions, suctioning with copious secretions or compromised consciousness, mechanical ventilation for respiratory failure, adequate nutritional support with supplemental feedings or total parenteral nutrition if necessary, monitoring of blood gases and general respiratory status; strict medical asepsis and universal precautions
Prevention/ Promotion	Prophylaxis with influenza vaccine and pneumococcal pneumonia vaccine in high-risk individuals and those over age 65 Smoking cessation Maintain proper nutrition, hygiene, rest, and exercise regimens
Education	Instruct on medication effects and side effects, deep-breathing techniques, precautions for prevention of spread

P

Poliomyelitis

An acute, communicable viral infection that affects the central nervous system (CNS), producing a range of manifestations from a subclinical or mild nonfebrile illness to aseptic meningitis, muscle weakness, and paralysis

Etiology and Incidence

Polio is caused by three distinct polio enteroviruses belonging to the Picornaviridae family and labeled types 1, 2, and 3. Type 1 is the most paralytogenic and the most likely to cause an epidemic. Polio has been all but eradicated in most developed countries because of widespread vaccination. In developing countries, however, the once rare disease has reached an incidence as high as that in the United States before a vaccine was developed. The mortality rate ranges from 1% to 10%, depending on the severity and type of disease. All current cases in the United States (under 10 per year) have been caused by the live attenuated virus in the Sabin (OPV) vaccine.

Pathophysiology

The poliovirus enters the mouth after contact with infected feces or oral or respiratory secretions. It multiplies in the lymphoid tissue of the throat and ileum, producing a follicular necrosis. The incubation period ranges from 5 to 35 days, averaging 7 to 14 days. A transient viremia of 3 to 5 days' duration occurs when the virus is transported via the bloodstream and autonomic nerve fiber endings to the CNS. The viremia disappears at the onset of disease symptoms. Paralysis results when extensive damage is inflicted on the motor neurons, resulting in atrophy of associated skeletal muscle fiber groups.

Clinical Manifestations

Most cases are subclinical and produce no signs or symptoms. Clinical disease may be either minor (abortive) or major. Major illness may or may not lead to paralysis. The person is infectious from the time of infection up to 6 weeks after infection.

Minor	Develops 3 to 5 days after exposure, accounts for 85% of clinical cases, occurs primarily in young children, no CNS involvement; slight fever, malaise, sore throat, headache, vomiting, anorexia, and abdominal pain lasting 24 to 72 hours
Major	Develops 7 to 14 days after exposure, primarily in older children and adults; fever, severe headache, stiff neck and back, deep muscle pain, paresthesia, or hyperesthesia
	May be followed by a loss of tendon reflexes and asymmetric weakness or paralysis, or may involve lower extremity, respiratory, facial, palatal, pharyngeal, or bladder muscles

Complications

Complications, which arise primarily from major paralytic disease, include respiratory failure, hypertension (HTN), cor pulmonale, soft tissue and skeletal deformities, and paralytic ileus. In paralytic polio, 50% of affected individuals recover with no residual effects, 25% have a mild disability, and 25% have a severe permanent residual disability. Recovery of muscle function takes 6 months to 2 years. A postpoliomyelitis syndrome has been identified, which occurs several years after the initial attack of polio. The syndrome is characterized by profound fatigue, muscle weakness, fasciculations, and muscle atrophy.

Diagnostic Tests

The definitive diagnosis is made through culture of throat washings or fecal material, or from convalescent serum antibody titers, which are four times higher than acute antibody titers.

Therapeutic Management

Surgery	Tracheostomy if necessary in respiratory paralysis
Medications	Mild sedatives for rest; analgesics for pain

General   *Mild:* Bed rest
              Major: Strict bed rest in acute phase; hot,
                moist packs for muscle spasm and pain;
                intermittent catheterization for urinary
                retention; assisted ventilation for respiratory
                paralysis; suctioning for pooling secretions;
                physical therapy for weakened or paralyzed
                extremities; IVs, tube feedings for those
                unable to swallow; monitoring for aspiration
                of secretions; long-term rehabilitation for
                those with permanent residual disability
              Note: All polio cases should be reported to
                the appropriate public health agency

Prevention/ Salk (IPV) vaccine is recommended for all
Promotion   infants and children and for individuals with
                underlying immunodeficiency disease as
                prophylaxis; Sabin (OPV) vaccine is
                recommended only for unvaccinated adults
                who are imminently traveling (within a
                month) to endemic or epidemic areas.

Education   Education for parents as to why Salk (IPV) is
                now vaccine of choice and the recommended
                vaccine schedule

Polycythemia

An increase in the number of circulating erythrocytes and hemoglobin concentration that is manifested in three forms: polycythemia vera, secondary polycythemia, and relative polycythemia

Etiology and Incidence

The cause of *polycythemia vera* is unknown, and the disorder is usually seen in older Jewish men. It occurs in 1 in 200,000 persons in the United States. *Secondary* polycythemia is a compensatory response to tissue hypoxia associated with underlying chronic obstructive pulmonary disease (COPD); hemoglobin abnormalities such as carboxyhemoglobinemia, which is seen in heavy smokers; congestive heart failure (CHF); congenital heart disease; or prolonged exposure to altitudes above 10,000 feet. The incidence is about 2 in 100,000 persons in the United States. *Relative* polycythemia is caused by fluid loss and dehydration and disappears when fluids are replaced.

Pathophysiology

Polycythemia vera involves rapid, uncontrolled cellular reproduction and maturation, which causes hyperplasia of all bone marrow cells and replaces bone marrow fat. Increased megakaryocytes may be present and form clumping patterns. Bone marrow iron is absent in about 90% of affected individuals. The cellular overproduction increases blood viscosity and blood volume, and organs and tissues become engorged with blood.

Clinical Manifestations

Polycythemia Vera	Weakness and fatigue; a feeling of fullness in the head, with headache, lightheadedness, and dizziness; visual disturbances (scotoma, double or blurred vision); dyspnea; nosebleeds; night sweats; epigastric and joint pain; later signs include pruritus, clubbing of digits, a reddened face with engorged retinal veins, and hepatosplenomegaly

| Secondary Polycythemia | Above manifestations plus hypoxemia in the absence of hepatosplenomegaly and hypertension (HTN) |
| Relative Polycythemia | Often individual has no complaints or vague complaints (e.g., headache, fatigue) with ruddy complexion and slight hypertension when recumbent |

Complications

Thrombosis, cerebrovascular accident (CVA), peptic ulcers, myeloid metaplasia, leukemia, and hemorrhage are common complications in polycythemia vera and result in the death of about 50% of untreated individuals within 18 months of the appearance of symptoms. The median survival rate in treated individuals is 7 to 15 years. Hemorrhage is the most common complication of secondary polycythemia. Hypercholesterolemia, hyperlipidemia, and hyperuricemia may complicate relative polycythemia.

Diagnostic Tests

Polycythemia Vera	Increased RBC mass and normal arterial oxygen saturation associated with splenomegaly or two of the following: thrombocytosis, leukocytosis, elevated leukocyte alkaline phosphatase, or elevated serum B_{12}; bone marrow shows panmyelosis
Secondary Polycythemia	Elevated erythrocytes, Hct, Hgb, mean corpuscular volume; absence of leukocytosis and thrombocytosis; erythroid hyperplasia of bone marrow
Relative Polycythemia	Normal or decreased RBC mass, elevated Hct, no leukocytosis, normal plasma volume; normal bone marrow studies

Therapeutic Management

| **Surgery** | Splenectomy to treat resistant splenomegaly |
| **Medications** | Chemotherapeutic agents to induce myelosuppression in some polycythemia vera |

	cases; allopurinol to treat hyperuricemia; antihistamines for pruritus; analgesics for joint pain; antacids for gastric hyperacidity
General	*Polycythemia vera:* Phlebotomy to reduce RBC mass; pheresis for removal of WBCs, RBCs, and platelets; exercise to promote circulation; monitoring for thrombus formation, hemorrhage, and ulcer formation
	Secondary polycythemia: Treatment of underlying causes
	Relative polycythemia: Fluid and electrolyte replacement, measures to prevent further fluid loss
Education	Education about chronic nature of disease, long-term phlebotomy treatment and complications if left untreated

P

Polyps

Common, benign, grapelike growths arising or protruding from mucous membrane tissue; the masses may be sessile or pedunculated and vary considerably in size. Polyps may appear as single growths or in clusters.

Etiology and Incidence

Polyps may be idiopathic or may be associated with an autosomal dominant trait (familial polyposis and Gardner's syndrome) or an underlying disease. Polyps are commonly found on the cervix, within the colon, in the nose, or on the vocal cords. The cause of each type of polyp differs depending on location. For example, *vocal cord* polyps often occur secondary to chronic voice abuse, inhalation of toxic irritants, smoking, and/or allergies. *Nasal polyps* are often the result of irritation of the mucous membrane from allergy or sinusitis. *Cervical polyps* are most often seen in women who use oral contraceptives and those approaching menopause. *Colon polyps* are often an autosomal dominant trait, which is often transmitted by an affected parent. The child of an affected parent has a 50% chance of acquiring colon polyps.

Incidence reports are highest in North America and Europe, and polyps have been noted on autopsy in as much as 50% of the population in the United States. The likelihood of acquiring polyps increases with age.

Pathophysiology

Normal cell proliferation and differentiation processes are altered, causing a proliferation of immature epithelial cells that accumulate to form a polyp tissue mass. Polyps are soft, pliable growths and may appear as single growths or in clusters. *Nasal polyps* are soft, pliable, nontender masses growing from the sinuses or nasal mucosa. *Vocal cord polyps* generally have a broad-base attachment to the vocal cords. This may interfere with voice tone. *Colon polyps* are often found as discrete mass lesions on the mucosal membrane of the colon. The lesions of familial polyposis may be considered precancerous adenomatous polyps. These polyps may increase in size and number until the entire colon is studded with hundreds of polyps. *Cervical polyps* generally arise from the endocervical tissue and are often bright red and vascular.

Risk Factors

Nasal	Chronic maxillary sinusitis, allergies, cystic fibrosis (CF)
Vocal Cord	Chronic overuse of voice, smoking, allergies
Cervical	Oral contraceptives, menopause
Colon	Family history

Clinical Manifestations

Nasal	May be asymptomatic or may have decreased air flow on the side of the polyp
Vocal Cord	Raspy voice
Colon	May be asymptomatic; often rectal bleeding is the first sign
	Other signs include diarrhea, increased mucus in the stools, and crampy abdominal pain
Cervical	Often are asymptomatic; may have some intermittent spotting or bleeding

Complications

Complications are dependent on location; nasal polyps may occlude airway, vocal polyps may affect voice, and colon polyps may become malignant.

Diagnostic Tests

Direct observation of the polyp is diagnostic. Methods of observation vary based on polyp location. Rectal examination, endoscopy, and/or barium enema are used to visualize rectal or colon polyps.

Therapeutic Management

Surgery	Most often polyps are surgically removed and sent for tissue evaluation
Medications	No routine medications
General	None

Prevention/ Promotion	Prophylactic proctocolectomy with ileostomy performed for inherited multiple polyposis syndrome
	Periodic clinical reevaluation for individuals with history of polyps
	Recommended sigmoidoscopy and/or colonoscopy screening schedules to detect colon polyps
Education	Education about colon polyps and relation to colon cancer and necessity for routine screening after age 49

Posttraumatic Stress Disorder (PTSD)

A syndrome of symptoms that occur in response to perceived severe physical or emotional trauma

Etiology and Incidence

PTSD may follow traumatic events such as rape, physical abuse, unintentional injuries, catastrophic illnesses, major losses, community violence, and all types of natural and human origin disasters. There is a relationship between intensity and duration of stress and severity of PTSD. Man-made disasters cause more intense reactions than natural disasters.

Prevalence of PTSD ranges from 1% to 14% of the general population in the United States. PTSD develops in up to 30% of disaster victims. It is thought that PTSD is underreported, since many individuals with PTSD fail to seek help. The group of individuals who have been most widely identified and studied are combat veterans of the Vietnam war. Veterans who were more involved in combat or who were prisoners of war are more likely to experience PTSD than other veterans.

Pathophysiology

There is no single explanation for PTSD. Theories and research demonstrate a causative interrelationship of biological and behavioral factors. Long-standing alterations in the biological response to stress may contribute to a number of complaints commonly expressed by individuals with PTSD. The most common biological studies on PTSD focus on hormone and neurotransmitter deregulation in PTSD: neurobiological response to danger, norepinephrine, hypothalamic-pituitary-adrenal axis (HPA), and opiates. Behavioral responses and experiences are also an integral component of the potential development of PTSD. Distorted perceptions of an event, inadequate coping skills, fear, and feelings of helplessness may all contribute to PTSD. The individual's interpretation of an event is a subjective process that may or may not reflect the actual reality of a situation. A distorted appraisal of a current event and a remembrance of the historic traumatic experience may interfere with the individual's ability to attach a healthy meaning to any single event. The individual has been fear conditioned, and this in turn prevents different and perhaps healthier interpretation of a similar yet nontraumatic event.

Risk Factors

Past traumatic event such as combat exposure, prisoner of war; rape, or sexual or physical assault

Contributing factors, such as unstable or problematic family members, domestic violence, early separation from family, family history of anxiety or antisocial behavior, physical and/or sexual abuse as a child, depression, substance abuse, emotional or behavioral problems, psychiatric instability

Clinical Manifestations

Hypervigilance/ Physiological Arousal	A feeling of continued danger or fear even though the individual is in a safe environment
Guilt	A feeling of survival or self-blame guilt because the individual survived
Dissociation	A sensation of being disconnected or separated from one's own feelings; this usually occurs because the feelings are very painful or negative
Depersonalization	A feeling of detachment from oneself and from one's interaction with others
Psychogenic Amnesia	Selective memory loss of a specific period related to the traumatic event or circumstance
Psychogenic Fugue	Sudden, unexpected travel from the individual's local home area to another geographical location
Flashbacks	Having a vivid image of the traumatic event or circumstance
Trigger Avoidance	Avoidance of any triggers, such as places, people, or things that may trigger a PTSD episode
Comorbidity	The coexistence of other disorders, such as substance abuse, generalized anxiety, depression, and antisocial or borderline personality

Complications

Complications include alcohol and substance abuse, depression, reenactment of trauma, self-inflicted violence, and suicide.

Diagnostic Tests

Historic presence of trauma or assault; clinical evaluation and structured interviews; repeated dysfunctional stress responses to similar triggers. The use of psychological testing and mental status exam—including use of tools, such as *The Mississippi Scale Post-Traumatic Stress Disorder* and *The Clinician-Administered Post-Traumatic Stress Disorder* test—when PTSD is suspected.

Therapeutic Management

Surgery	None
Medications	Medications, such as antianxiety agents; antidepressants may be used to treat secondary psychiatric signs and symptoms, such as anxiety, depression, and/or impulsive activities or thoughts
General	Individual and group psychotherapy; hypnotherapy, narcoanalysis, narcosynthesis
	Facilitate individual and family support
	Psychiatric hospitalization for dysfunctional activities of daily living (ADLs) or suicidal ideation and/or behavior
Prevention/ Promotion	Crisis intervention immediately after traumatic event in those prone to PTSD
Education	Education about disease, triggers, self-care

P

Preeclampsia and Eclampsia

Preeclampsia is a disorder occurring between the 20th week of pregnancy and the first week postpartum and is characterized by hypertension (HTN), proteinuria, and edema. *Eclampsia* is diagnosed when convulsions develop in a woman with preeclampsia or when the woman becomes comatose in the absence of any other underlying neurological disorder.

Etiology and Incidence

The cause of preeclampsia is unknown but is likely multifactorial. Current theories include an imbalance in vasoconstrictors and vasodilators, an abnormal trophoblastic invasion of the spinal arteries, or an increased sensitivity to angiotensin II by the muscular walls of the arteries. Immunological and genetic factors are also thought to play a role. The precise cause of eclampsia is also unknown but is in someway related to abnormalities in the autoregulation of cerebral blood flow. The incidence of preeclampsia ranges from 6.5% in multigravidas to 12% in primigravidas. Eclampsia develops in 2% to 4% of those individuals with preeclampsia. Fifty percent of diagnosed eclampsia occurs antepartum, 20% intrapartum, and 30% postpartum.

Pathophysiology

The primary pathological feature of *preeclampsia* is decreased placental perfusion that leads to production of endothelin, which produces vasospasms and endothelial cell damage. This leads to increased sensitivity to angiotensin II, fluid shifts to intracellular space, and intravascular coagulation, which in turn leads to generalized vasoconstriction and increased arterial pressure. Decreased perfusion also leads to glomerular and liver damage, generalized and pulmonary edema, cortical brain spasms, and hemolysis and platelet aggregation. The pathophysiology of eclampsia is not known.

Risk Factors

Preeclampsia	Primigravidas (85% of cases)
	Age (less than 20 or over 35)
	Grand multigravidas

	Large fetus or multiple fetuses
	Evidence of major uterine anomalies
	Morbid obesity (more than 100 lb above normal weight range)
	History of preeclampsia with previous pregnancies
	History of preexisting cardiovascular conditions, diabetes mellitus (DM), collagen vascular, or renal disease
	Familial tendencies (maternal or paternal line)
Eclampsia	Multifetal gestation
	Molar pregnancy
	Nonimmune hydrops fetalis
	Preexisting and/or uncontrolled HTN
	Preeclampsia
	Underlying renal disease
	Familial tendencies (mother or sister with eclampsia)

Clinical Manifestations

Mild Preeclampsia	Blood pressure (BP) of 140/90 or mean arterial pressure (MAP) greater than 105; proteinuria greater than 300 mg/dl in 24-hour urine; normal reflexes; urine output equals 30 ml/hr; absent or transient headache; no visual problems; nondependent edema of the hands and face
Severe Preeclampsia	BP of 160/90 or MAP greater than 105; proteinuria greater than 2 g/dl in 24-hour urine; hyperreflexia with possible ankle clonus; urine output of 20 ml/hr; severe occipital headache; photophobia; severe irritability; epigastric pain; late decelerations in fetal heart tones; signs may be accompanied by a sudden weight gain
Eclampsia	Seizure activity starting with facial twitching and spreading to a general clonic-tonic state with cessation of respiration and a postictal period of amnesia, agitation, and confusion

P

Complications

A major complication of preeclampsia is hemolysis, elevated liver enzymes, low platelet count (HELLP) syndrome, which can lead to abruptio placentae, acute renal failure (ARF), hepatic hematoma and rupture, preterm birth, and fetal and maternal death. Complications of eclampsia ❶ include placental abruption, aspiration pneumonia, pulmonary edema, renal failure, cardiopulmonary arrest, and coma and death.

Diagnostic Tests

The diagnosis of *preeclampsia* requires the presence of elevated blood pressure (two BP measurements in lateral recumbent position 6 hours apart of greater than 140/90 mm Hg, or MAP greater than 105 mm Hg), with proteinuria (greater than 300 mg protein on 24-hour urine). HELLP syndrome is a laboratory diagnosis manifested by intravascular hemolysis (elevated bilirubin, burr cells on peripheral smear), elevated liver enzymes (aspartate aminotransferase [AST] and alanine aminotransferase [ALT]) and low platelets (less than $100,000/mm^3$).

Therapeutic Management

Surgery	Delivery of infant for women with severe or unresponsive preeclampsia/eclampsia— vaginal delivery if cervix is ripe; Cesarean section if vaginal delivery is unlikely
Medications	*Severe preeclampsia:* ❶ IV magnesium sulfate or phenytoin for seizure prevention and to reduce BP, addition of hydralazine, labetalol, or nifedipine if inadequate response of BP; calcium gluconate as an antidote for excess magnesium sulfate; *diuretics are contraindicated because they reduce uteroplacental perfusion*; epidural anesthesia for pain control during labor or during Cesarean
	Eclampsia: ❶ Magnesium sulfate or phenytoin for seizures; sodium amobarbital for persistent seizures; reduce BP with labetalol, hydralazine, or nifedipine

General	*Mild preeclampsia:* Rest at home; increased fluid intake and normal salt intake; balanced diet; close monitoring of maternal BP, weight, and urine protein and assessment of fetal activity; emotional support; diversional activity
	Severe preeclampsia: ✪ Immediate hospitalization; quiet, darkened environment; bed rest, positioned on the left side to improve uteroplacental blood flow and increase urinary output; IV with balanced salt solution; monitoring of vital signs and reflexes; intake and output (I&O) measurements; monitoring for signs of increasing severity of preeclampsia/HELLP; continuous monitoring of fetal heart tones and fetal activity; seizure precautions; evaluation and preparation for delivery; careful monitoring and management in postpartum for possible eclampsia; emotional support
	Eclampsia: ✪ Maintain airway, adequate oxygenation, safety precautions during seizure activity; then follow general management for severe preeclampsia
Prevention/ Promotion	Careful management of DM and HTN during pregnancy
Education	Education about disease effects on mother and infant; instruction about effects, side effects of medication, management of the disease process

P

Premenstrual Syndrome (PMS)

A combination of affective and physical symptoms starting 7 to 10 days before menstruation and disappearing within a few hours to days after the onset of menstrual flow

Etiology and Incidence

The cause of PMS is unclear, but the disorder seems to be related to fluctuations in estrogen and progesterone. Excessive aldosterone, hypoglycemia, hyperprolactinemia, allergy to progesterone, changes in carbohydrate metabolism, and psychogenic factors have also been implicated. An estimated 50% of all women experience PMS sometime before menopause. Those over age 30 are at higher risk, and the severity often increases as a woman ages.

Pathophysiology

A fall in estrogen and progesterone is accompanied by an increase in aldosterone, ovarian steroids, and antidiuretic hormone (ADH). This promotes sodium and fluid retention and results in edema. Decreased estrogen levels may also reduce brain levels of monoamine oxidase, catecholamine, and serotonin, resulting in irritability, depression, and mood swings.

Clinical Manifestations

PMS is marked by a broad manifestation of signs and symptoms that may range from mild to severe.

Physical   Fatigue, edema, weight gain, oliguria, breast
                  fullness, headache, vertigo, syncope,
                  paresthesia, easy bruising, palpitations,
                  abdominal bloating, constipation, nausea,
                  vomiting, pelvic heaviness and cramping,
                  backache, acne, neurodermatitis, cystitis,
                  enuresis, aggravation of allergy, and asthma

Affective	Mood swings, depression, irritability, anxiety, outbursts of anger, lethargy, insomnia, decreased attention span, forgetfulness, crying, loss of motivation, confusion, change in sexual arousal

Complications

Extreme antisocial behavior that is potentially harmful to the woman or others is a complication of PMS.

Diagnostic Tests

Evaluation is based on the symptom pattern, which appears and disappears with the menstrual cycle. Conditions such as endometriosis, an ovarian cyst, pelvic infection, underlying thyroid disease, or a psychiatric disorder must be ruled out.

Therapeutic Management

Surgery	Endometrial ablation for severe, untreatable pain; oophorectomy for severe, unresponsive symptoms
Medications	Long-acting progestin to regulate cycles, gonadotropin-releasing hormone agonists or oral contraceptives to suppress ovulation, progesterone replacement, antiprostaglandins to reduce cramping, diuretics for edema, mild tranquilizers for agitation, antidepressants for depression, vitamin and calcium supplements
General	Restriction of sodium, caffeine, tobacco, alcohol, and refined sugar; increased intake of complex carbohydrates, protein, and fiber; consistent exercise program to release endorphins; stress reduction program; counseling, with partner involvement, to better understand and cope with symptoms
Education	Education about diet, exercise, and stress reduction techniques

P

Pressure Ulcer (Decubitus Ulcer, Bedsore)

Ischemic necrosis and ulceration of tissues that overlie a bony prominence and that have been subjected to prolonged external pressure from a supporting surface, such as a bed or wheelchair

Etiology and Incidence

Pressure sores are caused by prolonged pressure on tissue compressed between an internal body structure, such as bone and an external surface. The force and duration of the pressure directly determine the size of the ulcer. Almost two thirds of pressure ulcers develop in acute care settings, and 50% of those with ulcers are over age 70.

Pathophysiology

Pressure exerted over an area interferes with the blood supply to the tissue, producing ischemia and increasing capillary pressure. This leads to edema and multiple small-vessel thromboses and sets up an inflammatory reaction. If the pressure is not relieved, the ischemic tissue becomes necrotic and ulcerates.

Risk Factors

Immobilization
Sensory and motor deficits
Reduced circulation
Malnutrition
Anemia
Edema
Infection
Friction
Moisture
Incontinence
Shearing forces
Decreased tissue integrity or viability
Aging

Clinical Manifestations

Four grades or stages of ulcer formation are defined by the National Pressure Ulcer Advisory Panel Consensus Conference. These stages are classified by the degree of tissue damage observed and possess the following characteristic signs and symptoms:

Stage 1	Nonblanchable erythema of intact skin; in dark-skinned individuals, symptoms include skin discoloration with accompanying heat, edema, or hardness
Stage 2	Partial-thickness skin loss involving the epidermis or the dermis, including blisters, abrasions, and shallow craters
Stage 3	Full-thickness skin loss with damage or necrosis to subcutaneous tissue that may extend down to underlying fascia and appears as a deep crater
Stage 4	Full-thickness skin loss accompanied by extensive destruction, tissue necrosis, and damage to muscle, bone, or supporting structures (e.g., tendons, joint capsules)

Complications

Bacteremia and septicemia are common complications. Osteomyelitis, septic arthritis, and pathological fractures also can occur.

Diagnostic Tests

Clinical evaluation showing the characteristic picture described under Clinical Manifestations.

A history that shows one or more predisposing and contributing factors.

Therapeutic Management

Surgery	Sharp debridement to remove eschar and dead tissue in large ulcers

P

	Stage 3 or 4 ulcers that do not respond to conservative treatment: direct closure, skin grafting, skin flaps, muscle flaps, and free flaps
Medications	Topical applications (e.g., enzymatic ointments) to débride necrotic tissue, hydrophilic gels for reepithelialization, topical antibiotics to suppress infection; *do not use topical antiseptic agents (e.g., povidone-iodine, iodophor, hydrogen peroxide, sodium hypochlorite, and acetic acid) to clean ulcers because they are cytotoxic.*
General	Baseline and ongoing assessment of ulcer's (location, stage, size, necrosis, odor, exudate); elimination of pressure through frequent turning, special beds, mattress overlays, wheelchair pads filled with gels, air, water, sand, or other pressure-relieving ingredients; use of lifting devices to prevent shearing; dressings that keep wound moist and surrounding tissue dry (vapor permeable [Bioclusive, OpSite, Tegaderm], hypocolloid, hydrocolloid [Dermiflex, DuoDerm, Tegasorb]); careful cleansing at dressing change with saline or other nontoxic cleanser; débridement by irrigation with whirlpool baths; electrical stimulation to promote antibacterial effects and stimulate muscle protein synthesis; balanced nutrition; control of incontinence; use of drainage and secretion precautions
Prevention/ Promotion	Identification of high-risk individuals through systematic risk assessment
	Ulcer prevention protocol in high-risk patients (e.g., daily skin inspections; use of pressure relief mattress overlays and wheelchair cushions; use of lifting devices; clean, dry clothing, and bed linens free of wrinkles and treated with fabric softener; lotion on all skin surfaces, especially over bony prominences, to reduce friction)

	Prevent or correct nutritional deficits, multivitamin supplement
	Regular program of activity and exercise
Education	Education about cause, risk factors, early signs of ulcer formation, skin assessment and care; instruction in preventive measures (e.g., frequent use of pressure relief measures, such as turning, raising off buttocks, shifting weight when seated); education about adequate nutrition

P

Prostate Cancer

Adenocarcinomas account for most prostate cancers. The rest are transitional cell, squamous cell, endometrioid, or sarcomatous cancers.

(See also Cancer)

Etiology and Incidence

The cause is unknown but appears to be related to endogenous hormones. A genetic component may also play a role. Prostate cancer is the most commonly diagnosed cancer in men in the United States, with more than 220,000 cases reported annually. It is the second leading cause of cancer deaths in men, with nearly 29,000 deaths reported annually. It strikes those over age 50 most frequently (more than 85% are over age 65) and the incidence and mortality are higher in African-American men.

Pathophysiology

Adenocarcinomas usually begin in the lower posterior prostate and grow slowly to encompass the entire gland. The tumor spreads directly to the bladder and levator ani muscles and, via the lymphatic system, throughout the pelvis. Metastasis occurs through the bloodstream to the bones, liver, lungs, and kidneys.

Risk Factors

Age (70% of men over age 80 have evidence of disease)
Race (African Americans have twice the rate of Caucasians)
Familial history in first-degree relative
Diet with high fat intake (particularly saturated fats)

Clinical Manifestations

Early signs mimic benign prostatic hypertrophy (BPH); they include difficulty initiating and stopping the urinary stream, frequency and pain on urination, and a weak urinary stream.

Complications

Complications of advanced disease include thrombosis, pulmonary emboli (PE), retrograde ejaculation, and impotence. Prognosis is generally good and the overall 5-year survival rate is 97%.

Diagnostic Tests

Palpable nodules on digital rectal examination and an elevated prostate-specific antigen offer suspicions of a tumor. A needle biopsy is the definitive follow-up. Transrectal ultrasonography is used to assess size and shape of tumor. Testing for EZH2 protein in tumor tissue can aid in prognosis and help determine treatment course.

Therapeutic Management

Surgery	Prostatectomy for localized tumor, transurethral resection when the bladder is involved, bilateral orchiectomy for metastatic disease
Medications	Hormone therapy (diethylstilbestrol, lutenizing hormone–releasing hormone (LHRH) analogs, antiandrogens); chemotherapy for late-stage palliation
General	Radiation (external beam and/or interstitial implant) as a primary treatment alternative to surgery and for palliation; counseling for changes in sexual functioning; cryosurgical ablation
Prevention/ Promotion	Prostate-specific antigen (PSA) test and digital rectal evaluation annually for men who are 50 years of age or more or for high-risk men starting at 45 years of age
Education	Education about treatment side effects such as urinary incontinence and impotence, instruction in Kegel exercises to reduce incontinence; treatment options for impotence; importance of regular, long-term follow-up

P

Prostatic Hypertrophy, Benign

A progressive enlargement of the periurethral prostate gland

Etiology and Incidence

The cause of benign prostatic hypertrophy (BPH) is unknown but is thought to be related to hormonal changes as a man ages. It is most commonly seen in men over age 50. At least 50% of males over 50 and 80% of those over age 80 are affected. The incidence of BPH continues to rise as longevity increases.

Pathophysiology

Multiple fibroadenomatous nodules grow in the periurethral glands of the prostate, displacing the fibromuscular prostate. The lumen of the prostatic urethra becomes progressively compromised, and outflow of urine is obstructed.

Clinical Manifestations

A man may be asymptomatic for years before signs of progressive urinary frequency, urgency, nocturia, dribbling, and hesitancy occur. This is accompanied by a diminution in the size and force of the stream and a feeling of fullness in the bladder region after urination. Recurring urinary tract infections (UTIs) may be common.

Complications

Renal complications arise from prolonged obstruction. They can include hydronephrosis, renal infection, azotemia, renal calculi, uremia, and renal failure.

Diagnostic Tests

Digital Rectal Examination	Shows an enlarged, indurated, and tender prostate
System Assessment	Urinary frequency and urgency, interrupted and weak urine stream; straining and incomplete bladder emptying
Prostate-specific Antigen (PSA)	Elevated in 30% to 50% of cases

Post Void Residual	Assess degree of obstruction
Uroflowmetry	Decreased peak and mean flows
Cystoscopy/ Cystometrography	Allow visualization and assessment of the degree of urethral obstruction

Therapeutic Management

Surgery	Transurethral resection of the prostate is the definitive treatment of choice; alternatives include: intraurethral stent, balloon dilation, microwave therapy, cryotherapy, incisional resection laser ablation, and ultrasonic aspiration.
Medications	Alpha-antagonists or hormonal agents to reduce prostate's size (these may cause erectile dysfunction, loss of libido, feminization, and thromboembolism)
General	Intermittent catheterization; avoidance of alcohol, caffeine, foods and medications (cold and allergy remedies) that exacerbate symptoms; support and counseling for erectile dysfunction
Education	Postoperative instructions for managing incontinence, maintaining fluid balance, observing for UTI or wound infection, preventing constipation, refraining from heavy lifting
	General instructions to urinate every 2 to 3 hours to minimize urinary stasis

P

Prostatitis

An inflammation of the prostate gland; prostatitis may be classified as acute or chronic bacterial prostatitis, non-bacterial prostatitis, or prostatodynia.

Etiology and Incidence

Nonbacterial prostatitis has been associated with the presence of WBCs in prostatic secretions with no identifiable etiological agent. Acute and chronic bacterial prostatitis is caused by a gram-negative infection (e.g., *Escherichia coli, Proteus, Klebsiella, Pseudomonas,* and *Enterobacter)* of the prostate gland. Prostatodynia is caused by spasms in the neck of the bladder with no evidence of WBCs in prostate secretions. Prostatitis is a common condition, and it is estimated that more than 50% of men will experience some form of prostatitis in their lifetime. Nonbacterial prostatitis and prostatodynia are the most prevalent followed by chronic bacterial prostatitis. Acute prostatitis is uncommon.

Pathophysiology

The most common pattern of inflammation is a lymphocytic infiltrate in the stroma. The extent of the inflammation ranges from scattered lymphocytes to dense lymphoid nodules. Sheets, clusters, and occasional nodules of lymphocytes and scattered plasma cells are visible within the stroma. Infiltrates of inflammatory cells are restricted to the glandular epithelium and lumen. Inflammatory cells, such as neutrophils and macrophages, are typically found in the lumen. Neutrophils, lymphocytes, and/or macrophages are seen intraepithelially.

Risk Factors

Over 50 years of age
Male gender
Trauma (e.g., urethral instrumentation)
High-risk sexual behaviors (multiple partners, lack of condom use, and/or anal intercourse)
Sexual abstinence
Recurrent urinary tract infections (UTIs), urethritis, or epididymitis
Excessive alcohol intake

Clinical Manifestations

Acute Bacterial Prostatitis	Sudden onset of fever, chills, myalgia, arthralgia, and general malaise; localized discomfort or pain in the perineal area or low back and prostate; associated urinary symptoms include urgency, frequency, nocturia, diminished urine stream, dysuria, and a burning sensation in the urethra; pain in the testicles and with ejaculation. Firm, swollen prostate that is tender and warm to the touch; enlarged and tender inguinal lymph nodes; urethral discharge
Chronic Bacterial Prostatitis	Often asymptomatic; perianal pain; dysuria; irritative voiding; lower abdominal or back pain or pain on ejaculation; hematospermia; enlarged tender prostate, swollen scrotum, tender and enlarged inguinal lymph nodes, and urethral discharge
Nonbacterial Prostatitis/ Prostatodynia	Frequent urination; pain and/or burning with urination; low back pain; pain in testes and with ejaculation; pain with bowel movement; firm, tender, and swollen prostate; may be urethral discharge and scrotal swelling or tenderness

P

Complications

Complications include sterility, abscess, urinary retention, and sepsis

Diagnostic Tests

Diagnosis of nonbacterial prostatitis is made by demonstrating the presence of inflammatory cells in the expressed prostatic secretions in the presence of negative prostatic secretion and bladder cultures. Intravenous pyelogram (IVP) may be done to ensure bladder neck patency.

Clinical Evaluation	Revealing tender and/or enlarged prostate
Urinalysis and Urine Culture	For identification of infection, bacterial organisms
Blood Tests	To evaluate for systemic infection

Therapeutic Management

Surgery	Infrequent; however, transurethral resection of the prostate may be performed for chronic prostatitis if antibiotic therapy is not successful
Medications	Antiinfective agents (often IV for acute prostatitis) specific to cultured organism; stool softener for bowel movement discomfort; analgesics for pain; antipyretics for fever; suppressive therapy for refractory infection
General	Acute and chronic may necessitate urinary catheterization or suprapubic caterer; warm tub or sitz baths; increased fluid intake; counseling for sexual dysfunction
Prevention/ Promotion	Avoidance of high-risk sexual practices Adequate fluid intake Avoid alcohol excess Regular cleaning of genitals
Education	Education about cleanliness of the genitals, safe sex, and alcohol intake

Psoriasis

A recurrent chronic disease of the skin, characterized by dry, scaly plaques and papules of varying size

Etiology and Incidence
The cause is unknown but is thought to be related to genetic and environmental factors that trigger an overproduction of epidermal cells. The onset typically occurs between ages 10 and 60 with a bimodal peak incidence in adolescents and at 60 years of age. The disorder affects 2% to 4% of the U.S. population.

Pathophysiology
Three main pathological components are at work in psoriasis to varying degrees. An increased miotic rate causes rapid epidermal cell turnover and shortened transit time of the cell from the basal layer to the epidermis. Faulty keratinization of the horny layer causes easy desquamation and diminished protection for underlying tissue. Dilation of dermal vessels and intermittent discharge of leukocytes into the dermis cause hot, red skin.

Risk Factors
Familial tendencies (strong link to human leukocyte antigen [HLA] B13, B17, and B27)
Caucasian race

Clinical Manifestations
The onset is gradual, and the disorder is characterized by chronic exacerbation and remission. The scalp, elbows, knees, back, and buttocks are the most common sites. The nails, eyebrows, axillae, and anal and genital regions may also be affected. The lesions are well-defined, dry, nonpruritic papules or plaques overlaid with shiny silver scales, and they heal without scarring. The skin may be reddened and hot to touch. Affected nails are pitted, discolored, thickened, and crumbly.

Complications
Common complications include psoriatic arthritis and exfoliative psoriatic dermatitis, which can lead to crippling and general debility.

Diagnostic Tests

The diagnosis is based on evaluation of characteristic lesions.

Therapeutic Management

Surgery	None
Medications	Topical corticosteroids, keratolytics used in lotion, cream, ointment, or shampoo form to treat lesions; antineoplastic agents for severe recalcitrant disease
General	Short-wave or long-wave ultraviolet light therapy; lubricants to soften skin; exposure to sunlight but avoiding sunburn; stress-reduction programs; prevention of mechanical injury to skin; instruction that lesions are not communicable; counseling if body image is affected and to adapt to chronic nature of disease

Psychotic Disorders

(See Schizophrenia)

Pulmonary Embolism (PE) 🅠

Sudden blockage of a pulmonary artery by foreign matter, which impedes the blood flow to the lung tissue

Etiology and Incidence

The most common cause is a thrombus, which typically forms in the leg or pelvic vein but may be seen in other locations. Other causes include fat, amniotic fluid, air, and gas. PE is the third most common cardiovascular disease in the United States, and it causes approximately 50,000 deaths annually. It is the most common complication in hospitalized individuals, and approximately 5% of hospital deaths are attributable to PE.

Pathophysiology

Emboli in any form travel through the bloodstream and lodge in one or more pulmonary arteries. The area of the lung supplied by the affected artery becomes underperfused but is still ventilated. This results in physiological dead space or wasted ventilation and contributes to hyperventilation. Histamine release from the embolus produces reflex bronchoconstriction, leading to further hyperventilation. Depletion of alveolar surfactant results in diminished lung volume and compliance. If the clot is large enough and interferes greatly with pulmonary perfusion, it may result in pulmonary hypertension (HTN).

Risk Factors

History of thrombophlebitis, myocardial infarction (MI), severe
　　burns, congestive heart failure (CHF), venous insufficiency,
　　polycythemia vera, chronic pulmonary disease, autoimmune
　　hemolytic anemia, or cancer
Major surgery or fractures of pelvis or lower extremities
Pregnancy and childbirth
Prolonged immobility
History of chronic illness
Obesity
Use of oral contraceptives or estrogen supplements

Clinical Manifestations

The manifestations of a PE are nonspecific and vary in degree and intensity, depending on the size of the embolus, the extent of occlusion, the amount of collateral circulation, and preexisting cardiopulmonary function. Small emboli may be asymptomatic. The chief manifestation is sudden onset of unexplained dyspnea with rapid shallow breathing pattern. Other symptoms include anxiety, restlessness, tachypnea, sweating, cough, hemoptysis, chest pain, fever, and rales. Cyanosis may be present with a massive embolus.

Complications

Cardiac arrhythmias, cor pulmonale, atelectasis, shock, hepatic congestion, and necrosis are complications. Pulmonary infarction is an uncommon complication of PE that results in hemorrhagic consolidation and tissue necrosis distal to the occlusion. Death following a PE usually occurs within 1 to 2 hours of the initial event. Those with underlying cardiovascular or pulmonary disease and those with a large embolus are at greater risk of dying. Untreated individuals risk recurrent emboli and about a 50% chance of death.

Diagnostic Tests

The diagnosis is suggested by the clinical picture and confirmed by the following procedures:

Pulmonary Angiogram	Definitive test for emboli; visualization of intraarterial filling defects
Lung Perfusion/ Ventilation Scan	To detect perfusion defects and/or altered ventilation patterns
Blood Gases	Arterial hypoxemia (decreased PaO_2 and $PaCO_2$)
ECG	To rule out MI; a PE is characterized by tall, peaked P waves, depressed ST segments, T-wave inversions, and supraventricular tachyarrhythmias
CT Scan/MRI	Sensitive enough to detect most emboli
Chest X-ray	Unilateral elevation of the diaphragm, enlarged pulmonary artery, and pleural effusion 2 hours or longer after the event

Therapeutic Management

Surgery	Embolectomy for large emboli unresponsive to treatment; umbrella filter in inferior vena cava to trap multiple emboli before they reach the lung; interruption of blood flow through the inferior vena cava by ligation for multiple emboli
Medications	Anticoagulants to halt clot propagation (heparin is used in the acute phase and is replaced by Coumadin, which may be administered for 6 months to life; medications should overlap for 5 to 7 days to achieve effective blood levels of Coumadin); fibrinolytic enzymes may be used in place of anticoagulants for clot lysis, particularly of large clots; analgesics for pain; vasopressors, dopamine to treat hypotension
General	Oxygen therapy; bed rest in acute phase, followed by progressive mobilization; hemodynamic and cardiac monitoring; facilitation of breathing; intake and output (I&O) measurements to monitor renal function; observation for bleeding as a side effect of anticoagulants, and safety measures to prevent bleeding; antiembolism hose
Prevention/ Promotion	Avoidance or correction of modifiable risk factors, such as regular exercise of lower extremities on long air flights or other situations of prolonged immobility
Education	Information about long-term anticoagulant therapy; instruction in preventing pooled blood in the lower extremities

P

Pyelonephritis

An acute or chronic infection and inflammation of the kidney or renal pelvis
(See also Urinary Tract Infection)

Etiology and Incidence

Acute pyelonephritis is caused by a bacterial invasion that moves from the urethra to the bladder to the ureters to the kidney. The infecting bacteria are commonly normal intestinal and fecal flora that grow readily in urine. The annual incidence of pyelonephritis in the United States is 15 in 100,000; the annual nosocomial incidence rises to about 70 in 100,000. Chronic pyelonephritis most typically occurs as a result of repeated acute episodes but may also be caused by metastatic disease.

Pathophysiology

Bacteria ascend the urinary tract and colonize one or both kidneys. The kidney enlarges as the inflammatory process is activated, and parenchymal tissue is destroyed. Chronic inflammatory cells appear within a few days and medullary abscesses and papillary tissue necrosis occur. Patchy spots of infection develop and spread to the pelvic and caliceal epithelia and the cortex. If the process becomes chronic, atrophy, caliceal deformity, and parenchymal scarring occur.

Risk Factors

Individuals with a condition that interferes with the dynamics of normal urine flow are at greater risk. This includes those with underlying obstructions (strictures, calculi, tumors, and prostatic hypertrophy), neurogenic bladder, vesicoureteral reflux, diabetes, or renal disease; those who are sexually active or pregnant, and those undergoing medical or surgical procedures, such as catheterization or cystoscopy. Women are more susceptible than men because of the anatomical construction of the female urinary system.

Clinical Manifestations

The onset is fairly rapid and is characterized by dull, constant flank pain, chills, and fever. Concomitant signs of a lower urinary tract infection (UTI) (e.g., urinary frequency and dysuria) occur in about one third of individuals.

Complications

The most common complication of acute disease is septic shock or chronic pyelonephritis (or both). With chronic disease, there is a 2% to 3% chance of developing end-stage renal failure.

Diagnostic Tests

Clinical symptoms are confirmed by urinalysis, which shows antibody-coated bacteria, bacteriuria, WBC casts, and pyuria; a CBC shows an increase in WBCs. Renal function studies may assist in the diagnosis of chronic disease.

Therapeutic Management

Surgery	Correction of underlying obstructions
Medications	Oral or parenteral antiinfective drugs to combat infection; continuous suppression antiinfective therapy may be used to treat recurrent or chronic infection; antipyretics for fever
General	Increased fluid intake; urine cultures to track effectiveness of antiinfective drugs
Education	Instruction in preventing infection (cleansing perineum, proper wiping technique, adequate fluid intake, cleansing after sexual activity)

P

Rabies ⚠

An acute, viral, infectious, communicable disease of the central nervous system (CNS) characterized by CNS irritation, paralysis, and death

Etiology and Incidence

The causative agent is a neurotropic rhabdovirus, which is often present in the saliva of infected animals and is usually transmitted to humans through the bite of a rabid animal. Dogs are the most common source of infection, but bats, raccoons, skunks, foxes, cats, and cattle are all known to carry rabies. Rabies is fairly rare in the United States where vaccination has largely eliminated canine rabies. Rabid dogs are prevalent in Latin America, Africa, and Asia where they are a health risk to humans.

Pathophysiology

The virus travels from the site of entry via the peripheral nerves to the spinal cord and brain, where it incubates for 10 days to 1 year. It then multiplies and travels from the CNS through the efferent nerves to many body tissues, including the salivary glands, saliva, urine, cerebrospinal fluid (CSF), corneal cells, and skin. It causes vessel engorgement, edema, and punctate hemorrhages in the meninges and the brain, and diffuse degenerative changes occur in the neurons of the brain and spinal cord. Negri bodies may be formed in the hippocampus or neurons in the cerebellum, cortex, and spinal cord.

Clinical Manifestations

Signs and symptoms manifest in three stages: a prodrome (lasts 1 to 10 days), acute neurological or furious rabies (lasts 2 to 7 days), and paralytic or dumb rabies.

Incubation	Itching, hyperesthesia, and pain radiating from the bite wound
Prodrome	Headache, nausea, fever, chills, apathy, malaise, anxiety, irritability, restlessness, depression

Acute	Agitation, excessive salivation, marked motor activity followed by laryngeal and pharyngeal spasms, dysphagia, and hydrophobia; 1- to 5-minute periods of thrashing, hallucination, biting, seizures, and disorientation, followed by calmness and lucidity; autonomic hyperactivity with supraventricular arrhythmias, deregulated blood pressure (BP), and tachypnea
Paralytic	Progressive paralysis in an ascending fashion, with ensuing coma and death, usually within 12 days of symptom onset

Complications

⚑ Death is almost certain without prompt treatment. It is usually caused by fluid depletion and cardiovascular or respiratory collapse and may occur during the acute or paralytic stage.

Diagnostic Tests

Diagnosis is difficult in humans before the onset of symptoms, and virus isolation and antibody testing, although effective, may not show positive results until after the individual dies. An animal bite in humans should trigger immediate action. If the bite is from an apparently healthy domestic animal, the animal should be held for 10 days for observation in case of rabies symptoms. If the animal is rabid or suspected of being rabid, it should be killed immediately and its brain subjected to a fluorescent antibody test and viral isolation. If the bite is from a wild animal, such as a skunk, raccoon, bat, fox, or other carnivore, the animal should be considered rabid unless it is available for testing and test results are negative, or the geographic area is free of rabies.

Therapeutic Management

Surgery	None
Medications	Rabies vaccine (active immunity) and rabies immune globulin (passive immunity) administered prophylactically after a bite from an animal suspected of being or tested as rabid

General	Immediate cleansing of the wound with soap and water, flushing of deep puncture wounds as prophylaxis; once symptoms develop, treatment is supportive only to control respiratory, circulatory, and CNS damage; individual should be placed in isolation, and staff should use precautions in handling body secretions
Prevention/ Promotion	Preexposure vaccination should be considered for individuals at high risk for exposure to rabid animals (e.g., veterinarians, spelunkers, animal handlers, and laboratory workers who handle infected tissue)

Raynaud's Phenomenon

Episodic vasospasm of the small cutaneous arteries, usually in the fingers but occasionally in the toes, nose, or tongue, that results in intermittent pallor or cyanosis of the skin

Etiology and Incidence

When Raynaud's phenomenon is idiopathic, it is known as Raynaud's disease. There are multiple underlying conditions, such as connective tissue disorders, obstructive arterial disease, neurogenic lesions, trauma, or drug intoxication that cause secondary Raynaud's phenomenon. Attacks are often triggered by stress or cold or are seen in conjunction with migraines and angina. Raynaud's is found in 5% to 20% of the general U.S. population. The idiopathic type accounts for most of the reported cases and is most often seen in young women. An underlying condition, such as scleroderma or CREST syndrome, is often diagnosed after an initial diagnosis of Raynaud's disease.

Pathophysiology

The pathophysiology is not fully understood but involves a severe constriction of cutaneous vessels followed by vessel dilation and then a reactive hyperemia. Catecholamine release and prostaglandin metabolism are thought to play a role in the process. Vessels may thicken with advanced disease.

R

Risk Factors

Exposure to heavy metals

Drug side effects (beta-blockers, ergotamine, methylsergide, vinblastine, bleomycin, oral contraceptives)

Occupational trauma and/or pressure to fingertips (use of handheld vibratory tools, typists, pianists)

Underlying disease (connective tissue disorders, obstructive arterial disease, neurogenic lesions)

CREST syndrome

Carpal tunnel syndrome

Clinical Manifestations

Intermittent attacks lasting from a few minutes to hours cause the fingers to blanch, then become cyanotic, and finally turn red and throb with pain. In long-standing disease, the skin becomes smooth, shiny, and tight with a loss of subcutaneous tissue. Small, painful ulcers may appear on the tips of the fingers.

Complications

Recurring infection, ulceration, and gangrene of the fingertips are rare complications of severe Raynaud's disease.

Diagnostic Tests

The diagnosis is made from the clinical pattern and by abnormal perfusion patterns on digital plethysmography or peripheral arteriography.

Therapeutic Management

Surgery	Sympathectomy for individuals with progressive symptoms; amputation of gangrenous tissue
Medications	Reserpine to reduce vasoconstriction; alpha-adrenergic blocking agents and calcium antagonists to dilate peripheral vessels; use of prostaglandins is under study
General	Avoidance of exposure to cold and mechanical and chemical irritants; avoidance of nicotine, caffeine, and over-the-counter decongestants; stress-reduction programs, such as biofeedback; treatment of underlying causes in secondary disease
Prevention/ Promotion	Avoidance of modifiable risk factors
Education	Education about avoidance of known stressors and irritants

Renal Calculi (Kidney Stones)

The precipitation of normally occurring crystalline substances into irregularly shaped stones, which are deposited in the urinary tract, most commonly in the renal pelvis or calyces

Etiology and Incidence

The precise cause of renal calculi formation is unknown. Renal calculi are common, and about 1 in 1000 adults in the United States are hospitalized with them. Four of five individuals who develop calculi are men, and the peak onset is ages 20 to 30.

Pathophysiology

Certain conditions increase the supersaturation of urine with stone-forming salts, induce preformed salt nuclei, or reduce the production of crystal growth inhibitors. This allows the precipitation process to occur and stones to form, ranging in size from microscopic to several centimeters in diameter.

Risk Factors

Obstruction and stasis of urine
Urinary tract infection (UTI)
Dehydration and concentration of urine
Prolonged immobility
Vitamin A deficiency; dietary excess of vitamin D, calcium, vitamin C, protein, tea, or fruit juice
Underlying disease of the small bowel; an underlying metabolic disorder (e.g., hypercalcemia or hyperparathyroidism); and hereditary disease (e.g., cystinuria)
Anatomical abnormalities of the kidney or ureters

Clinical Manifestations

Many calculi are asymptomatic. If they obstruct the calyx, pelvis, or ureter, they cause severe pain that is typically described as traveling from the costovertebral angle to the flank and then to the suprapubic region and external genitalia. Back or abdominal pain, or both, may also be present. Chills, fever, nausea, vomiting, abdominal extension, and hematuria are also common.

Complications

Large stones can remain in the renal pelvis or calyx or lodge in the ureter and cause infection, necrosis, or obstruction, with subsequent hydronephrosis.

Diagnostic Tests

The diagnosis is based on clinical features plus an x-ray of the kidneys, ureter, and bladder, which demonstrates calculi, and a urinalysis, which may show hematuria, pyuria, and crystalline sludge in the sediment. Intravenous pyelography (IVP), ultrasound (US), and CT scans are also used to locate and visualize stones.

Therapeutic Management

Surgery	Pyelolithotomy or nephrolithotomy to remove large stones in kidney or ureterolithotomy to remove stones in the ureter that are not amenable to other treatment; nephrectomy when the kidney has been irreparably damaged
Medications	Percutaneous stone dissolution with chemical solvents to shrink large uric stones in preparation for other retrieval methods; antiinfective drugs to treat infection; narcotic analgesics for pain; diuretics to prevent urinary stasis; cholestyramine for prophylaxis; for hypercalciuria, allopurinol to reduce uric acid
General	Small, solitary calculi without infection or obstruction may be treated by increasing fluid intake to encourage passage; extracorporeal shock wave lithotripsy (ESWL) is the treatment of choice for stones less than 2 cm in diameter; percutaneous nephrolithotomy is used in conjunction with ESWL to remove stones larger than 2 cm; cystoscopy with basket extraction can be used to remove calculi less than 1 cm in diameter that are lodged in the ureter

Prevention/ Promotion	Increased fluid intake; treatment of underlying conditions; reduction of excess phosphorus, purine, and oxalates in diet
Education	Dietary instruction in restrictions of oxalate and purine intake; education about effects and side effects of medications; instruction in monitoring urine pH levels

R

Renal Failure, Acute

Sudden impairment of renal function marked by rapid, steadily increasing azotemia with or without oliguria

Etiology and Incidence

Acute renal failure (ARF) may be caused by: (1) prerenal factors that interfere with renal perfusion (e.g., fluid and electrolyte depletion, hemorrhage, septicemia, cardiac or liver failure, heat stroke, burn-induced fluid depletion, and myoglobinuria); (2) postrenal factors that cause obstruction (e.g., prostatism, calculi, and tumors of the bladder or pelvis); or (3) intrinsic renal factors that directly impair renal function (e.g., acute tubular injury, acute glomerulonephritis, disseminated intravascular coagulation [DIC], arterial or venous obstruction, tubulointerstitial nephritis, and intrarenal precipitation). About 1% of all hospital admissions in the United States are for ARF, and the mortality rate is about 50%. The most common cause is acute tubular necrosis. ARF caused by prerenal or postrenal factors is more treatable than ARF caused by intrinsic renal factors.

Pathophysiology

Prerenal azotemia results from inadequate renal perfusion. As the glomerular filtration rate (GFR) is reduced, sodium and water resorption is enhanced, causing oliguria. Urinary osmolarity is high, and urine sodium concentrations are low. Four mechanisms may be at work, either independently or in concert, in ARF caused by renal factors: (1) a decrease in renal blood flow; (2) a reduction in glomerular permeability; (3) tubular obstruction; and (4) diffusion of glomerular filtrate across injured tubular epithelium. Other mechanisms are unclear at present. Postrenal azotemia results from obstruction and subsequent glomerular or tubular dysfunction and mimics renally caused ARF in manifestation.

Risk Factors

Age (the very young and very old)
Dehydration
Underlying renal disease, diabetes mellitus (DM)
Hypotension

Sepsis, burns, jaundice

Recent surgery

Multiple organ system failure

Drug therapy (multiple drugs, aminoglycosides, angiotensins, angiotensin-converting enzyme [ACE] inhibitors, cyclosporin, cisplatin)

Exposure to heavy metals, radiographic contrast media

Clinical Manifestations

Prerenal	Nausea, vomiting, diarrhea, decreased tissue turgor, dry mucous membranes, bad taste in the mouth, oliguria, somnolence, fatigue, hypotension, tachycardia
Renal	Nocturia, fatigue, decreased mental acuity, fever, skin rash, edema, headache, anorexia, nausea, vomiting, oliguria or anuria, weight gain, rales, hypertension (HTN)
Postrenal	Renal signs plus difficulty voiding, changes in urine flow, possibly flank pain

Complications

ARF can lead to 🚫 renal shutdown, which affects all other body systems, and if left untreated leads to death. Even with treatment, pulmonary edema, hypertensive crisis, acidosis, hyperkalemia, and infection are common, and death occurs in as many as 50% of all diagnosed cases.

Diagnostic Tests

Diagnosis is directed to classification of the condition as prerenal, renal, or postrenal.

Urine	*Prerenal:* Decreased pH, urine sodium, and oliguria; increased specific gravity; normal results for creatinine and sediment
	Renal: Decreased specific gravity, increased urine sodium and creatinine, oliguria or normal volume, sediment contains casts, pyuria

	Postrenal: Normal specific gravity, urine sodium, and creatinine test results; sediment test results normal or hematuria possible
Serum	Decreased pH, calcium, and bicarbonate; increased potassium, chloride, phosphate, BUN, creatinine, and osmolality; sodium test results normal or decreased; Hgb and Hct elevated with dehydration and decreased with hypervolemia; decreased adhesiveness of platelets
US/CT Scan	Kidneys may be enlarged
Renal Scan/ IV Urogram	To visualize obstructions, tumors, and masses

Therapeutic Management

Surgery	Renal transplantation when cause is renal and unresponsive to other treatment
Medications	Alkalinizing agents for acidosis; potassium-removing resins for hyperkalemia; vasodilators, angiotensin antagonists, or calcium antagonists to treat HTN; diuretics in prerenal disease to increase perfusion unless oliguria is present; dopamine if vasopressor is needed; antiinfective drugs for associated infections (only antibiotics excreted primarily by the liver are used)
General	Limitation of all drugs that require renal excretion; balance of fluid intake and output (I&O), avoiding fluid overload; high-carbohydrate, low-protein feedings, essential amino acid replacement by IV and at least 100 g glucose per day; decreased potassium and sodium intake if levels are elevated; vitamin supplements; careful management of skin care to reduce dryness and prevent injury or infection; careful monitoring of I&O, weight, electrolytes, vital signs, cardiac status, and mental status; peritoneal or

	hemodialysis treatment of choice when milder measures fail
Education	Information about dietary and fluid restrictions, medications, and dialysis

Renal Failure, Chronic

Slow, insidious, and irreversible impairment of renal excretory and regulatory function

Etiology and Incidence

The causes of chronic renal failure (CRF) include chronic glomerular disease (e.g., glomerulonephritis); chronic infection (e.g., pyelonephritis or tuberculosis [TB]); congenital anomalies (e.g., polycystic kidneys); vascular disease (e.g., hypertension [HTN]); endocrine disease (e.g., diabetes mellitus [DM]); collagen disease (e.g., systemic lupus erythematosus [SLE]); obstructive processes (e.g., calculi); and nephrotoxins. The number of persons diagnosed with end-stage renal disease is increasing by about 8% a year in the United States. More than 250,000 patients receive renal dialysis treatments each year.

Pathophysiology

In CRF, the renal system experiences ischemia, inflammation, necrosis, fibrosis, sclerosis, and scarring. Nephrons are permanently destroyed, and the kidneys become unable to respond to excessive or decreased salt and fluid intake. Synthesis of erythropoietin diminishes, and the kidneys are unable to excrete end products of metabolism. CRF occurs in three stages: diminished renal reserve, then renal insufficiency, and finally renal failure and uremia. As failure is occurring, a number of substances that are normally excreted accumulate in the body, including nitrogenous waste, electrolytes, and uremic toxins. Eventually all organ systems are affected.

Clinical Manifestations

Individuals with diminished renal reserve are asymptomatic. Those with moderate renal insufficiency may have only vague symptoms such as nocturia or fatigue. Lassitude and decreased mental acuity are often the first signs of CRF. These may be followed by neuromuscular twitching, cramps, and seizure activity. Anorexia, nausea, vomiting, stomatitis, and a metallic taste in the mouth are uniformly present. Advanced disease symptoms include tissue wasting; itching, uremic frost, and yellow-brown discoloration of the skin; gastrointestinal (GI) bleeding; HTN; and coma.

Complications

All organ systems are affected by end-stage renal disease, and ◐ death is imminent without renal transplantation, although life may be prolonged with dialysis.

Diagnostic Tests

Urine	Acidic pH, low osmolality, fixed specific gravity, proteinuria, casts; WBCs and RBCs may be present in sediment
Serum	Decreased pH, bicarbonate, magnesium; increased potassium, sodium, hydrogen, phosphate, calcium ions; increased uric acid, BUN, osmolality; decreased iron and iron-binding capacity; decreased creatinine clearance
CBC	Decreased Hgb, Hct, and RBC survival time; reduced platelets and decreased adhesiveness
X-rays/US of Renal System	Small, contracted kidneys

Therapeutic Management

Surgery	Renal transplantation; insertion of Tenckhoff catheter for peritoneal dialysis; insertion of internal arteriovenous fistula for hemodialysis
Medications	Alkalinizing agents for acidosis; potassium-removing resins for hyperkalemia; antihypertensives for HTN; diuretics for edema and HTN; phosphate binders for hyperphosphatemia; antiinfective drugs for infection; anticonvulsants for seizures; antiemetics for nausea; H_2-receptor antagonists for GI irritation; antipruritics for itching; laxatives and stool softeners for constipation; calcium, iron, and vitamin replacements

General   Diet low in protein, sodium, potassium, and phosphate, high in calories and calcium, and supplemented with essential amino acids; balanced fluid intake and output; monitoring of intake and output (I&O), weight changes, vital signs, electrolytes, and cardiac and mental status; careful skin care; energy conservation with activities of daily living (ADLs); peritoneal dialysis or hemodialysis to treat end-stage disease; long-term emotional support, counseling for adaptation to chronic, potentially fatal disease

Education   Information about dietary and fluid restrictions, medications, skin care, energy conservation, and dialysis

Respiratory Distress Syndrome
(Hyaline Membrane Disease)

Self-limiting respiratory dysfunction that causes manifestations of respiratory distress in premature infants

Etiology and Incidence

Respiratory distress syndrome (RDS) is caused by a lack of pulmonary surfactant secondary to a developmental delay in lung maturation. It is seen almost exclusively in premature infants. It is the number one cause of infant death in the United States. Incidence rises as birth weight decreases. The incidence of RDS in infants weighing less than 1500 grams is 40% to 60%.

Pathophysiology

Premature infants are born with inadequate pulmonary surfactant production and abnormal surfactant composition and function. Lack of surfactant causes unequal inflation of the alveoli on inspiration and collapse of alveoli on expiration so that infants expend a great effort to inflate their lungs. This ventilation perfusion imbalance, loss of functional residual capacity, and progressive atelectasis lead to decreased oxygenation, cyanosis, and metabolic or respiratory alkalosis. This in turn leads to an increase in pulmonary vascular resistance, which can lead to a patent ductus arteriosus or foramen ovale. The immature development of the lung functions, numerous underdeveloped alveoli, limited pulmonary blood flow, an immature capillary network, weak respiratory muscles, and an overly compliant chest wall in premature infants all contribute to the problem.

R

Risk Factors

Premature infants (less than 37 weeks) of decreasing birth weight
Fetal asphyxia
Multiple births
Maternal factors (e.g., diabetes mellitus [DM], bleeding in third trimester, hypotension)
Male gender and/or Caucasian race of infant
Familial tendency

Clinical Manifestations

Signs and symptoms usually appear within 6 hours of birth and include rapid respirations, nostril flaring, expiratory grunting, chest retractions, labored breathing, frothing at lips, inspiratory crackles, cyanosis, and weak cry. These progress to apnea, flaccidity, unresponsiveness, mottling, peripheral edema, oliguria, hypotension, and bradycardia.

Complications

Possible complications include intraventricular hemorrhage, tension pneumothorax, retinopathy of prematurity, bronchopulmonary dysplasia, apnea, patent ductus arteriosus (PDA), congestive heart failure (CHF), neurological sequelae, necrotizing enterocolitis, pneumonia, sepsis, and/or death.

Diagnostic Tests

Clinical Evaluation	Evidence of clinical manifestations
X-rays	Diffuse granular pattern in bilateral lung fields indicating atelectasis, and bronchograms representing dilated air-filled bronchioles
Blood Gases	To determine extent of respiratory function and acid-base imbalances
Pulmonary Function Studies	To differentiate pulmonary and extrapulmonary illness and manage disease

Therapeutic Management

Surgery	None
Medications	Exogenous surfactant administered as soon as possible after birth
General	Supportive care in intensive care unit; warm, humidified oxygen by oxygen hood or mechanical ventilation; careful monitoring of respiratory, circulatory, acid-base, and electrolyte status; parenteral therapy for nutrition (*nipple and gavage feeding contraindicated*); parental support;

	long-term follow-up for neurological and respiratory sequelae
Prevention/ Promotion	Betamethasone injection to mother 24 to 48 hours before delivery of any premature infant 24 to 34 weeks in gestation; careful control of maternal DM; early and consistent prenatal care
Education	Education for parents about self-limiting nature of disease; information about available resources

Respiratory Syncytial Virus (RSV) Infection

(See Bronchiolitis/Respiratory Synctial Virus [RSV])

R

Retinal Detachment

Separation of the sensory layers of the retina from the pigmented epithelium

Etiology and Incidence

The most common cause is a hole or tear in the retina. Other causes may be seepage of vitreous fluid into the subretinal space as a result of inflammation, choroidal tumors, or systemic disease. Detachment may also occur as a result of vitreous traction placed on the inner lining of the retina from the contraction of fibrous band formations associated with diabetic retinopathy, sickle cell disease, or other retinal degeneration. Retinal detachment is most common after age 40 unless it is associated with trauma.

Pathophysiology

As vitreous fluid fills the subretinal space, the sensory layers of the retina progressively pull away from the pigmented epithelium. Separation may occur suddenly or may develop slowly over years.

Risk Factors

Degenerative changes associated with aging
Myopia
Cataract surgery
Trauma
Gender (twice as common in males)
History of retinopathy of prematurity, diabetic retinopathy

Clinical Manifestations

Retinal detachment may be totally asymptomatic until the macular area is invaded, reducing central vision and often fracturing images. Lightning flashes or floaters also may be present, particularly if separation is fairly rapid.

Complications

Untreated detachments may lead to severe vision impairment or blindness.

Diagnostic Tests

The diagnosis is made by indirect ophthalmoscopy, which reveals tears, breaks, and detachment.

Therapeutic Management

Surgery	Photocoagulation, diathermy, or cryothermy to burn or freeze tear margins and to promote inflammation and scarring to seal the hole or tear *Scleral buckle:* An implant is used to encircle the eyeball, indent the sclera, and draw it flat against the retina in cases of large or multiple holes or tears
Medications	Mydriatics to dilate the pupil before and after surgery, prophylactic antiinfective drugs to prevent uveitis, steroids to control inflammation, antacids to prevent gastric irritation from steroids, narcotic analgesics to aid in maintaining sustained positions with scleral buckle, stool softeners for 4 to 6 weeks to prevent constipation
General	Eye patches 1 to 2 days after surgery to promote rest of the eyes; with scleral buckle, strict bed rest and specific head positioning to promote adhesion (position is maintained with foam wedges for 4 to 5 days); orientation measures if eyes are bilaterally patched; avoidance of heavy lifting, vigorous exercise, and head jarring
Prevention/ Promotion	Use of protective eyewear to prevent trauma in hazardous occupational settings
Education	Instruction in avoidance of heavy lifting, bending, head jarring, straining at stool, and vigorous exercise for 6 to 8 weeks after repair

R

Rheumatic Fever (RF)

A nonsuppurative, acute inflammatory complication from a group A streptococcal infection characterized by lesions in the connective tissue of the joints, heart, central nervous system (CNS), and subcutaneous tissue.

Etiology and Incidence

The causative agent of RF is a group A streptococcus, and the disease usually is a delayed complication of an upper respiratory infection (URI). The role of predisposing host and environmental factors is unclear. Malnutrition and overcrowding seem to be factors. However, recent outbreaks in the United States tend to be among white middle-class children and young adults. An autoimmune theory and genetic predisposition have also been hypothesized. More than 2 million cases are reported annually in the United States, and more than 5000 deaths occur from the disease. Children are most susceptible, and the disease is twice as common among females.

Pathophysiology

A week to a month after a streptococcal throat infection, the streptococcal agent begins to damage the cardiac connective tissue by forming lesions that fragment the collagen fibers, infiltrate cellular lymphocytes, and leave fibrin deposits. Aschoff's nodules (bullous hemorrhagic lesions) then develop, surrounded by large mononuclear and polymorphonuclear leukocytes, and the result is pericarditis, myocarditis, and left-sided endocarditis. The leaflets and chordae of the heart valves are infiltrated and thicken, resulting in stenosis and insufficiency. Joint tissue is infiltrated by lesions and Aschoff's nodules, causing a polyarthritis that is reversible and migratory, favors large joints, and lasts 1 to 2 days in the affected joint before moving on. Subcutaneous nodules may form under the skin over bony prominences, and a transient nonpruritic rash (erythema marginatum) may form on the trunk and proximal regions of the extremities. The CNS may also become involved, since streptococcal antigens cause cross-reactive antibodies to bind to the nerve tissue, where damage is caused by lymphocytes. After the damage occurs, as long as 6 months may lapse before the onset of chorea, which causes involuntary, purposeless, nonrepetitive movements that subside without neurological deficit in 3 to 6 months.

Clinical Manifestations

The five major manifestations of RF (carditis, polyarthritis, subcutaneous nodules, erythema marginatum, and chorea) can appear alone or in combination, producing a number of clinical disease patterns. Signs and symptoms of each of the major manifestations are given below.

General	Low-grade fever, anorexia, malaise, pallor, weight loss, abdominal pain that mimics appendicitis
Carditis	Tachycardia, gallop rhythm, effusion, diastolic murmurs, cardiac enlargement, pericardial friction rubs, congestive heart failure (CHF), high-pitched apical murmur of mitral regurgitation, low-pitched apical middiastolic flow murmur, diastolic murmur from aortic regurgitation, mitral and aortic stenotic murmurs with chronic valvular disease
Polyarthritis	Heat, swelling, redness, and severe tenderness of major joints, with migration from joint to joint, lasting 1 to 2 days and then moving on for about 1 month
Subcutaneous Nodules	Firm, painless nodules 0.5 to 1 cm in diameter that are found in crops over bony prominences and that persist 1 to 2 weeks before resolving gradually
Erythema Marginatum	Nonpruritic macular eruptions on the trunk and proximal extremities; individual lesions clear within hours, but the rash may persist for months
Chorea	Involuntary, purposeless, rapid movements of the extremities, facial grimaces, speech disturbances, muscle weakness, and emotional lability

R

These conditions develop up to 6 months after other symptoms and last about 2 weeks before gradually subsiding.

Complications

Rheumatic heart disease caused by damage to mitral and aortic valves is the most common complication and may eventually lead to death. Individuals who have RF are susceptible to recurrent bouts of the disorder.

Diagnostic Tests

The diagnosis is made using the guidelines of the American Heart Association. These include evidence of a previous streptococcal A infection, the presence of two of the five major manifestations or one major and two general manifestations, and a positive C-reactive protein serum test or an elevated erythrocyte sedimentation rate.

Therapeutic Management

Surgery	None
Medications	Antiinfective drugs specific for group A streptococci during RF and afterward for prophylaxis; antipyretics for fever; nonsteroidal antiinflammatory drugs (NSAIDs) for polyarthritis; corticosteroids for carditis; diuretics and digitalis for signs of CHF; sedation for chorea
General	Bed rest, then limited activity for carditis; nonstimulating environment for chorea; oxygen and restriction of sodium for cardiac failure
Education	Education about the recurrent nature of RF and the importance of (1) long-term prophylactic treatment and (2) notifying health care personnel (dentists, physicians, nurses) about rheumatic history before treatment for other conditions

Rocky Mountain Spotted Fever

An acute, febrile, infectious, rash-producing disease

Etiology and Incidence

The cause is the *Rickettsia rickettsii* organism, which is transmitted through the bite of an adult *Ixodes* tick. The disease is seen most often from May to September, when adult ticks are active and humans are likely to be outdoors in tick-infested areas. The incidence is highest in children under age 15 and in those who frequent tick-infested areas for work or recreation. It is most prevalent in the Southeastern United States followed by the South Central United States.

Pathophysiology

The organism enters humans through a prolonged bite (4 to 6 hours) by an adult tick. *R. rickettsii* then localizes and proliferates in the vascular endothelium of small and medium blood vessels, producing widespread swelling and degeneration that result in thrombi and vasculitis and affect the skin, subcutaneous tissue, heart, lungs, kidneys, liver, spleen, and central nervous system (CNS).

Clinical Manifestations

The incubation time between bite and symptoms ranges from 3 to 12 days. The shorter the incubation period, the more severe the manifestations. The onset is abrupt and is marked by a severe headache; intermittent fever; chills; pain and aching in the back, bones, muscles, and joints; anorexia; nausea; vomiting; a thick, white covering on the tongue; and a nonproductive cough. Skin eruptions develop on the wrists, ankles, and forehead within 2 to 5 days of symptom onset, and the rash spreads to the entire body, including the palms, soles, and scalp, within 2 days. The lesions become petechial and coalesce into hemorrhagic areas that ulcerate and peel; restlessness, insomnia, delirium, and coma may ensue.

R

Complications

Untreated cases lead to complications such as pneumonia; tissue necrosis, with gangrene of the digits; disseminated intravascular coagulation (DIC); circulatory failure; renal failure; and cardiac arrest with sudden death.

Diagnostic Tests

The diagnosis is made through a history of a tick bite, a pattern of symptoms, and blood cultures that isolate the causative agent. Immunofluorescent tests that detect the organism in a punch biopsy of affected cutaneous tissue are also used.

Therapeutic Management

Surgery	None
Medications	Antiinfective, rickettsiostatic drugs until individual is afebrile; antiinfective drugs in combination with corticosteroids if treatment is started later in the disease process; analgesics for pain; antipyretics for fever; *aspirin is avoided because it can cause hemorrhage*
General	Rest; fluid and electrolyte replacement; meticulous mouth and skin care; monitoring for complications
Prevention/ Promotion	Use of tick repellent and long pants tucked inside boots in tick-infested areas; careful skin inspection after work or play in tick-infested areas; inspection of pets who play in wooded or infested areas

Rubella (German Measles)

A mild, febrile, highly communicable viral disease characterized by a diffuse, punctate, macular rash

Etiology and Incidence

Rubella is caused by a ribonucleic acid (RNA) virus, which is spread by airborne droplets or direct contact with nasopharyngeal secretions. The disease is communicable from a week before the rash appears to 5 days after the rash disappears. Rubella is common in childhood, but it also affects adults who were not infected during childhood. Infection confers lifelong immunity. Epidemics are seen during the spring of each year, and major epidemics occur in 6- to 9-year cycles. The incidence declined dramatically after the advent and widespread use of a vaccine in the 1960s, and less than 250 cases are reported annually in the United States.

Pathophysiology

The virus invades the nasopharynx and travels to the lymph glands, causing lymphadenopathy. After 5 to 7 days, it enters the bloodstream, causing a viremia and stimulating an immune response that results in a skin rash. The rash lasts about 3 days. Subclinical infection may remain for as long as 5 days after the rash disappears.

R

Clinical Manifestations

Prodrome	Swollen suboccipital, postauricular, and postcervical glands; fever, sore throat, cough, fatigue
Rash	Tiny reddish spots on the soft palate on the last day of prodrome or the first day of the rash; light pink to red, discrete, maculopapular rash that starts on the face and trunk and spreads to the upper and lower extremities
Post rash	Headache, mild conjunctivitis

Complications

Complications include transitory arthritis, encephalitis, purpura, and congenital rubella syndrome. Congenital rubella syndrome occurs in an infant born to a woman who contracts rubella during the first trimester of pregnancy. The result can be abortion, stillbirth, or congenital rubella. The syndrome develops in about 25% of exposed infants, who have such defects as cataracts, deafness, microcephaly, mental retardation, heart defects, hepatosplenomegaly, jaundice, and bone defects. Many die within 6 months of birth.

Diagnostic Tests

The diagnosis is made on the appearance of the rash plus a positive culture of pharyngeal secretions and a fourfold increase in specific antibodies.

Therapeutic Management

Surgery	None
Medications	Antipyretics for fever; analgesics for discomfort
General	Isolation from pregnant women
Prevention/ Promotion	Active immunization in all persons over age 12 months with no evidence of immunity, except those who have a compromised immune system or who are pregnant

Rubeola (Red Measles)

A highly contagious, acute viral disease characterized by Koplik's spots and a spreading maculopapular rash

Etiology and Incidence

Rubeola is caused by a paramyxovirus and is spread by airborne droplets or direct contact with nasopharyngeal secretions. The disease is communicable from 4 days before the rash appears until the rash disappears. Before the advent of a vaccine in the 1960s, epidemics were seen every 2 or 3 years among small and school-age children in the United States. Now outbreaks occur primarily in previously immunized adolescents and adults and in unimmunized children. Slightly more than 500 cases are reported annually in the United States. Infection confers lifelong immunity.

Pathophysiology

The virus invades the nasopharynx and the respiratory epithelium, incubates, and multiplies there for about 7 to 14 days. It spreads via the lymphatics, producing hyperplasia and viremia, which spreads by means of the leukocytes to the reticuloendothelial system. The reticuloendothelial cells necrose and set up a secondary viremia, which infects the respiratory mucosa and produces edema. Two to 4 days after the respiratory invasion, the virus travels to and invades the cells of the epidermis and oral epithelium—stimulating a cell-mediated response and producing Koplik's spots—followed in 1 to 2 days by a skin rash. The rash lasts 4 to 7 days before fading.

R

Clinical Manifestations

Prodrome	Fever, coryza, hacking cough, conjunctivitis, photophobia, lymphadenopathy
Rash	Koplik's spots on the buccal mucosa 2 to 4 days after prodrome onset; irregular maculopapular rash starts on face and neck and spreads to trunk and extremities
Post rash	Brownish desquamation

Complications

Complications include secondary bacterial infections (e.g., otitis media or pneumonia); viral pneumonia; and encephalitis and delayed, subacute, sclerosing panencephalitis.

Diagnostic Tests

The diagnosis is made on the basis of the symptom pattern plus a positive culture of pharyngeal or conjunctival secretions or of blood or urine, plus a fourfold increase in specific antibodies.

Therapeutic Management

Surgery	None
Medications	Antipyretics for fever; vitamin A supplementation; prophylactic antiinfective drugs to prevent secondary bacterial infection in high-risk children
General	Bed rest in a quiet, darkened room during prodrome; isolation during prodrome and rash; skin care; tepid baths; cool mist vaporizer
Prevention/ Promotion	Active immunization for persons over age 15 months except those with compromised immune systems; passive immunization (immune globulin) for high-risk contacts
Education	Instructions to parents to monitor for complications

Scabies

A transmissible parasitic infestation of the skin characterized by burrows, intense itching, and excoriations

Etiology and Incidence

Scabies is caused by the *Sarcoptes scabiei* mite and is easily transmitted by skin-to-skin contact. The mite cannot live long off the human body and is rarely transmitted in any other fashion. Incidence is worldwide and flourishes in areas where overcrowding and poor sanitation are common. Scabies is also common in institutionalized settings such as hospitals and nursing homes.

Pathophysiology

The impregnated female mite burrows under a superficial layer of skin, forming a tiny tunnel. She extends the tunnel daily as she deposits feces and two or three eggs to incubate and hatch. After 20 days, she dies. The eggs hatch and form adult mites within 10 days.

Risk Factors

Overcrowded conditions
Poor sanitation and/or hygiene

Clinical Manifestations

The individual is asymptomatic for 30 to 60 days after initial contact unless he or she has been previously sensitized. In those cases, symptoms appear within 48 hours. The first symptom is severe itching that is most intense at night. The burrows are seen as very fine, wavy dark lines, which range from a few millimeters to 1 cm in length. They are seen primarily in finger webs, on the palms, on flexor wrist and elbow surfaces, in the axillary folds, around the areolae in girls and women and on the genitals in boys and men, on the buttocks, and around restrictive clothing lines. In infants, they may be seen on the face. Scratching causes excoriation, papules, pustules, crusting, and secondary superimposed bacterial infections.

Complications

The individual may have a post scabies pruritus that is self-limiting. Refractory cases may be seen in immunocompromised individuals and those with underlying skin conditions.

Diagnostic Tests

The diagnosis is made from visualization of the lesions and scrapings that show the mite on microscopic examination.

Therapeutic Management

Surgery	None
Medications	Permethrin cream applied to entire body for 24 hours as a scabicide; corticosteroid cream for itching, which may take 1 or 2 week's to subside; systemic antiinfective drugs for persistent secondary infections. Oral ivermectin has recently been approved to treat scabies and is particularly effective for secondary excoriations.
General	Examination of all close contacts for infestation; treatment of all members in the household, including pets; cool soaks or compresses to reduce itching
Prevention/ Promotion	Use of prophylactic scabicide for all exposed individuals including staff in institutional settings
Education	Education about scabies infestation and instruction on proper use of scabicide creams (e.g., application to all body surfaces, leaving cream on for required number of hours)

Scarlet Fever

An acute, contagious bacterial disease characterized by a skin rash and a strawberry tongue

Etiology and Incidence

The cause of scarlet fever is a circulating erythrotoxin that is produced by a group A beta-hemolytic streptococcus. Scarlet fever is spread by airborne droplets, contact with nasopharyngeal secretions, or ingestion of contaminated milk or other food. It is communicable from the point of infection through the active disease phase and postdisease in individuals with sinusitis or otitis media. The disease is seen predominantly in children ages 5 to 15.

Pathophysiology

The invading streptococcus releases an erythrogenic toxin that stimulates a sensitivity reaction in the individual. The result is widespread dilation of small capillaries and toxic injury to the vascular epithelium, particularly in the kidneys, liver, and heart.

Clinical Manifestations

Signs and symptoms appear 1 to 3 days after exposure to the agent, starting with a prodromal period.

Prodrome	Abrupt high fever, chills, tachycardia, nausea, vomiting, headache, abdominal pain, malaise, sore throat
Enanthema	Enlarged, reddened tonsils covered with patchy exudate; red, edematous pharynx; after the first day, the tongue is coated and white with red, swollen papillae (white strawberry tongue) until the white coat sloughs off on the fourth day, leaving a red strawberry tongue; red punctate lesions on the palate

S

Exanthema	A rash appears 12 hours after prodromal symptoms. The rash displays as pinhead-size red lesions, which rapidly cover the body except for the face. The rash concentrates in the axial folds, on the neck, and in the groin and lasts 4 to 10 days; the face is flushed on the cheeks with a circumoral pallor; after a week, desquamation and peeling begin on the palms and soles.

Complications

Complications include otitis media, sinusitis, peritonsillar abscess, and severe, disseminated toxic or septic disease (fulminating scarlet fever), which may cause septicemia and hepatic damage.

Diagnostic Tests

The diagnosis is made from clinical signs and a positive Schultz-Charlton reaction skin test or a positive throat culture.

Therapeutic Management

Surgery	None
Medications	Antiinfective drugs to combat the streptococcal agent, antipyretics for fever, analgesics for pain
General	Bed rest while febrile, respiratory precautions for 24 hours after initiation of antibiotics, adequate fluids, gargles and throat washes for sore throat, room humidification for comfort
Education	Instructions on prevention of spread of disease

Schizophrenia

A complex illness characterized by loss of contact with reality, hallucinations, delusions, behavioral disturbances, and disrupted social function

Etiology and Incidence

The specific causes of schizophrenia are unknown but changes in the structure and neurochemistry of the brain, neurophysiological changes, endocrine factors, viral and/or immune factors, and genetic factors have all been implicated in the cause of schizophrenia. The prevalence of schizophrenia in the United States is about 1% of the general population. Onset typically occurs in adolescence or early adulthood, with the disease developing in males earlier than females.

Pathophysiology

The precise pathophysiological mechanisms that occur in schizophrenia are not known. However, there are a number of documented brain abnormalities (structural, functional, and chemical) in individuals with schizophrenia, including increased cortical folding in the prefrontal cortex, decreased volume of gray matter, excess dopaminergic and serotonin activity, and abnormal activity in the cholinergic, glutamatergic, GABAergic, and neuropeptide systems. These changes are present long before the appearance of symptomatology, and it is unclear whether these changes are genetically or environmentally linked or both.

Risk Factors

Deficits in information processing, attention, and sensory
  inhibitions in young children
Familial tendency

Clinical Manifestations

Characteristics vary in type and severity and onset may be sudden or insidious. Symptomatic periods may be episodic or continuous. Typical characteristics are divided into prodromal

S

(pre/early), positive (excess/distortion of normal function), and negative (reduction/loss of normal function) symptoms and are listed below.

Prodromal	Withdrawal, social isolation, reduced interest or initiative, elaborate speech, magical thinking, unusual perceptual experiences, strange behaviors
Positive	Psychosis evidenced by distortions of thought content (delusions) and/or perceptual distortion (hallucinations); disorganization evidenced by disorganized speech and behavior
Negative	Restricted emotional expression (flattened affect), poverty of speech (alogia), apathy, decreased ability to experience pleasure (anhedonia), difficulty naming or describing emotions (alexithymia), lack of interest in relationships (asocial)

Complications

Symptoms greatly impair the ability to function, interfering with work, relationships, and self-care and leading to social isolation. Deterioration in function is marked in first 5 years with a plateau effect later in the disease process. Suicide is the major cause of premature death in schizophrenics. Comorbid substance abuse is a significant problem for about 50% of individuals with schizophrenia and signals the likelihood of a poor outcome.

Diagnostic Tests

Clinical History and Evaluation	Diagnostic criteria established by DSM-IV require two or more of the following: delusions, hallucinations, disorganized speech or behavior, catatonia, or negative symptoms for at least a month with evidence of prodromal manifestations or social, occupational, or self-care impairments for at least 6 months.

Neurological Evaluation	May exhibit soft signs, such as astereognosis, agraphesthesia, dysdiadochokinesia, muscle twitching, increased eye blinks, impaired fine motor movements, abnormal smooth pursuit eye movements
CT Scan/ MRI	Structural brain abnormalities, medial and superior lobe abnormalities seen with positive manifestations; frontal, cortical, and ventricular system abnormalities seen with negative manifestations

Therapeutic Management

Surgery	None
Medications	Antipsychotics (particularly atypical drugs such as risperidone, olanzapine, quetiapine, and ziprasidone) for control of delusions/hallucinations; sedatives for agitation; antiparkinsonian agents to treat tardive dyskinesia
General	Hospital milieu for early disease stages, crisis care for periods of high risk of harm (suicide and/or violence); supportive psychotherapy; psychosocial skill training; vocational rehabilitation; occupational therapy for activities of daily living (ADLs); community support services to promote self-care; supervised living arrangements; family therapy and/or support and respite care; specialized programs and structured living environments for dual diagnosis patients (schizophrenia and substance abuse)
Prevention/ Promotion	Long-term prophylaxis with antipsychotic drugs for individuals who have had one schizophrenic episode
Education	Individual and family education about disease process; psychosis identification; early symptoms of relapse; effects and side effects of medications; importance of long-term compliance with treatment regimen;

S

instruction in coping strategies to increase daily functioning; information and referral to community support systems that can aid in individual and family coping with the disease process (e.g., National Alliance for the Mentally Ill).

Scoliosis

A complex spinal deformity involving lateral curvature, spinal rotation, and kyphosis or lordosis

Etiology and Incidence

The cause varies by the type of defect. Congenital defects may be caused by a formation or segmentation failure of the vertebra. Neuromuscular defects occur because of an underlying disease process (e.g., polio, cerebral palsy, or muscular dystrophy) or because of spinal cord trauma or tumors. Functional defects occur as a result of discrepancies in leg length. However, 80% to 90% of all scoliosis cases have no apparent cause and are labeled idiopathic. Genetic factors are implicated in these cases.

The prevalence of scoliosis is 4 cases per 1000 persons in the United States. Idiopathic scoliosis usually becomes noticeable during a preadolescent growth spurt and is most commonly found in adolescent girls. Young boys comprise 100% of the cases associated with Duchenne's muscular dystrophy (DMD).

Pathophysiology

The spine begins to show a lateral convex curve in the thoracic, lumbar, or thoracolumbar regions. This is accompanied by a rotation of the vertebral column around its own axis with displacement of attached ribs and overlying paraspinal musculature on the convex side of the curvature, creating a depression on the concave side. A kyphosis of the thoracic spine and/or lordosis of the lumbar spine dictated by the location of the lateral curvature also occurs.

Clinical Manifestations

Visible lateral curvature of the spine, unevenness of shoulders, ill-fitting clothes (e.g., uneven hems)

Complications

Untreated scoliosis may lead to progressive curvature with increasing deformity, premature degenerative joint disease, and cardiorespiratory compromise.

Diagnostic Testing

Clinical Evaluation	Presence of curvature of spine
Standing Radiographs	Confirm and establish degree of curvature
CT/MRI	Used in non-idiopathic evaluation

Therapeutic Management

Surgery	Spinal instrumentation and fixation for severe curves (greater than 40° to 45°) in idiopathic scoliosis and in all curves from neuromuscular causes
	Spinal fusion or hemivertebrae excision in congenital scoliosis
Medicines	Analgesia for postoperative pain or back pain associated with severe curvature
General	*Idiopathic:* Bracing to slow the progression of curvature during growth period; exercise used in conjunction with bracing to strengthen spinal and abdominal muscles; postoperative care: immobilization is dependent on type of instrumentation; scrupulous skin care and pressure-relieving mattresses to prevent pressure sores; range of motion (ROM); physical therapy; emotional support, diversionary activity, and involvement in peer group activity
	Functional: Correction of underlying defect (e.g., shoe orthotic for leg length discrepancies)
Education	Education about correction processes and time involved; instruction in application and removal of brace apparatus, hygiene and skin care; preoperative/postoperative instruction (e.g., cough and deep breathing, log rolling, and cast care); information on community resources, such as National Scoliosis Foundation

Seborrhea

(See Dermatitis [Eczema])

Seizure Disorders (Convulsions, Epilepsy)

Paroxysmal episodes of sudden, involuntary muscle contractions and alterations in consciousness, behavior, sensation, and autonomic functioning; the episodes may be partial (simple or complex), generalized (absence, myoclonic, tonic, clonic, or tonic-clonic) or unclassified. Seizures are labeled epilepsy if they are recurring and caused by a chronic underlying condition.

Etiology and Incidence

The cause of seizures may be idiopathic or symptomatic. Identified causes include pathological processes in the brain (e.g., vascular anomalies or lesions, space-occupying lesions, trauma, acute cerebral edema, infection, degeneration, and neuronal injury); endogenous or exogenous toxic substances (e.g., uremia, lead ingestion, alcohol intoxication, or phenothiazides); metabolic disturbances; febrile states; developmental abnormalities; or birth defects. A seizure disorder develops in more than 180,000 persons in the United States annually. Nearly 2.3 million persons in the United States have diagnosed epilepsy.

Pathophysiology

Seizures result from a generalized disturbance in cerebral function. An internal or external stimulus causes abnormal hypersynchronous discharges in a focal area in the cerebrum that spread throughout the cerebrum. During the seizure, neuropeptides and neurotransmitters are released and blood flow is increased. Extracellular concentrations of potassium are increased, and concentrations of calcium are decreased. Changes occur in pH and use of glucose increases. It is

S

hypothesized that the seizure ceases when the neuronal cell membrane hyperpolarizes and causes the neuronal cells to cease firing, suppressing the surface potentials of the cerebrum. Partial seizures begin locally with a specific aberration of sensory, motor, or psychic origin, reflecting the cerebellar origin of the seizure. A complex partial seizure progresses to impairment of consciousness. A generalized seizure affects both consciousness and motor function from the onset. Absence seizures last 10 to 30 seconds and involve twitching and loss of contact. Myoclonic seizures involve intermittent contraction of muscles without loss of consciousness. Tonic seizures are marked by prolonged involuntary muscle contraction with a 30- to 60-second loss of consciousness. Clonic seizures involve intermittent muscle contractions and loss of consciousness for several minutes. Tonic-clonic seizures involve loss of consciousness with sustained muscle contractions, followed by intermittent muscle contractions and then a limp body state.

Clinical Manifestations

Simple Partial	*Motor:* Recurrent involuntary muscle contractions of one body part (e.g., face, finger, hand, or arm) that may spread to other, same-side body parts
	Sensory: Auditory or visual hallucinations, paresthesia, vertigo
	Psychic: Sensation of déjà vu, complex hallucinations or illusions, unwarranted anger or fear, pupillary dilation, sweating
Complex Partial	*Onset:* May have aura before onset
	Motor: Automatisms (patting body parts, smacking lips, aimless walking, or picking at clothes), unintelligible muttering, staggering gait
	Sensory: 1 to 2 minutes of loss of contact with surroundings, hallucinations
Generalized	*Absence:* Transient loss of consciousness, flickering of eyelids, or intermittent jerking of hands
	Myoclonic: Rapid, jerky movements in extremities or over entire body, which may cause a fall

Tonic: Sudden abnormal dystonic posture, deviation of eyes, and head to one side

Clonic: Symmetric jerking of extremities for several minutes with loss of consciousness

Tonic-clonic: Aura of epigastric discomfort, outcry, loss of consciousness, cyanosis, fall; tonic then clonic contractions, then limpness, sleep, headache, muscle soreness, confusion, and lethargy; loss of bowel and bladder control

Complications

Complications may occur as a result of the onset of seizure activity and can include injury from a fall or from jerking, and airway occlusion and aspiration. A condition known as 🔾 *status epilepticus,* in which motor sensory or psychic seizures follow one another with no intervening periods of consciousness, is a medical emergency. Failure to get immediate treatment can lead to hypoxia, hyperthermia, hypoglycemia, acidosis, and death.

Diagnostic Tests

The presence of seizures is diagnosed by clinical history and evaluation. The diagnostic priority is to distinguish idiopathic seizure activity from symptomatic activity.

CT/MRI/PET	Structural changes
Skull X-ray	Evidence of fractures, shift in calcified pineal gland, bony erosion, separated sutures
Cerebral Angiography	Vascular abnormalities, subdural hematoma
Echoencephalography	Midline shifts in brain structures
Urine	To detect medication toxicity
Serum	Hypoglycemia, electrolyte imbalance, increased BUN, increased blood alcohol levels

S

EEG   *Tonic-clonic:* High, fast voltage
                              spiked in all leads
                            Absence: 3 per second, rounded,
                              spiked wave complexes in all leads
                            Complex partial: Square-topped, 4
                              to 6 per second spike wave
                              complexes over involved lobe
                            Inherited pattern: 2.5 to 3 per
                              second spike and wave pattern;
                              presence of delta waves indicates
                              destroyed brain tissue

Therapeutic Management

Surgery   Resection of epileptic focus or stereotactic
                    lesions in the brain
Medications   Anticonvulsants to prevent or control seizure
                    activity
General   *During seizure:* Safety precautions to prevent
                    injury (e.g., loosen restrictive clothing, roll
                    on side to prevent aspiration, place a small
                    pillow under the head, ease from a standing
                    or sitting position to the floor)

     🔴 *Do not place a finger or other object into the
                    person's mouth to protect or straighten the
                    tongue. It is unnecessary and dangerous. Do
                    not try to hold the person still because you may
                    injure the individual or yourself.*

     Maintain a patent airway; note frequency,
                    type, time, involved body parts, and length
                    of seizure; monitor vital signs and
                    neurological status; reorient individual as
                    seizure ceases. Encourage normal lifestyle,
                    moderate exercise, and participation in
                    sports with proper safeguards. A driver's
                    license is permitted in most states if the
                    person is seizure-free for 1 year. Person
                    needs individual and family support to adapt
                    to seizure disorder.

Prevention/ Promotion	Eliminate causative or precipitating factors (e.g., alcohol, fatigue, loss of sleep, poor eating habits, bright lights, and excessive stress)
	Promotion of general safety measures (e.g., wearing bicycle helmets, stress reduction techniques)
	Prophylactic use of antiseizure medications to prevent recurrence in epilepsy
	Regular laboratory monitoring of anticonvulsant blood levels
Education	Education about disease, effects and side effects of medication, and importance of taking medications as directed and not deleting doses; instruction in relaxation and biofeedback techniques; instruction in first aid during and after seizure activity; instruction to wear a medical alert tag; information on community resources, such as Epilepsy Foundation of America

S

Severe Acute Respiratory Syndrome (SARS)

A serious viral infection of the respiratory tract first identified in late 2002 in China

Etiology and Incidence

The cause of SARS is a new strain of corona virus (SARS-CoV). As of July 2003, there have been 8437 recognized cases of SARS in 17 countries across 5 continents including 45 cases in the United States. There have been 813 reported deaths, with none in the United States. The infection seems to involve primarily adults aged 25 to 70 years, with rare infections among children and the elderly.

Pathophysiology

SARS appears to be spread through droplet transmission. Spread through other means, such as contact and transfer from contaminated surfaces, is not yet known. Clinical data suggests that individuals are infectious when they have symptoms, but whether they are infectious before symptoms appear is unknown. Precise pathophysiology after inhalation is also unknown but is believed to mimic pneumonia.

Risk Factors

Pollution (study reports that SARS deaths doubled for patients residing in polluted areas)

Likely that factors such as smoking, chronic lung diseases, and immune compromise pose an increased risk

Clinical Manifestations

The incubation period appears to range from 2 to 10 days. Early signs are rapid onset of fever (greater than 100.4° F), headache, chills, rigors, and achiness. Upper respiratory symptoms (e.g., runny nose and sore throat) are unlikely. After a period of 3 to 7 days lower respiratory symptoms, such as shortness of breath and a dry cough, develop. Nausea, vomiting, and diarrhea are seen in about 25% of cases. In the next 7 days, mild cases show an abatement of symptoms, and about 20% of patients show a progressive respiratory deterioration with severe dyspnea, hypoxemia, and adult respiratory distress syndrome (ARDS). More than half of these patients have required mechanical ventilation.

Complications

Patients with progressive deterioration are at high risk of respiratory failure and death. High initial levels of lactate dehydrogenase (LDH) and absolute neutrophil counts and an age greater than 60 appear to be predictors of severe disease and death.

Diagnostic Tests

Clinical Evaluation	Centers for Disease Control and Prevention (CDC) clinical criteria:
	Early illness: Presence of two or more of the following features: fever (might be subjective), chills, rigors, myalgia, headache, diarrhea, sore throat, or rhinorrhea
	Mild to moderate illness: History of fever equal to 100.4° F and one or more symptoms of lower respiratory tract illness (cough, dyspnea, and shortness of breath [SOB])
	Severe illness: Radiographic evidence of pulmonary infiltrates or ARDS or autopsy findings consistent with pathological conditions of pneumonia or ARDS without identifiable cause and no alternative diagnosis
Clinical History	CDC epidemiological criteria:
	Possible exposure: Travel to location with recent transmission of SARS up to 10 days before symptom appearance and/or close contact with a person with respiratory illness and history of travel
	Likely exposure: Close contact with person with confirmed SARS and/or close contact with a person with respiratory illness for whom a chain of transmission can be linked to a confirmed case of SARS 10 days before appearance of symptoms

S

Laboratory   Tests to detect SARS-CoV are being refined so lab criteria are changing. The following are general criteria for lab confirmation: detection of serum antibody to SARS-CoV by a test validated by CDC (e.g., enzyme immunoassay), or isolation in cell culture of SARS-CoV, or detection of SARS-CoV ribonucleic acid (RNA) by a reverse transcription polymerase chain reaction (PCR) test validated by CDC and confirmed in a reference laboratory.

Therapeutic Management

Surgery   Tracheostomy if indicated for maintaining patent airway or for mechanical ventilation

Medications   Analgesics for pain; in vitro tests with interferon have shown promise; pulsed steroids may shorten course of disease

General   Immediate isolation (droplet, contact, and respiratory) for anyone suspected of having SARS; supportive care (e.g., rest, humidification, hydration, nutritional support, oxygen if indicated, and mechanical ventilation if indicated). All suspected cases should be reported to the local public health authorities/state health department and CDC.

Prevention/ Promotion   Various vaccines are currently in animal and human trials

Vigilance for early signs or symptoms among those in close contact with SARS cases

Education   Education about isolation procedures for patients, family, and staff

Sexually Transmitted Diseases (STDs)

Infectious diseases that are transmitted primarily through sexual contact

Etiology and Incidence

STDs are caused by bacteria or viruses. An estimated 65 million individuals in the United States are currently infected with one or more STDs. Fifteen million cases are diagnosed annually.

Pathophysiology

Most infections begin as lesions of some form on the genitalia or other sexually exposed membranes in the rectum, mouth, or pharynx. Wide dissemination to other body areas can then occur. All STDs have a latent or subclinical phase. In this phase, an asymptomatic individual harbors the bacteria or virus and can transmit the disease even before they are aware that they have an STD.

For detailed information on specific STDs, see the following:

Chlamydia trachomatis Infections

Genital Warts (Condyloma Acuminatum)

Gonorrhea

Herpes Simplex Infections (Fever Blisters, Genital Herpes)

Human Immunodeficiency Virus (HIV) Infection/Acquired Immunodeficiency Syndrome (AIDS)

Syphilis

S

Shingles (Herpes Zoster)

An acute central nervous system (CNS) infection involving the dorsal root ganglia that is characterized by vesicular eruption and neuralgic pain in various areas of the skin

Etiology and Incidence

Shingles is caused by the varicella-zoster virus, the same virus that causes chickenpox. It is theorized that the virus lies dormant in the dorsal root ganglia after a chickenpox outbreak and is reactivated by local trauma, acute illness, emotional stress, systemic disease (particularly Hodgkin's disease), immune system compromise, or immunosuppressive therapy. About 10% to 20% of the U.S. population will suffer an outbreak of shingles during their lifetime. The disease is more likely to develop in individuals over age 50 and in immunocompromised individuals or persons with human immunodeficiency virus (HIV).

Pathophysiology

The reactivated virus travels from the dorsal root ganglia down the sensory nerve and inflames and infects the skin of the affected ganglion.

Clinical Manifestations

Prodrome	Chills, fever, malaise, gastrointestinal (GI) upset 3 to 4 days before eruption
Eruptive Phase	Crops of vesicles on an erythematous base appear on the skin above the affected dermatome with hyperesthesia, severe pain, burning, and itching. After day 5, the lesions dry out and crust over and may scar as they heal.
Postherpetic Phase	Neuralgia that may persist for months or years

Complications

Herpes zoster ophthalmicus may result in vision loss. A generalized outbreak of shingles may lead to acute urinary retention and unilateral paralysis of the diaphragm. In rare cases, shingles may be complicated by CNS infection, muscle atrophy, transient paralysis, and ascending myelitis.

Diagnostic Tests

Physical Examination	Characteristic lesions
Cytological Smear	Direct identification of multinucleated cells
Culture	Varicella virus in vesicular fluid

Therapeutic Management

Surgery	Rhizotomy for severe, persistent, unresponsive pain
Medications	Topical and oral analgesics for pain; antipruritics for itching; antiviral agents for immunocompromised individuals, the elderly, and those with ophthalmological involvement during eruptive phase to accelerate healing and reduce neuralgia; corticosteroids for older individuals if no contraindications; use of anticonvulsants, antidepressants, neuroleptic agents for severe and/or persistent postherpetic neuralgia; sympathetic blocks for unresponsive cases
General	Wet compresses on lesions, avoidance of scratching and spread to other body regions, cryotherapy or transcutaneous electrical nerve stimulation for neuralgia; hospitalization and treatment with IV acyclovir in disseminated herpes

S

Sickle Cell Disease

An inherited, autosomal recessive disorder that results in chronic hemolytic anemia characterized by sickle-shaped red blood cells

Etiology and Incidence

Sickle cell disease results from a genetic mutation in a hemoglobin molecule that is transmitted from parent to child. If two persons carrying the trait have children, the child has a 1 in 4 chance of developing the disease and a 1 in 2 chance of being a carrier. The disease is most prevalent in tropical Africa and in those of African descent. People from the Mediterranean region, Puerto Rico, Turkey, India, and the Middle East may also have the disorder. Between 45,000 and 75,000 African-Americans have the disease and 2.5 million more carry the trait.

Pathophysiology

The erythrocytes of individuals with sickle cell disease contain more hemoglobin (Hgb) S than Hgb A. Consequently, the erythrocytes become rigid, rough, elongated, and crescent shaped when oxygen tension decreases. Hypoxic conditions or elevated blood viscosity causes a decrease in oxygen tension. These "sickled" cells are easily destroyed as they enter the smaller blood vessels in the body. They accumulate in the capillaries, impairing circulation and causing pain, tissue and organ infarction, and hypoxia, which in turn causes more sickling.

Clinical Manifestations

Signs and symptoms are seldom seen before age 6 months. When they do occur, manifestations are the result of anemia, chronic disease, and vaso-occlusive events known as sickle cell crises.

| General | Characteristically the individual has a history of chronic fatigue, dyspnea, joint swelling and aching, chest pain, ischemic leg ulcers, and multiple infections. Jaundice or pallor, tachycardia, hepatomegaly, and cardiomegaly also may be present. Children tend to be small for their age, and growth or puberty may be delayed. Adults tend to have narrow shoulders and hips, long extremities, a curved spine, and a barrel chest. |
| Sickle Cell Crisis | Sleepiness, difficulty staying awake; severe abdominal, thoracic, muscular, or bone pain; dark urine, hematuria; pale lips, tongue, palms, and nail beds; lethargy; listlessness; irritability; fever (these conditions last days to weeks) |

Complications

Sickle cell anemia causes systemwide, long-term complications, which include multiple infections, hemolytic anemia, chronic obstructive pulmonary disease (COPD), congestive heart failure (CHF), retinopathy, neuropathy, myocardial infarction (MI), cerebrovascular accident (CVA), pulmonary emboli (PE), splenic failure, and renal failure. These complications eventually lead to death. The average life span for an individual with sickle cell anemia is currently about 40 years.

S

Diagnostic Tests

Stained Blood Smear	Visualization of sickled cells
Sickle Cell Prep	Sickling noted after deoxygenation
Turbidity Tube Test	A mix of blood and Sickledex in a turbid solution indicates presence of Hgb S
Electrophoresis	Presence of Hgb S and Hgb A indicates sickle cell trait; presence of only Hgb S indicates sickle cell anemia
Blood	Decreased erythrocyte life span

Therapeutic Management

Surgery	None
Medications	Nonsteroidal antiinflammatory drugs (NSAIDs) analgesics for pain, continuous IV narcotics for severe pain during crisis; hydroxyurea to reduce crisis and provide an increment in Hgb content; iron supplements for low folic acid level
General	Blood transfusions are given in aplastic crisis or before general anesthesia and surgery; chronic transfusion therapy for those under age 18 who have had a stroke, individuals with recalcitrant leg ulcers, and pregnant individuals. Allogeneic stem cell transplants have been a successful cure in some individuals but death rate is approximately 10%.
	Crisis: Hospitalization with rest, hydration; oxygen; monitoring of vital signs; cardiovascular, fluid and electrolyte, and blood gas monitoring; monitoring for signs of renal involvement, PE, and vessel occlusion
	Other: Early, aggressive treatment of infection, dehydration, vomiting, and diarrhea; support groups and counseling for long-term adaptation to chronic disease
Prevention/ Promotion	Routine screening of all newborns with Sickledex test
	Genetic screening and counseling for high-risk individuals and carriers
	For those with sickle cell disease: avoidance of factors that may precipitate a crisis (e.g., avoidance of dehydration, strenuous exercise, exercise in high altitudes, and smoking); protection of extremities from cold; health promotion activities, such as adequate hydration and balanced diet, balance of rest and exercise; measures to prevent infection, such as regular hand washing, antiinfective drugs starting at age 4 months for

	prophylaxis against infection; pneumococcal and influenza vaccines for prophylaxis against influenza and pneumonia
Education	Education about disease, difference between sickle cell trait and disease, plans to prevent sickling crises; importance of prompt and aggressive treatment for any signs of infection; information on community resources

S

Sinusitis

An acute or chronic inflammatory process affecting the paranasal sinuses

Etiology and Incidence

Sinusitis is caused by bacteria (streptococci, staphylococci, pneumococci, and *Haemophilus influenzae*); viruses (rhinovirus, influenza virus, and parainfluenza virus); and fungi (aspergilli, Dematiaceae, Mucoraceae, *Penicillium* spp.). Onset often occurs after an acute respiratory infection but may also be triggered by a dental procedure or gum infection, allergic rhinitis, diving or swimming episode, or sudden drop in temperature. Sinusitis may also be associated with anatomical abnormalities of the nose. Fungally induced sinusitis most often is seen in immunosuppressed individuals, such as those with acquired immunodeficiency syndrome (AIDS), leukemia, lymphoma, or multiple myeloma, or in persons with poorly controlled diabetes mellitus (DM). More than 35 million cases are reported in the United States annually, and the rates are higher among women and those living in the southern United States.

Pathophysiology

Some factor precipitates a swollen nasal mucous membrane, which obstructs the ostium of the paranasal sinus. The oxygen in the sinus is absorbed into the blood vessels in the mucous membrane and sets up a negative pressure (vacuum) in the sinus, inducing pain. If the vacuum is maintained, a transudate is formed from the mucous membrane and fills the sinus, serving as a medium for transient bacteria, viruses, or fungi. Serum and leukocytes then rush to combat the resulting infection, causing a painful positive pressure in the obstructed sinus. The mucous membrane becomes hyperemic and edematous.

Clinical Manifestations

Signs and symptoms include tender, swollen areas over the involved sinus; malaise and slight fever with rhinorrhea, and seropurulent or mucopurulent drainage. Pain is specific to the sinus. Maxillary sinusitis causes pain in the maxillary area, toothache, and frontal headache. Frontal sinusitis causes frontal pain and headache. Ethmoid sinusitis causes pain behind the eyes and a splitting frontal headache. Pain from sphenoid sinusitis occurs in the occipital region.

Complications

Repeated sinus attacks may lead to permanent damage to the mucosal lining and a condition known as chronic suppurative sinusitis. Frontal sinusitis may lead to severe intracranial complications, including brain abscesses, which may prove fatal. Fungal sinusitis, particularly in severely immunosuppressed individuals, can be fatal.

Diagnostic Tests

Culture	Causative organism in sinus discharge
Transillumination	Involved sinus produces a dark shadow (a normal sinus is light)
Sinus X-rays/CT Scans	To determine extent of sinus involvement

Therapeutic Management

Surgery	Endoscopy to create nasal window in acute maxillary sinusitis; Caldwell-Luc procedure for chronic maxillary sinusitis; ethmoidectomy for ethmoid or sphenoid sinusitis; creation of an osteoplastic flap to drain frontal sinus; débridement of tissue in fungally induced sinusitis
Medications	Antiinfective drugs specific to causative agent, analgesics for pain and headache, antihistamines to reduce secretions, nasal spray vasoconstrictors to open nasal passages, adrenergics for chronic sinusitis
General	Irrigation and drainage of affected sinus; steam inhalation to promote drainage; hot, moist compresses to nose to relieve pain and congestion
Prevention/ Promotion	Avoidance of smoking and other nasal irritants and allergens

S

Skin Cancer

Skin cancers can be divided into two groups: melanomas and non melanomas. Three distinct types of nevi (moles) give rise to melanomas: common acquired, dysplastic, and congenital melanocytic. They produce four types of melanoma: superficial spreading (70%), nodular (15%), lentigo maligna (5% to 10%), and acral-lentiginous (less than 10%). Non melanomas are typically either basal cell (80%) or squamous cell (20%) in origin.

Etiology and Incidence

Environmental factors such as ultraviolet radiation and chronic sun exposure in direct interaction with skin type are directly linked to the development of non melanoma skin cancer. Immunosuppression is also an identified risk factor. The precise cause of melanoma is unknown, though ultraviolet radiation in interplay with hereditary factors (chromosomal abnormalities) and immune incompetence is strongly suspected.

Skin cancer is the most common of all malignancies. An estimated 560,000 cases are diagnosed annually in the United States alone. More than 500,000 of these are non melanomas (400,000 basal cell, 100,000 squamous cell), 54,000 of these are melanomas, and nearly 5000 are other non epithelial skin types. The incidence of melanoma is increasing by approximately 4% a year. More than 9800 deaths are attributed to skin cancer each year, and 7600 of these are from malignant melanomas.

Pathophysiology

Basal cell carcinomas vary considerably in appearance but usually begin as a small, shiny, flesh-colored nodule on the skin. The carcinoma enlarges slowly and develops a pearly border with telangiectases on the surface. It often bleeds, crusts, and then bleeds again in a chronic cycle. It rarely metastasizes but does invade adjacent tissue structures. Squamous cell carcinomas are usually scaly and crusty or nodular, warty, and raised and often develop in keratotic tissue or old scars. They eventually ulcerate and invade the underlying tissue. They rarely metastasize, but when they do, the lungs are the most common site. Malignant melanomas arise from a mole that begins to show changes in size, color, shape, and consistency. They begin by growing on the epidermis and then invade the dermis and subcutaneous tissue. Once this occurs, the tumor metastasizes fairly rapidly through the vascular and lymphatic systems. Common metastatic sites include the bones, brain, liver, and lungs.

Risk Factors

Non melanoma	Fair complexion, light hair, blue eyes (i.e., skin that burns easily and is difficult to tan)
	Occupations that necessitate prolonged sun exposure
	Albinism
	Long-term x-ray exposure
	Occupational exposure to radium, arsenic, coal tar, and creosote
	Family history of the disease
	History of chronic irritation or inflammatory diseases of the skin (e.g., leprosy, lupus, granulomas, ulcers, burn scars)
	Immunodeficiencies
	Genetically inherited syndromes (e.g., xeroderma pigmentosum, familial dysplastic nevus syndrome, Bazex's syndrome)
Melanoma	Large number of moles greater than 2 mm (more than 120 moles between 1 and 5 mm; more than 5 moles greater than 5 mm)
	Large number of moles on buttocks or raised moles on arms
	Moles that are atypical (e.g., asymmetrical or with no clear border)
	Tendency to freckle
	History of one or more blistering sunburns
	Extensive exposure to sunlight in early childhood
	History of non melanoma skin cancer, acne, or dysplastic nevus

S

Clinical Manifestations

A skin lesion that does not go away and that grows larger over time or a mole that changes appearance is a possible sign, as are itchiness, scaling, oozing, bleeding from a mole or lesion, and changes in sensation. For melanomas, four manifestations are key in early detection and are known as the ABCD rule.

Melanomas tend to be *asymmetrical,* with a notched or indistinct *border,* variegated in *color,* and a *diameter* of greater than 6 mm.

Complications

The prognosis for non melanoma carcinomas is excellent with intervention because metastasis is rare. The long-term prognosis for melanomas is tied to the thickness of the tumor at the time of diagnosis. Tumors more than 3-mm deep carry a survival rate of less than 50%. Metastasized disease reduces the survival rate dramatically. Common complications include scarring and disfigurement at the site of tumor removal.

Diagnostic Tests

Tissue biopsy and a histological evaluation form the basis for a definitive diagnosis.

Therapeutic Management

Surgery	Excision is the treatment of choice for melanoma. Excision, cryosurgery, electrodesiccation and curettage, and Mohs' chemosurgery are used for non melanomas.
Medications	Topical chemotherapeutic agents to treat premalignant actinic keratosis; interferon to treat recurrent or advanced basal cell carcinoma; hyperthermic regional perfusions in combination with surgery to treat melanomas
General	Radiation in combination with surgery for extensive non melanomas; radiation may be used instead of surgery in elderly patients or to treat non melanomatous lesions of the nose, eyelids, or lips (melanomas are radioresistant)
Prevention/ Promotion	Avoidance of excessive tanning and sun/ tanning bed exposure
	Liberal use of sunscreens with UVA and UVB protection, use of protective clothing when in the sun
	Routine, regular skin inspections using a partner for early detection

Sleep Apnea Syndrome

A group of disorders in which breathing ceases for multiple short periods of time during sleep, disrupting normal ventilation and sleep patterns; it can be classified as *obstructive, central, or mixed*.

Etiology and Incidence

Obstructive sleep apnea (OSA) is caused by narrowing and/or blockage of the upper airway in the presence of airflow drive. Common narrowing or blocking factors include obesity, enlarged tongue or tonsils, underdevelopment of the jaw, hypothyroidism, and use of substances that relax musculature at bedtime (e.g., sedatives and alcohol). *Central* sleep apnea (CSA) is caused by loss of ventilatory effort as a result of some physiological or pathophysiological event. Precipitating events are voluminous and include neurological disorders (particularly those that affect the brainstem); conditions such as congestive heart failure (CHF) and diabetes mellitus (DM); abnormalities in the respiratory control system; and exposure to extreme altitude. Most individuals with central apnea also have some obstructive overlay *(mixed)*.

OSA is the most common form of sleep apnea (greater than 95%) and is seen in 2% to 5% of the general population in the United States. The most frequently affected are obese men over 65 years of age, but OAS is present across all age groups including children. Men are twice as likely as women to be affected. The incidence of CSA is fairly low (less than 5% of all sleep apnea cases).

Pathophysiology

OSA: there is a narrowing of one or more sites along the retropalatal, retroglossal, or hypopharyngeal regions of the upper airway and decreased effectiveness of the phasic inspiratory muscles, which lead to a collapse of the pharynx during the drive to breathe. This leads to multiple (greater than 20) periods of apnea (equal to 10 seconds) each hour during the sleep cycle. These apneas cause pressure fluctuations in the airway, which over time cause pharyngeal muscle damage and hypertrophy. These further compromise the airway and set up a cycle of deterioration and worsening OAS.

S

CSA: the precise pathophysiological mechanisms are not clear. However, pauses occur in respiration, and there is no evidence of ventilatory effort or electromyographic (EMG) activity of the respiratory muscles during the period of apnea. After breathing resumes, there is a return to normal muscular activity, thus implying some transitory loss of neuronal input resulting in a loss of ventilatory drive.

Risk Factors

OAS	Obesity, aging, male gender, smoking, postmenopausal, positive family history, alcohol ingestion, sedative and/or tranquilizer use, supine sleeping position, low vital capacity, nasal congestion, respiratory allergies, use of antihistamines, underlying disease (e.g., Marfan syndrome, tonsillitis, Down syndrome, acromegaly), other diseases (e.g., asthma, chronic obstructive pulmonary disease (COPD), Parkinson's, neurodegenerative disorders, myopathies, neuropathies, hypothyroidism, [DM, arthritis in women])

Clinical Manifestations

OAS	*Nocturnal:* Heavy snoring, witnessed apnea, choking, dyspnea, restlessness, nocturia, diaphoresis, reflux, drooling
	Daytime: Sleepiness, fatigue, morning headache, poor concentration, decreased sex drive, impotence, decreased attention, depression, clumsiness, personality changes
CSA	Clinical manifestations vary by whether the underlying cause of the CSA produces hypoventilation.
	Hypercapnic: Respiratory failure, cor pulmonale, polycythemia, snoring
	Nonhypercapnic: Insomnia or restlessness, intermittent mild snoring, awakenings with feelings of choking or dyspnea

Complications

Complications include slowed mentation, cardiac arrhythmias, heart failure, hypertension (HTN), myocardial infarction (MI), and stroke.

Diagnostic Tests

Clinical Evaluation	Presence of common clinical manifestations; evidence of airway narrowing or obstructions, such as enlarged tongue, dental malocclusion, craniofacial deformities, enlarged tonsils, nasal-septal deviation; measurements of palatal height, maxillary and mandibular intermolar distance, and overjet for evidence of narrow upper airway
Polysomnography	Used for definitive diagnosis of all forms of sleep apnea and to determine frequency and severity of the apnea
Esophageal Balloon/ Respiratory Inductive	To assess and confirm lack of respiratory effort in suspected CSA plethysmography

Therapeutic Management

Surgery	Uvulopalatopharyngoplasty (standard or laser guided) in significant obstruction of retropalatal airway; nasal septoplasty in nasoseptal deformity; radiofrequency ablation of upper airways and/or tongue to reduce tissue mass; adenotonsillectomy for enlarged tonsils; tracheostomy in life-threatening cases unresponsive to other treatment
Medications	Acetazolamide to shift Pco_2 apnea threshold in some forms of CSA; fluticasone nasal inhaler beneficial in children with mild OSA

S

General	Continuous positive airway pressure (CPAP) primary treatment of choice for all forms of sleep apnea; weight loss, removable custom dental appliances, special pillows during sleep for OSA; low flow oxygen, treatment of underlying causes in CSA; atrial overdrive pacing for individuals with nocturnal dysrhythmias
Prevention/ Promotion	Weight loss if obese; eliminate use of alcohol, sedatives, tranquilizers, and antihistamines before bedtime; use of side or prone sleep position; prompt treatment of nasal infections and respiratory allergies
	Routine screening for habitual snoring during health maintenance visits for all children and adults
Education	Instruction in use and maintenance of CPAP machine; education about importance of long-term follow-up and periodic reevaluation with polysomnography

Smallpox

An acute viral communicable disease characterized by severe constitutional symptoms and a classic pustular rash

Etiology and Incidence

The cause is the *variola* virus, which invades the body through the respiratory membranes. There are two strains of the virus; the most virulent is known as *variola major* and a less virulent strain is known as *variola minor*. There have been no reported cases of smallpox in the world since 1977 in large part because of a worldwide vaccination program, which ended in 1980. The United States ceased routine vaccination in 1972. Recent concerns about the use of smallpox stockpiles in terrorist activities have raised the specter of recurrence of this epidemic disease. Because immunity declines over time, most people are now susceptible in varying degrees to the smallpox virus.

Pathophysiology

The virus enters the body by means of direct droplet contact or inhalation through the respiratory system. The virus invades the respiratory mucosa and multiplies in the regional lymph nodes before localizing in small blood vessels in the dermis and oropharyngeal mucosa. Individuals become infectious after the appearance of a classic pustular rash and remain infectious for 7 to 10 days, with declining infectiousness after a crust forms over the skin lesions and no infectiousness after the crusts fall off.

Clinical Manifestations

The incubation period is 7 to 17 days after exposure. After the incubation period, initial prodromal symptoms include high fever, severe fatigue, headache, and backache. A centrifugal rash with flat red lesions (most prominent on face, oral mucosa, and extremities) follows in 2 to 3 days. They become vesicular and then pustular and begin to crust early in the second week. The lesions are domed, firm to the touch, and umbilicated. All lesions are in the same stage of development.

Complications

Complications include residual scarring, pneumonia, blepharitis, conjunctivitis, and corneal ulceration, and the mortality rate is about 30%. There are two variant forms (hemorrhagic and malignant), which are almost uniformly fatal.

Diagnostic Tests

Diagnosis is made primarily by clinical evaluation of the characteristic lesions and confirmed by electron microscopy, Giemsa staining, or viral culture of lesion scrapings. Lab tests should only be performed in high-containment (BL-4) facilities. Polymerase chain reaction (PCR) techniques can differentiate the viral strains.

Therapeutic Management

Surgery	None
Medications	Analgesics for pain; antiinfectives for secondary infection; topical idoxuridine for corneal lesions
General	Strict respiratory and contact isolation during infectious stages; supportive therapy, adequate hydration; mandatory reporting to local health authority in all suspected cases
Prevention/ Promotion	Preexposure vaccination for individuals at high risk (lab technicians, health care workers, mortuary attendants, armed forces combatants)
	Postexposure vaccination to close contacts of infected individual
	Strict isolation of identified cases

Spina Bifida

A developmental malformation of the spine, in which the posterior vertebral laminae fail to close, leaving the meninges and spinal cord exposed. The three common types are: (1) spina bifida occulta, in which the only defect is vertebral and the meninges and spinal cord are normal; (2) spina bifida with meningocele, in which the meninges protrude through the vertebral opening, forming a cyst filled with cerebrospinal fluid (CSF) and covered with skin; (3) spina bifida with myelomeningocele, in which the protruding cyst also contains a portion of the spinal cord and spinal nerves and is covered by a thin membrane.

Etiology and Incidence

The cause is unclear, but the most recent hypothesis suggests a genetic predisposition involving a polygenic interaction with environmental factors, such as maternal malnutrition, alcohol, organic solvents, drugs, toxins, or potato blight. This interaction precipitates a faulty closure of the neural groove on day 28 of gestation. The geographic distribution and incidence of spina bifida vary widely, but it is the most common developmental defect of the central nervous system (CNS). It occurs in approximately 0.3 of every 1000 live births in the United States, and the incidence has been steadily declining in recent decades. It is more common in infants of European descent, females, and those in poverty.

Pathophysiology

During the normal formative stages of the nervous system, a decided depression known as a neural groove appears on the dorsal ectoderm of the embryo at approximately 20 days of gestation. The groove deepens rapidly, spreads laterally, and then fuses dorsally to form the neural tube. Neural tube formation begins in the cervical region and advances caudally and cephalically until day 28 of gestation, when both ends of the tube seal themselves off. Spina bifida occurs when the neural tube fails to close or when a closed tube splits as a result of abnormal CSF pressure.

Clinical Manifestations

Manifestations vary widely, depending on the degree and location of the spinal defect. Sensory and motor disturbances parallel one another.

Occulta	Typically asymptomatic; dimple or hair growth on the skin over the malformed vertebra; weakness in feet, bowel, or bladder sphincter possible as child grows if defect goes undetected and uncorrected
Meningocele	External cystic sac seen on spinal cord at birth; hydrocephalus possible; weakness in legs or bowel and bladder sphincters is rare if defect is surgically corrected
Myelomeningocele	*At birth:* Round, raised, poorly epithelialized sac on spinal cord, which may be bluish and may be leaking or ruptured; hydrocephalus; loss of partial or total motor and sensory control below the level of the lesion; poor anal sphincter and detrusor tone; possible rectal prolapse; constant urine dribbling or urinary retention; possible joint deformities and kyphosis formed in utero *Developing in childhood:* Clubfeet, contractures in ankles, knees, and hips; hip dislocations; scoliosis; decreasing ability to ambulate; incontinence; urinary tract infections (UTIs); constipation; skin breakdown; obesity

Complications

An immediate complication, often seen after birth with a leaking or ruptured sac, is meningitis. Other immediate complications include hypoxia and hemorrhage. Other congenital abnormalities, such as cardiac or gastrointestinal (GI) malformations, may also be present. Long-term complications are associated with motor and sensory disability and include respiratory infection and failure, renal infection and failure, permanent skeletal deformities, and decubiti. In the 1950s most individuals with myelomeningocele died in infancy. Now most have a near normal life expectancy with careful and consistent health care.

Diagnostic Tests

Clinical Evaluation	Pigmented spots, hairy patches, and spinal sinuses seen at birth may indicate spina bifida occulta; motor and sensory function tests determine level of injury in myelomeningocele; palpation of fontanelles and increasing head circumference indicate hydrocephalus.
US/CT Scan/ MRI	To detect abnormalities of head or spine or both
Myelography	Spinal defects
IVP	To detect abnormalities in renal system
Urodynamics	To assess detrusor and sphincter function
Fetal US	May detect major myelomeningocele defects
Alpha-fetoprotein	Elevated at 16 to 18 weeks' gestation

Therapeutic Management

S

Surgery	Repair and closure of defect within 24 to 72 hours after birth; ventriculoperitoneal shunt to treat hydrocephalus; shunt revisions as child ages or if shunt is not patent or functional; corrective orthopedic procedures for contractures, clubfeet, scoliosis (spinal instrumentation), hip dislocations; vesicostomy for vesicourethral reflux; augmentation enterocystoplasty to increase bladder capacity and reduce bladder

	pressure; placement of artificial urinary sphincter or ureteral sling to aid bladder emptying; urinary diversion to control chronic urine leakage and retention
Medications	Collagen injection in sphincter submucosa to control bladder incontinence; stool softeners and laxatives for constipation; antispasmodics to treat bladder spasms; antiinfective drugs for UTI
General	*Initial care:* Monitoring for associated defects and complications; measures to prevent infections; monitoring of patency and functioning of ventriculoperitoneal shunt; adequate hydration and nutrition; normal infant stimulation; meticulous skin care; proper positioning and body alignment; monitoring of intake and output; emotional support of family; teaching parents to hold, feed, and stimulate infant and any special techniques needed for care; physical therapy and range-of-motion (ROM) exercises; safety measures for decreased sensation
	Long term: Consistent medical monitoring by neurologists/neurosurgeons for shunt function and revision and spinal cord tethering; orthopedic surgeons for treatment of contractures, gait analysis, and bracing; urologists for bladder and kidney function; pediatricians for minor infections, bowel program, and coordination; physical therapists for maintenance of ROM, prevention of contractures, gait training, strengthening, and endurance; occupational therapists for activities of daily living (ADLs); intermittent catheterization for bladder control; weight-maintenance diet to prevent obesity and maintain ambulation; counseling for long-term adaptation; case management for long-term support of individual, family, and school; coordination of ongoing care

Prevention/ Promotion	American Academy of Pediatrics recommends that all women of childbearing age take a 0.4-mg supplement of folic acid a day and that women contemplating pregnancy take 4.0 mg daily 1 month before conception through the first trimester of pregnancy. This can reduce the chances of a neural tube defect by at least 50%.
	Use preventive measures to guard against development of latex allergies in children with spina bifida.
Education	Education about disease and functional management; instruction in home positioning, ROM, stretching, skin care, feeding, bowel and bladder programs, shunt care and management; information about community resources; education about high risks for and common signs and symptoms of latex allergy; methods to establish a latex-free environment

Spinal Cord Injury (Paraplegia, Quadriplegia)

An insult to the spinal cord that results in alteration of autonomic, motor, and sensory function below the level of injury; paraplegia involves the lower extremities; quadriplegia involves all extremities. Injury to the cord may result in incomplete or total transection.

Etiology and Incidence

Spinal cord injury (SCI) may be caused by external trauma or internal disease or degeneration. Common traumatic causes of spinal cord injury include vehicle accidents (48%), falls (21%), acts of violence (15%), and sports injuries (14%). Metastatic carcinoma, spinal cord tumors, spondylosis, and vertebral disk degeneration are common nontraumatic causes of spinal cord injury. The worldwide incidence of SCI is about 55 persons per million per year with about 35 individuals per million of those surviving the acute insult. About 10,000 cases occur in the United States annually, and 250,000 individuals are living with SCI in the United States today. About 55% of individuals are quadriplegic, and the remaining 45% are paraplegic. Traumatic injury occurs most often in young adult men 18 to 25 years of age, whereas nontraumatic injury is more common in individuals of both genders who are over age 50.

Pathophysiology

Injury may be direct or indirect. Direct injuries involve compression or transection of the cord by the causal agent (e.g., bone fragments, bullets, or other external debris in the cord; external severing of the cord; tumor growth on the cord, or bony overgrowth of the spine that squeezes the cord). Tissue necroses around the site of injury. Indirect injury involves compression, overstretching, rotation, wedging, or misalignment of the cord, which results in edema, swelling, and localized hemorrhage. This in turn reduces vascular perfusion, decreases oxygen tension, and increases the norepinephrine concentration, producing ischemia and tissue necrosis. Necrotic tissue is removed by body functions within a month of injury and is gradually replaced by connective scar tissue and glial fibers.

Clinical Manifestations

Manifestations differ by level and completeness of injury.

Initial Phase (Spinal Shock)	Partial or complete flaccid paralysis below injury level; partial or complete loss of proprioception, pain, touch, pressure, temperature, spinal reflexes, vasomotor tone, and visceral and somatic sensation below injury level; loss of ability to perspire below injury level; dysfunction of bowel and bladder; impaired or absent respiration if injury is above C5; bradycardia; hypotension
🔵 Autonomic Hyperreflexia	Onset occurs after resolution of spinal shock and return of reflex activity; affects mostly those with an injury at T6 or above; paroxysmal hypertension (HTN), bradycardia, pounding headache, profuse sweating and flushing above injury level, nausea, nasal stuffiness
Long Term	Muscle spasms, exaggerated deep tendon reflexes, contractures, hyperesthesia immediately above injury level, paresthesia, neuropathic pain; impotence, trophic ulcers, dry skin, nail changes, skin breakdown

Complications

The immediate complications are generally life threatening and include respiratory failure, hemorrhage, and cardiac failure. Long-term complications include pneumonia and atelectasis, cardiovascular disease, orthostatic hypotension, severe bradycardia, hyperkalemia, deep vein thrombosis, pulmonary embolism (PE), gastric atony, ileus, bladder and kidney infections, decubiti, pathological fractures, heterotrophic ossification, degeneration of upper extremity joints, emotional debility, and suicide.

Diagnostic Tests

Clinical Evaluation	Absence of reflexes, flaccidity, loss of sensation below injury level; evaluation of dermatomes and muscles to determine level of injury
Spinal X-rays	Vertebral fractures, bony overgrowth
CT Scans/ MRI	Evidence of cord compression and edema or tumor formation
LP/ Myelography	Spinal blockage

Therapeutic Management

Surgery	*Initial:* Laminectomy or fusion for decompression and stabilization, wound débridement, placement of cervical tongs or halo traction for stabilization, tracheotomy for mechanical ventilation if needed
	Long term: Myotomies, tenotomies, rhizotomies, and muscle transplantation to treat spasticity; contracture release; débridement of decubiti; spinal instrumentation to halt scoliosis; penile implant for impotence; colostomy for atonic colon; urinary diversion for incontinence or retention; implant of an intrathecal baclofen pump to control spasticity
Medications	*Initial:* Massive corticosteroid therapy to improve outcome, vasopressors for shock; prophylactic antiinfective drugs for open wounds, analgesics for pain, anticoagulants to prevent emboli and thrombus formation, antihypertensives for hyperreflexia, antianxiety agents to reduce emotional stress
	Long term: Muscle relaxants for spasms, stool softeners and laxatives for constipation, anticholinergics for bladder spasticity

General   *Initial:* Spinal stabilization with backboard or cervical collar on initial transport; mechanical ventilation if necessary; cardiac monitoring; blood gases; intake and output (I&O); vital signs and neurological vital signs; maintain skeletal traction and body alignment; reposition, turn every 2 hours; passive range-of-motion (PROM) exercises; footboard; all activities of daily living (ADLs) performed for person; monitor bowel and bladder function; monitor skin integrity; avoid temperature extremes

Long term: Bowel training using digital stimulation, gravity, high-fiber diet, regularity, adequate hydration

Bladder training using intermittent catheterization

Physical therapy to diminish orthostatic hypotension, increase strength and endurance, decrease muscle spasticity, prevent contractures, teach functional mobility skills (e.g., transfer techniques, wheelchair manipulation)

Occupational therapy to aid adaptation of ADLs (e.g., feeding, bathing, hygiene, grooming, dressing) and to learn use of adaptive equipment

Respiratory therapy to increase vital capacity and tidal volume

Recreational therapy to enhance quality of life

Speech therapy if injury is high enough to affect swallowing or when permanent ventilation necessitates alternative communication systems

Case management for needed resources, procuring and maintaining adaptive equipment (e.g., wheelchairs, electric beds, standers, exercise equipment) and supplies

Long-term medical follow-up by physical medicine, urology, gastroenterology, and respiratory specialists to reduce and/or treat complications

S

	Vocational training
	Counseling of individual and family for support and adaptation
Prevention/ Promotion	Daily skin inspections; use of pressure relief devices, positioning and lifting exercises to prevent skin breakdown
	Diligent use of bowel and bladder programs to prevent bowel obstruction and urinary tract infection
	Regular exercise and weight-bearing program to prevent pathological fracture, deep vein thrombosis
	Influenza and pneumonia vaccines to prevent respiratory complications
	Early recognition and treatment of urinary tract and respiratory problems to prevent complications
Education	Education about recognition of hyperreflexia manifestations; instruction on management of body temperature, injury prevention, bowel and bladder programs, skin inspection, pressure relief, decubitus ulcer prevention, prevention or early treatment of urinary tract and upper respiratory infections (UTIs and URIs); information about availability of advanced wheelchair skills/driver training programs, adaptive equipment; information on available community resources, such as wheelchair sports programs and the National Spinal Cord Injury Association

Stomach Cancer (Gastric Cancer)

Most malignant lesions of the stomach (95%) are adeno-carcinomas. The rest are lymphomas and leiomyosarcomas.

Etiology and Incidence

The precise cause of stomach cancer is unknown, but chronic *Helicobacter pylori* infection, gastritis, gastric atrophy, and genetics are believed to be interactive factors. Food preservation and preparation factors, such as smoking and salting, may also be implicated. The incidence varies worldwide. Stomach cancer is the most common malignancy in Japan, and the incidence is also extremely high in Iceland and Chile. The number of cases has declined significantly in Western Europe and the United States. More than 22,000 new cases are seen in the United States each year, with more than 12,000 deaths reported per year. The incidence is higher in men than in women (3:2 ratio). It occurs most often in individuals ages 50 to 70. The peak decade is for men in their 70s and women in their 80s.

Pathophysiology

Cancer cells usually begin to grow in the distal end of the stomach in the lesser curvature. The cells form a tumor that spreads along the mucosa, eventually invading and moving through the stomach wall. The tumor then spreads directly to surrounding structures, such as the spleen, esophagus, pancreas, colon, duodenum, and peritoneum. The cancer is also spread via the lymphatic system to regional nodes and via the blood-stream to the liver.

S

Risk Factors

Ingestion of nitrosamines and other food preservatives used in salting, pickling, smoking

Lack of refrigeration or poor food preparation techniques

Use of well water with high nitrate concentrations or *H. pylori* bacteria colonies

Smoking and/or alcohol abuse

History of gastric atrophy, chronic gastritis, gastric surgery or *H. pylori* infection, celiac sprue, pernicious anemia, or late onset immunoglobulin deficiency

Occupational exposure to heavy metals, rubber, or asbestos

Familial tendency (mutations in E-cadherin gene)

Type A personality features

Clinical Manifestations

No specific symptoms appear in the early stages. Most people have generalized gastrointestinal (GI) complaints, such as indigestion, burping, and fullness after eating. Later signs may include vomiting, dysphagia, anorexia, weight loss, and back pain.

Complications

The prognosis for long-term survival is poor (12%, 5-year survival rate), primarily because most cases are diagnosed after metastasis has occurred. Complications include malnutrition and GI obstruction.

Diagnostic Tests

Double-contrast x-ray studies of the stomach can delineate suspicious lesions. The definitive diagnosis is made by endoscopy with brush biopsy. CT scans and carcinoembryonic antigen (CEA) and carbohydrate antigen (CA) 19-9 may help detect and monitor progression of malignancy.

Therapeutic Management

Surgery	Excision of the tumor and regional lymph nodes; subtotal or total gastric resection or gastrectomy for resection for cure, depending on tumor location; gastroenterostomy for palliation
Medications	Systemic chemotherapy to treat advanced metastatic disease; vitamin B_{12} replacement after gastrectomy
General	Radiation for palliation of GI obstruction; supportive care for individual and family, hospice care
Prevention/ Promotion	Avoidance/reduction of modifiable risk factors Prophylactic gastrectomy for carriers of germ-line truncating CDH1 gene mutations and a family history of gastric cancer

| **Education** | Instruction about eating small, frequent meals to prevent dumping syndrome after gastrectomy |
| | Education about chemotherapy, radiation regimen effects and side effects; information on community resources |

Stomatitis

An inflammation or ulceration of the mouth that may be locally or systemically induced

Etiology and Incidence

Causes of stomatitis are multiple and include viral or bacterial infection; drugs or toxic agents (barbiturates, antibiotics, chemotherapy, radiation, lead, mercury, acids, and heavy metals); trauma from cheek biting, mouth breathing, or ill-fitting orthodontia; overuse of tobacco or alcohol; sensitivity to toothpaste, mouthwash, food dyes, or preservatives and spices; poor nutrition; and poor oral hygiene. Thrush, a common form of stomatitis, is seen in more than 80% of individuals with human immunodeficiency virus (HIV) or acquired immuno-deficiency syndrome (AIDS). Canker sores are also common and are commonly seen in adolescence or young adulthood. Herpetic stomatitis, the most common virally induced stomatitis, is seen in infants and small children. Mechanically induced stomatitis is often seen in older individuals with dentures that are difficult to fit because of continuing deterioration of gum and bone. Necrotizing ulceration is often seen in individuals using certain antibiotics and in people who have depressed immune systems.

Pathophysiology

The pathophysiology depends on the cause, but it involves a process that creates tissue inflammation in the oral mucosa or gums. These inflammatory changes lead to redness, ulceration, and fissures in the mouth.

Risk Factors

Side effects from use of prescribed drugs (e.g., antibiotics, barbiturates, inhaled steroids, immunosuppressants, chemo-therapeutics)

Tobacco use (cigarettes, chewing tobacco)

Alcohol abuse

Exposure to radiation, lead, mercury, acids, heavy metals

Trauma from cheek biting, mouth breathing, or ill-fitting orthodontia

Sensitivity to toothpaste, mouthwash, food dyes, preservatives, and spices

Poor nutrition

Poor oral hygiene

History of cancer, HIV, AIDS, iron-deficiency anemia, gastrointestinal (GI) disease, diabetes mellitus (DM)

Clinical Manifestations

Manifestations vary by type of stomatitis.

Allergic	Shiny erythema with slight edema, itching, drying, burning
Thrush	White, raised, milk-curd patches; bleeding; dryness of the mouth; diminished taste; pain; fever; lymphadenopathy
Gingivitis	Redness, swelling, bleeding of gums; gum retraction from teeth
Herpetic	Ulcers 3 to 4 cm in diameter scattered over mucous membranes; swollen, inflamed gums; enlarged lymph nodes
Canker Sores	Small, yellowish, hardened, painful sores with red, raised margins that often appear singly or in groups on the lips or in the corner of the mouth
Necrotizing	Necrotic ulceration of mucous membranes with severe pain, increased salivation, and inability to eat; fetid breath; bleeding gums; difficulty talking and swallowing; pseudomembrane on ulcers

S

Complications

Tissue sloughing from necrosis may create craters and other altered tissue topography.

Diagnostic Tests

The diagnosis is made on the clinical history and a physical examination. Cultures or smears may aid in identification of the causative organism in cases arising from infection.

Therapeutic Management

Surgery	None
Medications	Topical anesthetics for pain; antiinfective drugs (topical and systemic) for bacterial or fungally induced stomatitis; topical or systemic corticosteroids or acyclovir for herpetic lesions
General	Meticulous oral hygiene; mild mouthwashes for comfort; treatment of underlying causes; bland, soft, pureed, or liquid diet if eating is a problem
Prevention/ Promotion	Reduce/avoid modifiable risk factors (e.g., stop drugs, alcohol, and tobacco products; avoid toxins; refit orthodontics, eliminate allergens)
	Regular meticulous dental hygiene and dental maintenance
	Balanced diet
Education	Instruction on proper oral hygiene and dental care

Streptococcal Disease

(See Rheumatic Fever, Scarlet Fever)

Stroke

(See Cerebrovascular Accident [CVA] [Stroke])

Substance Abuse and/or Dependence

A recurring pattern of substance use despite adverse physical, mental, social, and/or legal consequences is termed substance abuse. Substance dependence occurs when there are manifestations of physiological tolerance, physiological withdrawal, and/or the inability to control the amount or to discontinue the substance. Substances of abuse include alcohol, amphetamines, anabolic steroids, barbiturates, cannabinoids, cocaine, heroin, inhalants, lysergic acid diethylamide, methamphetamines, narcotic analgesics, nicotine, opium, phencyclidine, etc.

Etiology and Incidence

Etiology of substance abuse is unclear but appears to be multifactorial and includes the interaction of genetic, environmental, and social factors. Incidence of substance abuse is difficult to determine and estimates of abuse range from 10% to 40% of the adult population in the United States. Substance use is definitely on the rise in the United States, presents a major public health problem, and has increasing consequences for the national economy.

Pathophysiology

Substance abuse and the development of dependencies is a complex and poorly understood process. It is a process influenced by the properties of the substances used; the user's predisposing characteristics including physical makeup, genetic predisposition, personality, socioeconomic class, and culture; and external influences, such as family, peers, and environmental and social stressors.

Risk Factors

Familial or past personal history of substance abuse
Male gender, adolescent/young adult
Mental disorders (e.g., depression, anxiety, antisocial personality disorder)
Chronic physical disorder, pain syndromes, or disability
Accessibility, peer pressure

Instability in relationships or divorce, death of spouse, retirement, household income, unemployment
Academic problems, school dropout
Criminal involvement
Lack of support network

Clinical Manifestations

Erratic performance or failure to perform normal roles and functions at home, school, or work. In addition, each type of substance may present with different clinical manifestations.

Alcohol	Alcohol odor on the breath or clothing, decreased alertness, impaired judgment, nausea, vomiting, staggering, slurred speech, emotional impulsivity, uncharacteristic behavior, delayed reaction times, dizziness, confusion, agitation, stupor, hangover
Amphetamines/ Stimulants	Euphoria, agitation, irritability, hyperactivity, chest pain, insomnia, sweating, elevated blood pressure (BP), headache, chills, fever, confusion, impaired judgment, paranoid behavior, seizures, possible death
Cocaine/Crack	Impulsivity, compulsivity, hyperactivity, disinhibition, hypervigilance, anxiety, irritability, dilated pupils, sweating, slow pulse, increased BP, slowed shallow breathing, rhinitis, nose bleeds
Hallucinogens	Bizarre behavior, mood swings, agitation, aggression, paranoia, feelings of depersonalization, dilated pupils, sweating, hypertension (HTN), tachycardia, flushing, tremors, nystagmus, violent outbursts, convulsions, possible death
Heroin/Opiates	Euphoria with tranquility, slowed reaction, drowsiness, impaired function with psychomotor retardation, watery eyes, constricted pupils, shallow slow breathing, decreased muscle tone, increased pulse and BP

Inhalants	Giddiness, silliness, drowsiness, disorientation, slurred speech, headache, nausea, vomiting, increased vital signs, stupor, delirium, coma
Marijuana	Giddiness, laughter, lightheadedness, slow movements, drowsiness, increased appetite, red eyes, increased vital signs
Sedatives	Slurred speech; motor impairment; disorientation; drowsiness; clammy skin; depression; unconsciousness; slow, shallow respirations; weak, rapid pulse

Complications

Secondary medical problems (e.g., hepatitis, human immuno-deficiency virus [HIV], tuberculosis [TB], infections, malnutrition); depression; schizophrenia; suicide; violence; poor marital and social adjustment may occur. Overdoses can result in seizures, arrhythmias, cardiac or respiratory arrest, coma, and death.

Diagnostic Tests

Clinical history and use of substance abuse screening tests
Toxicology and blood levels for suspected abused substances

Therapeutic Management

| **Surgery** | Surgery may be required for treatment of secondary conditions that occur as a result of addiction. |
| **Medications** | Medications (e.g., Antabuse, methadone, naltrexone, clonidine, valproic acid, buspirone, buprenorphine, nicotine replacement) for detoxification of specific substances; adjunct medications (e.g., thiamine, fluoxetine, lithium, sedatives) and medications for specific secondary problems related to substance abuse |

S

General	Detoxification and treatment of physiological complications (e.g., malnutrition, fluid deficit, infection) are the first level of treatment. Therapy, support groups, substance abuse and/or rehabilitation programs, self-help groups, community reinforcement for psychosocial intervention. Support groups for family members; monitoring for infectious disease and other complications. Hospitalization for severe withdrawal symptoms, psychiatric comorbidities, or suicide threat
Prevention/ Promotion	Early identification and aggressive intervention Avoidance of trigger stimuli or uncoupling triggers from substance ingestion
Education	Education about long-term effects and chronic relapsing nature of disease; information about available community resources, programs, and self-help groups

Sudden Infant Death Syndrome (SIDS)

The sudden, unexplained death of an infant under age 1 that remains unexplained after a complete postmortem examination

Etiology and Incidence

The cause of SIDS is unknown. One widely accepted hypothesis is that it is related to brainstem abnormalities in the neurological regulation of cardiorespiratory control, which leaves the infant more vulnerable to various internal and external forces after birth. Despite a 50% decrease in incidence since 1992, SIDS remains the leading cause of death in infants aged 1 month to 1 year, with 3500 deaths annually in the United States. Males are affected more often than females, as are Native Americans and African-Americans and Hispanics. The incidence is higher in the winter, with January the peak month of occurrence.

Pathophysiology

The pathophysiology is unknown, but pathology results on autopsy are consistent and include findings of pulmonary edema and intrathoracic hemorrhages.

Risk Factors

Maternal factors during pregnancy, such as less than 20 years of age, smoking, substance use (cocaine, heroin, methadone), anemia, less than 20-lb weight gain, lack of prenatal care, urinary tract/vaginal infection, multiparity, multiple births (three or greater), short intervals between conception

Infant factors, such as prematurity, low birth weight, intrauterine growth retardation, low Apgar scores, central nervous system (CNS) or respiratory disturbances, prone sleeping position, use of soft bedding, pillows, excess blankets, swaddling, overheating or chilling, exposure to cigarette smoke, bottle feeding

S

Clinical Manifestations

The infant is usually found dead in the bed or crib. The bed-clothes tend to be disheveled, and the infant is often huddled in a corner face down with the covers over the head. The infant's hands are often clutching the sheets. Frothy, blood-tinged fluid is in the mouth and nose, and stool and urine fill the diaper.

Apnea of infancy (AOI), which presents as an apparent life-threatening event (ALTE) with apnea, cyanosis, choking, gagging, hypotonia requiring intervention and/or resuscitation can be a precursor to SIDS and is seen in about 7% of all SIDS deaths.

Complications

The syndrome is fatal.

Diagnostic Tests

The diagnosis is confirmed by postmortem evaluation, including examination of the site of death.

Therapeutic Management

Management focuses on helping the family to cope and on preventing the disorder in infants seen as high risk.

Surgery	None
Medications	Respiratory stimulant medications for high-risk infants to prevent SIDS
General	Intensive psychological and emotional support of the family—from the time of health care contact—for at least 1 year, including time to say good-bye to the infant at the emergency center, arranging transportation home, an immediate home visit to allow family to talk and to discuss SIDS (written supplemental material is desirable), support group and counseling referrals, follow-up home visits
	Complete investigation of suspected SIDS deaths, including autopsy and investigation of death scene

Prevention/ Promotion	Maternal actions while pregnant: good prenatal care, cessation of smoking, cessation of substance use
	Identification and use of home monitoring devices with infants with high-risk profiles (prematurity with apnea, excessive periodic breathing, one or more episodes of an ALTE requiring resuscitation, history of two or more infants with SIDS in family)
	Use supine sleeping position for all infants using a firm mattress and no pillows or soft bedding materials
	Avoid co-sleeping arrangements
	Breastfeeding
	Routine well-baby checks and immunizations
Education	Instruction for use of home apnea monitors and resuscitation measures in high-risk infants
	Information about available community resources, such as National SIDS Alliance, American SIDS Institute

S

Suicide

Suicide is self-inflicted death. Attempted suicide refers to nonlethal attention-seeking gestures and potentially lethal self-inflicted acts that do not result in death.

Etiology and Incidence

Suicide appears to be caused by a combination of psychiatric crisis and social circumstance. The incidence of death from suicide is greater than 30,500 per year, making it the eleventh leading cause of death in the United States. Individuals with a mental or substance abuse disorder account for 90% of these deaths. Rates are highest among adolescents and the elderly. Females make more suicide attempts (3:1 ratio), and males complete more suicides (3:1 ratio).

Pathophysiology

Major depression generally precedes a suicide attempt. Methods used in suicide and attempted suicide differ greatly. Overdose and wrist cutting are the two leading mechanisms used in attempted suicide, and firearms and hanging are the two most commonly used methods in completed suicides.

Risk Factors

Demographics	Male gender, adolescent or geriatric, Caucasian or American Indian, single or divorced, family history
Psychiatric	Mood disorders (depression, bipolar); substance abuse; psychosis (hallucinations, delusions); organic mental syndromes (Alzheimer's, delirium and/or dementia) prior suicide attempts; feelings of hopelessness about future
Psychological	Recent loss of significant other, job; loss of social supports or economic resources; important dates (anniversaries, holidays, birthdays)

| Medical | Diagnosis of terminal illness, chronic intractable pain, chronic disabling disease or disability |

Clinical Manifestations

Suicidal ideation with organized plan and intent; tools at hand to carry out the event (e.g., gun, medication, etc.), discusses the plan with others, affairs put in order, giving away personal possessions, says good-bye to others; symptoms of major depression (change in sleep patterns, loss of interest, lack of energy, inability to concentrate, anorexia); delusions, hallucinations

Complications

Severe disability with unsuccessful attempt, death with successful attempt.

Diagnostic Tests

Clinical Suicide Risk Assessment	Standardized risk assessment using one of the standardized evaluation tools (*Hopelessness Scale, Suicide Assessment Scale, and others*)
Laboratory Tests	Clinical tests for depression: thyrotropin-releasing hormone (TRH) test, dexamethasone suppression test (DST), sleep and waking EEG, thyroid function test

S

Therapeutic Management

Surgery	None
Medications	Antidepressants and other medications that treat underlying cause
	Caution: Provide medications only as prescribed. Do not leave excess medications with individual. Keep all medications in a safe environment away from depressed individual.

General	Ensure that the individual is in a safe and protected environment. Provide frequent checks to ensure that the individual is safe. Do not leave excess medications or other items with individual that may be used to harm self. Provide counseling to determine underlying cause of depression and feelings of suicide.
Prevention/ Promotion	Screening/assessment for high-risk individuals Provision of crisis hotlines Mobilize support systems Take all suicide threats seriously
Education	Information on available community resources and support systems; family instructions about suicidal behaviors and steps to take if behaviors present in high-risk individuals

Syphilis

A contagious, sexually transmitted systemic disease characterized by sequential clinical stages with intervening years of symptomless latency

Etiology and Incidence

Syphilis is caused by the *Treponema pallidum* spirochete. The primary mode of transmission is sexual contact, although the disease may be transmitted transplacentally from an infected mother to her fetus. Syphilis is transmissible by blood in the incubation period and through intimate sexual contact in the primary and secondary stages. It occurs worldwide and is on the increase, particularly in women and neonates. The incidence in the United States is showing a slight rise in the 2000s after a decade of steady decline, and more than 35,000 cases are reported each year in the United States. The peak incidence occurs among African-American males age 30 to 39 with multiple sex partners. A striking relationship exists between syphilis and human immunodeficiency virus (HIV)–positive individuals; one fourth of the syphilitic population in some urban clinics also have HIV.

Pathophysiology

Syphilis occurs in five distinct stages: incubation, primary, secondary, latency, and late (tertiary). Incubation lasts 10 days to 10 weeks and begins with penetration of a mucous membrane by *T. pallidum*. Some spirochetes remain at the site, whereas others migrate to regional lymph nodes and then across all organ systems. The inflammatory response in the endothelial tissue produces perivascular infiltration of lymphocytes and plasma cells, causing edema of the endothelium and endarteritis in the capillaries and terminal arterioles. Vessels thicken as fibroblasts proliferate and cause fibrosis and necrosis. The primary stage is marked by the appearance of a single lesion (chancre) at the site of infection. Serum infiltration and accumulation in the associated connective tissue produce a firm, hard lesion. The lesion heals spontaneously in 1 to 5 weeks. Satellite lesions may form in adjacent tissue or in regional lymph nodes. Nodes are swollen and nontender. The secondary stage begins as the primary stage disappears and generally lasts 2 to 6 weeks. Parenchymal, systemic, and mucocutaneous processes occur throughout the body. After the second stage a 1- to 40-year latency period ensues, followed by the late stage, in which the cardiovascular and nervous systems degenerate.

Risk Factors

Unprotected sexual contact (vaginal, anal, oral) with an infected partner

Sharing needles with an infected individual when using IV drugs

Multiple sex partners

Infants of infected mothers

History of sexually transmitted disease (STDs), HIV, acquired immunodeficiency syndrome (AIDS)

Clinical Manifestations

The disease can appear at any stage without manifestations from the previous stages.

Incubation	Asymptomatic; report of sexual contact with infected partner
Primary	Single lesion starting as a red papule and eroding into a painless ulcer that exudes a clear fluid; red areola around lesion; common sites include penis, anus, rectum, vulva, cervix, perineum, lips, tongue, buccal mucosa, and tonsils; swollen regional lymph nodes
Secondary	Symmetric, pale red (in whites) or pigmented (in blacks) macules, papules, or pustules that predominate on flexor and volar body surfaces, particularly the palms and the soles of the feet; grayish-white erosive patches on mucous membranes; patchy hair loss; generalized swelling of lymph nodes
Latency	May see early mucocutaneous relapse signs but seldom after first year; asymptomatic period that may last rest of individual's lifetime or may move at any time to late stage

Late	Lesions (gummas) of skin, bone, viscera, heart, and nervous system; lesions are indolent, increase slowly in size, and resolve slowly to painless ulcerations that scar on healing; deep, boring pain in bones with lump over involved site; dilation of ascending aorta with aortic insufficiency; meningovascular signs (e.g., headache, dizziness, confusion, lassitude, insomnia, stiff neck, blurred vision, aphasia, hemiplegia); mental deterioration, dementia, delusions; locomotor ataxia; body tremors; urinary retention; impotence; joint degeneration

Complications

Complications occur as a result of untreated disease; they include periostitis, Charcot's arthropathy, aortic regurgitation or aneurysm, meningitis, and widespread damage to the central nervous system (CNS), resulting in paresis or dementia paralytica.

Diagnostic Tests

Serology	Positive venereal disease research laboratory (VDRL), rapid plasma reagin, automated reagin, or reagin screen tests useful for screening in primary and secondary stages (many false positive results with these tests); tests for fluorescent treponemal antibody (absorbed) and T. pallidum agglutination and microhemagglutination done to confirm positive screening tests (they become reactive in the early primary stage and remain reactive in late-stage disease)
Darkfield Microscopy	Result from evaluation of exudate from lesion is positive for T. pallidum in primary and secondary stages
Lumbar Puncture	Positive cerebrospinal fluid (CSF) VDRL in latent syphilis

S

Therapeutic Management

Surgery	None
Medications	Antiinfective drugs to kill spirochete are effective at all stages
General	Mandatory report to local health authority, tracking of all sexual contacts, refraining from sexual activity until result from evaluation of exudates is negative, repeat serological testing after treatment
Prevention/ Promotion	Examination and treatment of all potentially exposed sex partners
	Use of condoms to prevent spread of infection/reinfection
Education	Instruction about STDs and the importance of completing the full antibiotic course and of returning for all follow-up examinations

Temporomandibular Joint (TMJ) Syndrome

A group of disorders of the TMJ structure characterized by pain, muscle spasm, and changes in jaw movement

Etiology and Incidence
There are multiple causes for TMJ disorders. The most common cause is from teeth grinding and/or jaw clenching often related to stress. Other causes include internal derangements of the intraarticular disk; congenital and developmental anomalies (agenesis); degenerative joint diseases (arthritis, ankylosis, neoplasms, or lupus); fractures and dislocations from trauma; orthodontic surgery; and intraarticular steroid injections. An estimated 15% of the United States population has some type of TMJ disorder. It is more prevalent in females and usually occurs between the ages of 20 and 50.

Pathophysiology
The precise pathophysiological process is dictated by the causative agent. Teeth grinding and jaw clenching habits set up increased muscle tonus, which induces muscle fatigue and spasm. Congenital and developmental anomalies and fractures and dislocations produce a shift in the mandible and a severe malocclusion, which leads to asymmetric jaw movements, muscle spasms, and pain. Underlying disease processes lead to inflammation and infection in the joint, which limit jaw movement and cause pain.

T

Risk Factors
Teeth grinding/jaw clenching
Emotional stress
Internal derangement of the intraarticular disk
Agenesis
Underlying degenerative joint disease (arthritis, ankylosis, neoplasms, or lupus)
Jaw fractures/dislocations
Mouth surgery/intraarticular steroid injections

Clinical Manifestations

Common signs and symptoms include muscle spasm and pain at the joint, temples, mandible, or masticatory muscles that worsen with jaw movement or finger pressure on the joint. Cracking, clicking, and popping sounds may occur with jaw movement. Pain may be referred to the neck and shoulders and may be accompanied by headache, tinnitus, and earache.

Complications

Freezing of the joint may be a complication.

Diagnostic Tests

X-rays	To evaluate joint and determine predisposing factor
Occlusion Analysis	To evaluate bite
CT Scan/MRI	To detect soft tissue abnormalities and degenerative changes
Kinesiography	To assess degree of mandibular jaw dysfunction

Therapeutic Management

Surgery	Arthroscopy to debride joint, lyse adhesions, or reposition or remove disk if condition is unresponsive to more conservative management; jaw reconstruction to correct facial deformities and realign jaw; condylectomy to remove condyle; osteotomy to excise bony overgrowth
Medications	Nonsteroidal antiinflammatory drugs (NSAIDs) for symptom relief; muscle relaxants for spasm; antianxiety agents if disorder is stress related; intraarticular joint injection of corticosteroids for degenerative disease

General	Nightguard, bite plate to prevent grinding and clenching; splint to realign malocclusion; moist heat and ultrasound to induce muscle relaxation and enhance analgesia; cold to reduce muscle spasm and inflammation; jaw exercises to stretch muscles; biofeedback or relaxation exercises to relieve stress; soft diet to rest mastication muscles
Prevention/ Promotion	Daily stress management techniques (exercise, biofeedback, meditation)
	Diagnosis and management of teeth grinding before TMJ occurs
Education	Instruction about use of mouth guards, splints; referral for stress management

T

Tendinitis, Tenosynovitis

An inflammation of the tendon (tendinitis) and lining of the tendon sheath (tenosynovitis) characterized by pain on movement of the associated joint; the most commonly affected sites are the shoulder, elbow, wrist, index finger, hip, and ankle.

Etiology and Incidence

The cause is thought to be mechanical overload and/or repetitive microtrauma to a musculotendinous unit. Certain individuals are more susceptible to tendon injury because of a variety of predisposing intrinsic (anatomic, systemic, age related) and extrinsic (workplace, sports, equipment) factors.

Pathophysiology

Repetitive microtrauma damages the fibers in the common extensor tendon of the involved joint, causing extravasation of tissue fluid and setting up an inflammatory process. Over time, healing builds fibrous, inelastic tissue and scarring, which often bind the tendon and sheath together, limiting joint motion.

Risk Factors

Anatomic (muscle imbalance/weakness/inflexibility, misaligned tendons/joints)

Aging (increased stiffness/degeneration/calcification of tendons, decreased vascularity)

Systemic (underlying disease, such as rheumatoid arthritis, gout, sclerosis, disseminated gonococcal infections; pregnancy; obesity)

Repetitive motion (excessive duration, frequency, or intensity) of a tendon group

Improper body mechanics or technique

Poorly fitting athletic gear, such as shoes, protective gear; poor playing surface, such as artificial turf

Occupations that require repetitive motions, awkward positions, vibrations, and/or forceful sudden exertions

Clinical Manifestations

The involved tendons usually show visible swelling; the joint may be tender and hot to the touch; motion of the joint causes pain. Joint motion may be restricted because of pain and edema.

Complications

Rupture of the tendon is a possible complication.

Diagnostic Tests

The diagnosis is based on a history of repetitive motion or underlying disease and physical examination of the joint. Radiology may show calcium deposits in the tendon or tendon sheath. Ultrasound is used to evaluate tendon inflammation, thickening, or tears.

Therapeutic Management

Surgery	Removal of calcium deposits in cases unresponsive to other treatment; release of fibro-osseous tunnels associated with de Quervain's disease; tenosynovectomy for chronic inflammation associated with rheumatoid arthritis; repair of Achilles tendon ruptures
Medications	Analgesics/antiinflammatories to relieve pain; corticosteroid injections in major tendons (e.g., Achilles, patellar) are *contraindicated* because of risk for spontaneous rupture
General	Cold to joint for acute inflammation; moist heat compresses to joint for chronic inflammation; rest, elevation, and/or immobilization of joint with controlled progressive exercise program as acute inflammation subsides

T

Prevention/ Promotion	Use of exercises to achieve balance in muscle development/strength
	Use of appropriate warm-up and cool-down techniques when engaging in physical activity
	Use of proper sports equipment and clothing
	Use of proper body mechanics and technique
	Improved ergonomic design in the workplace
	Avoidance of overexertion, sudden exertion
Education	Instruction in timing for icing vs. heating, immobilization vs. progressive exercise; written instructions with illustration for progressive exercise program

Testicular Cancer

Most carcinomas of the testes are germ cell in origin and are either seminomas or nonseminomas.

Etiology and Incidence

The cause of testicular cancer is unknown, although it occurs 40 times more often in men with undescended or atrophic testicles and is believed to be tied to genetic factors. There is a wide geographic difference in reported incidence, with Scandinavia, Switzerland, and Germany reporting the highest per capita rates. Rates are lowest in Africa and Asia. Testicular cancer accounts for 1% to 2% of all cancer in men in the United States, with about 7600 cases and 400 deaths reported per year. However, it is the most common solid malignancy in males under age 30. It is also seen in infants and men over age 60. Caucasians are much more susceptible than African-Americans. Male offspring of mothers who received diethylstilbestrol during pregnancy are at greater risk.

Pathophysiology

The cells arise from the primordial germ cell and grow within the testis itself. The cancer forms a solid mass and then metastasizes via regional lymph nodes to the retroperitoneum and distantly to the lungs.

Risk Factors

Caucasian race
Ages 15 to 35
Undescended testis (not surgically corrected)
Diethylstilbestrol exposure of mother during pregnancy
History of testicular atrophy (Klinefelter's syndrome, viral orchitis), human immunodeficiency virus (HIV), or acquired immunodeficiency syndrome (AIDS)
Familial tendency

Clinical Manifestations

The most common presenting sign is a firm scrotal mass with or without local tenderness and pain.

Complications

The prognosis is excellent if the condition is treated before metastasis occurs in the lymph nodes. Ureteral and bowel obstructions are complications.

Diagnostic Tests

Palpation, ultrasound, and CT scans are used to locate suggestive lesions. Alpha-fetoprotein and human chorionic gonadotropin serum markers are elevated. A biopsy through orchiectomy is used for definitive diagnosis.

Therapeutic Management

Surgery	Inguinal orchiectomy with or without transabdominal retroperitoneal lymph node dissection is the primary treatment; testicular implants
Medications	Chemotherapy (cisplatin alone or in combination) to promote regression of tumors, making them more amenable to surgery
General	Radiation to treat seminomas; counseling for altered sexual functioning, infertility; referral for sperm banking for future children; follow-up examinations, chest x-rays, CT scans, and monitoring of tumor marker levels
Prevention/ Promotion	Regular testicular self-examination
Education	Education about chemotherapy side effects; sexuality, sexual function, infertility post-treatment; instruction in regular skin inspections for dysplastic nevi, testicular exam for second cancer growth

Tetanus (Lockjaw) ⓘ

An acute infectious disease of the central nervous system (CNS) characterized by intermittent tonic spasms of the voluntary muscles

Etiology and Incidence

Tetanus is caused by the tetanospasmin exotoxin produced by the spore-forming *Clostridium tetani* bacillus. The organism enters the body through a wound contaminated with soil and feces containing viable spores. The incidence is sporadic, and the disease occurs worldwide. It is rare in developed countries, where immunization is common. In developing countries, newborns are at particular risk as the unhealed umbilical cord serves as a convenient port of entry.

Pathophysiology

The bacillus spores enter and multiply in a skin wound to produce the tetanospasmin toxin. The toxin travels to the CNS via the bloodstream and peripheral motor nerves, and binds to ganglioside membranes, blocking release of an inhibitory transmitter. This induces a hyperexcitability in the motor neurons, which results in tonic rigidity and spasms of the voluntary muscles. Once bound, an antitoxin cannot neutralize the toxin.

Clinical Manifestations

The incubation period ranges from 2 to 50 days, with an average of 5 to 10 days before symptoms occur. The most common symptom is stiffness of the jaw. Others include irritability, restlessness, headache, fever, sore throat, stiff neck, and difficulty swallowing. As the disease progresses, the person has difficulty opening the mouth, facial spasms, and rigidity with a fixed grin; opisthotonos; painful, generalized tonic spasms; profuse sweating; cyanosis; and exaggerated reflexes.

T

Complications

The worldwide mortality rate is 50%, and prognosis is poor when the incubation period is short and the symptoms progress rapidly. Complications include cardiac and pulmonary failure, and muscle rupture.

Diagnostic Tests

The diagnosis is made through history and physical examination. Blood and wound cultures and tetanus antibody tests are commonly negative.

Therapeutic Management

Surgery	Débridement of deep penetrating wounds; tracheotomy if necessary for prolonged respiratory management
Medications	Muscle relaxants to treat rigidity and spasm; antiinfective drugs for infection; analgesics for pain
General	Prompt, thorough débridement of wound; intubation and mechanical ventilation if necessary; tube feedings or hyperalimentation to manage nutrition; catheterization to manage urinary retention; coughing, turning, and deep breathing to prevent pneumonia; cardiac and hemodynamic monitoring; adequate fluids and electrolytes
Prevention/ Promotion	Tetanus toxoid with subsequent booster shots for primary immunity; tetanus antitoxin or tetanus immune globulin given at time of penetrating injury with no history of recent vaccination; immediate cleansing of all open wounds
Education	Instruction in the importance of maintaining immunization, with routine booster every 10 years

Thrombocytopenic Purpura

A platelet disorder with a falling platelet count, leading to bleeding into the skin, mucous membranes, internal cavities, and organs. There are two types: immune thrombocytopenic purpura (ITP) and thrombotic thrombocytopenic purpura (TTP).

Etiology and Incidence

ITP is the most common form and is an autoimmune disease caused by the production of autoantibodies to platelet membrane antigens. ITP incidence is about 100 cases per 1 million individuals annually in the United States. Women constitute about three fourths of the diagnosed cases, and ITP occurs most frequently in children aged 2 to 4 and in women under age 40.

TTP is a rare disorder affecting primarily females over age 10 and the precise causes are unknown, but it is associated with platelet agglutination precipitated by endothelial injury, infectious agent, drug side effects, malignancy, pregnancy, allogenic bone marrow transplant, or neurologic disorder.

Pathophysiology

In ITP, the platelets are coated with antibodies. These platelets function normally until reaching the spleen where they are mistaken for a foreign invader and destroyed. Survival rate for the coated platelets is only 1 to 3 days—normal survival 8 to 10 days—so the number of platelets falls.

In TTP, the platelets aggregate as the result of some precipitating event. These aggregates form microthrombi, which deposit in the arterioles and capillaries and produce simultaneous bleeding and clotting.

Clinical Manifestations

Common manifestations include petechiae and ecchymoses on the skin, particularly the lower extremities; easy bruising; bleeding from the nose and gums; melena; hematemesis; heavy menses and breakthrough bleeding; hematuria.

Complications

Complications include hemorrhage into organs such as the brain, gastrointestinal (GI) tract, or heart, which can be fatal without treatment.

Diagnostic Tests

Other platelet disorders must be ruled out

Platelets	Count decreased; size and morphological appearance may be abnormal in TTP
Platelet Survival	To help distinguish between ineffective and inappropriate platelet production
Bone Marrow	Abundance of megakaryocytes
Bleeding Time	Prolonged while coagulation time is normal
Capillary Fragility	Increased

Therapeutic Management

Surgery	Splenectomy for severe unresponsive thrombocytopenia
Medications	Corticosteroids to enhance platelet production and promote capillary integrity; immunosuppressants when disease does not respond to steroids; immune globulin to prepare severely thrombocytic individuals for surgery; discontinuing any drug that may be causing or contributing to the disorder
General	Platelet transfusions for severe bleeding; plasma exchange or plasmapheresis in TTP; safety precautions to prevent bruising; balance of rest and activity; monitoring of platelet counts and bleeding episodes
Education	Education about trauma prevention and safety precautions, avoidance of contact sports, Valsalva's maneuver; instruction in gentle coughing, sneezing, and nose blowing; necessity for increased fluid intake, and balanced periods of rest and exercise; instruction in infection precautions for those

taking immunosuppressants; education about avoiding anticoagulant over-the-counter medications, such as aspirin/aspirin products and other nonsteroidal antiinflammatory drugs (NSAIDs).

T

Thrombosis, Venous
(Phlebothrombosis, Thrombophlebitis)

An abnormal vascular condition in which a thrombus develops in a vein; *thrombophlebitis* refers to a thrombus accompanied by inflammation of the vein (phlebitis). *Phlebothrombosis* refers to a thrombus with minimal inflammation. Dislodgment and migration of a thrombus are known as *thromboembolism*.

(See also Pulmonary Embolism)

Etiology and Incidence

A number of factors acting in concert contribute to thrombus formation, including intimal damage to the vein from indwelling catheters, injection of irritating substances or septic phlebitis; hypercoagulability related to underlying disorders (idiopathic thrombocytopenic purpura, malignancies, blood dyscrasias) and use of oral contraceptives; and stasis from prolonged immobilization, incorrectly applied casts, or postpartum or postoperative states. Venous thrombosis is the most commonly seen venous disorder except for varicose veins. Individuals at greatest risk are postoperative patients and those receiving IV therapy.

Pathophysiology

Most thrombi begin forming in the valve cusps of deep calf veins. Tissue thromboplastin is released and forms thrombin and fibrin, which trap RBCs to form a clot. The clot continues to enlarge until it eventually occludes the lumen of the vessel. It may break off and migrate to the systemic circulation.

Clinical Manifestations

Deep Veins	Calf pain and tenderness; positive Homans' sign (calf pain on foot dorsiflexion) in about 50% of cases; dilated superficial veins; edema; increased size of involved extremity; redness and warmth over vein site
Superficial Veins	Redness, warmth, and tenderness over affected vein, which is visible and palpable

Complications

Chronic venous insufficiency and pulmonary embolus (PE) are the most common complications of thrombosis. (See Pulmonary Embolus.)

Diagnostic Tests

A physical examination is the primary diagnostic tool in detecting venous thrombosis and in distinguishing arterial from venous obstructions. Noninvasive tests include ultrasonography and plethysmography, which show reduced blood flow. Contrast venography is the most accurate and the confirming diagnostic tool.

Therapeutic Management

Surgery	Ligation, clipping, plication, and thrombectomy when thrombosis fails to respond to conservative therapy; extravascular vena cava interruption with possible placement of intracaval filter when emboli are probable
Medications	*Superficial:* Nonsteroidal antiinflammatory drugs (NSAIDs) for pain and inflammation
	Deep vein: Fibrinolytics to lyse clots; anticoagulants (heparin for acute treatment, warfarin for maintenance) to augment thrombolysis; antiplatelets and/or low molecular weight heparin to prevent thrombus formation; analgesics for pain *(aspirin is contraindicated because it interferes with platelet function)*
General	*Superficial:* Moist compresses to treat discomfort
	Deep vein: Bed rest with elevation of affected extremity above the level of the heart; warm, moist packs; antiembolism hose when ambulatory; monitoring of prothrombin time and partial thromboplastin time during anticoagulant therapy; monitoring for signs of PE

T

Prevention/ Promotion	Avoidance or correction of modifiable risk factors, such as regular exercise of lower extremities during periods of prolonged activity (e.g., air flights, car trips, bed rest); use of support stockings; prophylaxis with baby aspirin
Education	Information about anticoagulant therapy and bleeding precautions; instruction in preventing pooled blood in the lower extremities

Thrush

(See Stomatitis)

Thyroid Cancer

Papillary carcinomas are the most common type of thyroid cancer (60% to 70%). Follicular carcinomas account for 15% to 20% of diagnosed cases, anaplastic carcinomas for 10%, and medullary carcinomas for less than 5%.

Etiology and Incidence

There is a strong link between radiation therapy to the neck region (a popular childhood treatment to shrink tonsils, adenoids, and thymus glands in the 1950s) and papillary cancer of the thyroid. Other suspected precursors of thyroid cancer include prolonged secretion of thyroid-stimulating hormone (TSH), iodine deficiencies, and chronic goiter. Familial predisposition (autosomal dominant trait) is strongly suspected in medullary cancer. About 22,000 cases of thyroid cancer are diagnosed, and about 1400 deaths are reported in the United States each year. It can occur at any age, although anaplastic carcinoma is seen almost exclusively in the elderly. Thyroid cancer is three times more common in women than in men.

Pathophysiology

Papillary and follicular carcinomas begin in the epithelial cells of the thyroid, growing slowly and forming nodules in the gland. Papillary tumors are usually nonencapsulated, extend to adjacent tissue beyond the thyroid, and metastasize to local cervical lymph nodes. Distant metastasis is rare. Follicular tumors are encapsulated, invade local tissue and cervical nodes, and metastasize to distant sites (e.g., lungs, bone) through the bloodstream.

Anaplastic carcinomas arise from the epithelium of the thyroid and are characterized by rapid, painful invasive growth to the trachea and major blood vessels, with metastasis to the bones and liver. Medullary carcinoma arises from the parafollicular cells of the thyroid and causes excessive secretion of calcitonin, lowering serum calcium and phosphate levels. Amyloid and calcium deposits are common. The tumor grows rapidly and metastasizes through lymphatics to cervical and mediastinal nodes and to the liver, lungs, and bone, leaving dense calcifications in its wake.

Risk Factors

History of radiation to thyroid gland (papillary cancer)
History of prolonged secretion of TSH, or chronic goiter
Use of steroids
Diet deficient in iodine or very high in iodine
Female gender (three times as common in females)
Familial predisposition (medullary cancer)
Advanced age (anaplastic cancer)

Clinical Manifestations

The most common presenting sign is a palpable, symptomless lump in the neck. Hoarseness and cervical lymphadenopathy may also be present.

Complications

The prognosis is excellent for papillary and follicular cancers if they are treated before distant metastasis occurs. Medullary and anaplastic cancers have a much higher death rate. Medullary tumors are treated successfully only if detected very early, before any tissue invasion is evident; anaplastic tumors are resistant to treatment and spread so rapidly they often cause death within 6 months of diagnosis. Complications include dysphagia, stridor, and tracheal obstruction.

Diagnostic Tests

Thyroid scan and/or high-resolution ultrasound are used to identify and visualize the size and extent of the tumor and calcifications. A calcitonin assay for elevated levels of calcitonin is a reliable indicator for medullary carcinoma. The definitive diagnosis is made through fine needle aspiration biopsy.

Therapeutic Management

Surgery	Thyroidectomy with or without lymph node dissection as primary treatment; lobectomy with isthmectomy in papillary tumors less than 2 cm and no irradiation history; modified radical neck resection for recurrence or metastasis

Medications	Palliative treatment in widespread disease; thyroid hormone as replacement therapy and to suppress TSH production
General	Radioactive iodine ablation as adjuvant to surgery or alone for palliation
Prevention/ Promotion	Deoxyribonucleic acid (DNA) screening for individuals with familial history of medullary cancer
	Regular thyroid evaluation as part of a cancer-related health examination
Education	Instruction about lifelong use of thyroid replacement hormones after surgery

T

Tinnitus

The perception of sound in the absence of an acoustic stimulus, which may be intermittent, continuous, or pulsatile

Etiology and Incidence

The cause is unknown, but tinnitus occurs as a symptom in nearly every disorder of the ear. Contributory factors include obstruction of the external ear canal; infection and inflammation; use of certain drugs (salicylates, quinine, aminoglycoside antibiotics, thiazide diuretics); exposure to certain toxins (carbon monoxide, heavy metals, alcohol); damage to cranial nerve VIII; underlying cardiovascular disease, anemia, or hypothyroidism; acoustic or head trauma. An estimated 30 million individuals in the United States are thought to suffer from tinnitus.

Pathophysiology

The pathophysiological mechanisms of tinnitus remain obscure.

Clinical Manifestations

The primary manifestation is a sound variously described as ringing, roaring, sizzling, whistling, humming, buzzing, hissing, or clicking. It may be intermittent, continuous, or pulsatile and may be accompanied by a hearing loss.

Complications

Tinnitus that is loud, high pitched, and continuous has been known to drive some individuals to attempt suicide if treatment fails.

Diagnostic Tests

An audiological evaluation is done to rule out underlying systemic disease or disease of the ear known to produce tinnitus. The evaluation will also reveal any hearing loss. Measurements of tone masking also are done. Pulsatile tinnitus calls for a work-up of the vascular system for aneurysm, obstruction, and neoplasm.

Therapeutic Management

Surgery	None
Medications	Antianxiety agents, benzodiazepines, antidepressants may help
General	Correction of any associated hearing loss; treatment of underlying disease; tinnitus retraining (habituation) using counseling with low-level broad band noise exposure; use of background noise to mask tinnitus; use of a tinnitus masker worn in the ear to produce a more pleasant sound
Prevention/ Promotion	Cessation/avoidance of causative drugs or toxins
	Prompt treatment of ear infections
	Prevention of wax build-up in ear canal
	Regular dental maintenance
	Use of protective ear gear in noisy occupational settings
Education	Information about community resources, such as American Tinnitus Association

T

Tonsillitis

An inflammation of the palatine tonsils

Etiology and Incidence

Tonsils normally filter out bacteria and other microorganisms to prevent infections to the body. If they become overwhelmed by bacteria or viral infection, they may become enlarged, causing tonsillitis. *Streptococcus* (β-hemolytic streptococci group A) is the most common cause of tonsillitis. Tonsillitis may be acute or chronic and occurs most often in children.

Pathophysiology

The classic symptoms of tonsillitis are a sore throat, swollen tonsils, and enlarged and tender anterior cervical lymph nodes. The tonsils are swollen, reddened, and inflamed with pus or exudate (often yellow pustules). Some cases may have referred pain to the ears. If the exudate is scraped from the tonsils, bleeding may result.

Risk Factors

Children with frequent colds, pharyngitis
Winter season

Clinical Manifestations

Symptoms include moderate to severe sore throat lasting longer than 2 days; difficulty swallowing; pain referred to the ears; enlarged anterior cervical nodes; fever and chills; headache; muscle and joint pain; anorexia; increased secretions from the throat; enlarged, reddened, inflamed tonsils; pus or exudate on the tonsils; halitosis; or edematous or inflamed uvula. Symptoms often last 2 to 3 days after treatment is initiated.

Complications

If not treated, the following can occur: peritonsillar abscess, airway occlusion, rheumatic fever and subsequent cardiovascular disorders, kidney failure, or poststreptococcal glomerulonephritis.

Diagnostic Tests

Direct inspection of the tonsils for enlargement, redness, inflammation, infection. Throat culture to isolate organisms.

Therapeutic Management

Surgery	Tonsillectomy if tonsillitis is severe, recurs often, or does not respond to antibiotics
Medications	Antiinfective agents if cause is bacterial
General	Rest; warm, bland fluids or very cold fluids may alleviate discomfort; saltwater gargles, adequate fluids
Education	Education about signs of hemorrhage and prevention (limit activity, discourage coughing, clearing throat; avoid throat irritants; gargles); instruction to treat any sign of bleeding as medical emergency

T

Tourette's Syndrome

A chronic, hereditary neuromuscular disorder characterized by multiple motor and vocal tics that begin in childhood

Etiology and Incidence

Tourette's syndrome (TS) is an autosomal dominant genetic
disorder probably caused by the interaction of multiple genes
with the environment. The genetic cause is closely aligned with
obsessive compulsive disorder (OCD), attention deficit hyperactivity disorder (ADHD), and a variety of anxiety disorders. More
than 80% of those with TS have at least one of these additional
disorders, and 40% eventually develop OCD. The incidence of
TS is 5 to 10 cases per 10,000, and an estimated 1 million
persons in the United States are living with the disorder. The
predominant age of onset is between 2 and 15 years of age, and
males are affected three to four times as often as females.

Pathophysiology

The pathogenesis of TS is unclear, but current research suggests
that genetic abnormalities affect the brain's metabolism
of neurotransmitters, such as dopamine, serotonin, and
norepinephrine.

Risk Factors

Dominant mode genetic transmission (offspring of person with
   TS has 50% chance of inheriting genes)
Male gender

Clinical Manifestations

There is a wide variation in manifestation and severity of the tic
symptoms. The tics worsen with stress, are more severe during
the daytime, are less severe with physical activity, and seldom
occur during sleep. Tics may persist for months then disappear
only to reappear in a new constellation. Severity usually lessens
in adulthood.

First symptoms are usually facial tics (e.g., eye blinks, nose
twitches, grimaces). Other motor (e.g., head jerking, neck
stretching, body twisting, and foot stamping) and verbal (e.g.,
throat clearing, barking, yelping, coughing, shouting) tics may

be seen. Complex vocal tics are also seen and include use of obscenities (coprolalia) or obscene gestures (copropraxia); constant repetition of other's words (echolalia) or own words (palilalia); excessive touching and obsessive repetition of behaviors. Comorbid presentation of OCD, ADHD, or anxiety disorders is also seen.

Complications

Some persons with very severe TS may demonstrate self-destructive behavior (e.g., lip/cheek biting, head banging, eye gouging). These manifestations are rare. TS sufferers may also display orthopedic or neurological sequelae from years of forceful neck jerks, head turning, or knee bending movements.

Diagnostic Tests

Family History	Evidence of TS in family
Clinical History	Using DSM IV criteria: presence of multiple motor tics and one or more verbal tics for at least 1 year with no tic-free period of greater than 3 months beginning before age 18 and not caused by a medical condition or substance use

Therapeutic Management

Surgery	None
Medications	Low-dose dopamine-blocking neuroleptics (risperidone, haloperidol, pimozide) if tics interfere with activities of daily living (ADLs); clonidine often used when comorbid diagnosis of ADHD exists.
General	Coordinated multidisciplinary approach; supportive individual and family therapy to facilitate adaptation and coping; structured home environments with clear expectations; structured classroom settings with low student-pupil ratios, additional time for assignment completion and availability of computer aids; monitoring for associated disorders such as ADHD or OCD

T

Prevention/ Stress reduction techniques
Promotion
Education   Comprehensive education plan involving the
individual, family, school personnel, and
classmates about features of the disease;
information about community resources,
such as Tourette' Syndrome Association.

Toxic Shock Syndrome (TSS)

An acute bacterial infection that may progress rapidly to severe shock

Etiology and Incidence

Staphylococcus aureus and group A streptococci are the known etiologic agents. The syndrome was first reported in children and adolescents in 1978. In 1980 a large number of cases occurred in young menstruating women who used tampons. Changes in the composition of tampons and their use have drastically reduced the incidence in this group. Cases have subsequently been detected in nonmenstruating vaginal conditions, after surgery, in concert with various focal infections, and with presence of other foreign substances in the body. Incidence is currently about 1 to 2 cases per 100,000 persons in the United States. Reported mortality rates range from less than 1% in staphylococcal TSS to 30% to 70% in streptococcal TSS.

Pathophysiology

The causative agent produces exotoxins when certain host and environmental factors are favorable. Individuals who develop TSS have insufficient levels of antitoxin antibodies and are unable to rebuff the exotoxins. These exotoxins are absorbed into the bloodstream through inflamed, traumatized, or infected membranes, or tissue sites. The absorbed toxins set up a cascading reaction by inducing the production of cytokines, interleukins, and tumor necrosis factors, which produce immunosuppression, systemic vasculitis, growth of opportunistic gram-negative organisms, and multisystem organ involvement.

Risk Factors

Foreign bodies (e.g., tampons, diaphragms, cervical caps or contraceptive sponges, pulmonary embolism (PE) tubes, nasal packing)

Childbirth, puerperal sepsis, mastitis

Surgical procedures (e.g., orthopedic, abdominal, nasal/sinus, gynecologic, urinary)

Focal infections (e.g., abrasions, abscesses, bites, burns, cysts, cellulitis, furuncles)

T

Underlying diseases, such as acquired immunodeficiency syndrome (AIDS), influenza

Clinical Manifestations

The onset is sudden and marked by high fever, headache, sore throat, nonpurulent conjunctivitis, lethargy, confusion, vomiting, diarrhea, and a sunburnlike skin rash. Within 48 hours the syndrome progresses to syncope, orthostatic hypotension, diminished urine output, and shock. Peripheral and pulmonary edema, hepatitis, and myolysis then occur. After 3 to 7 days, the skin sloughs off on the palms and soles. Tissue necrosis is common in streptococcal TSS.

Complications

TSS can lead to residual neurological or psychological deficit, disseminated intravascular coagulation (DIC), gangrene, renal failure, respiratory failure, and death.

Diagnostic Tests

The Centers for Disease Control and Prevention (CDC) has set up the following revised diagnostic criteria for TSS: Fever = 102° F; diffuse macular erythema; desquamation 1 to 2 weeks after onset; systolic = 90 mm Hg or drop in diastolic = 15 mm Hg from lying to sitting.

At least three of the following conditions must be present on a clinical evaluation or laboratory test: (1) gastrointestinal (GI) effects, including vomiting and profuse, watery diarrhea; (2) muscular effects, with severe myalgia and a fivefold increase in serum creatine phosphokinase; (3) mucous membrane effects; (4) renal involvement, with BUN or serum creatinine at least double normal levels; (5) hepatocellular damage, with serum bilirubin, alanine aminotransferase (ALT), and aspartate aminotransferase (AST) double the normal levels; (6) blood involvement, with thrombocytopenia and a platelet count under $100,000/mm^3$; and (7) central nervous system (CNS) effects, such as confusion without focal signs.

Negative laboratory test results (if performed) are expected on blood, throat, and cerebrospinal fluid (CSF) cultures with a rise in titer to Rocky Mountain spotted fever, leptospirosis, or rubeolain staphylococcus TSS. There must be a positive culture for streptococcal TSS. Streptococcal TSS also requires two or more of the following on clinical examination: renal impairment; coagulopathy, liver abnormalities, adult respiratory distress syndrome (ARDS), extensive tissue necrosis, and erythematous rash.

Therapeutic Management

Surgery	Tracheostomy if necessary for ventilation; debridement of wounds; removal of dead tissue; amputation for gangrene
Medications	Antiinfective drugs for streptococcal TSS, *S. aureus* in menstrual TSS to prevent recurrence and to treat secondary infection; vasopressors for hypotension; antidiarrheal drugs and antiemetics to reduce diarrhea and vomiting; analgesics for pain; IV pooled immune globulin if unresponsive to other therapy.
General	Immediate removal of bacteria source (tampons, nasal packs, or other foreign bodies); immediate treatment for septic shock if indicated: aggressive fluid (IV crystalloids) and electrolyte (K^+, Ca^+) replacement; replacement with packed RBCs and/or coagulation factors, hemodynamic monitoring, monitor intake and output (I&O), and central venous pressure (CVP); Foley catheter; universal precautions for secretions and discharges; vital signs, neural vital signs, and reorientation for confusion; safety measures to prevent falls from orthostatic hypotension; mechanical ventilation and/or renal dialysis if necessary; hyperbaric oxygen for necrotizing fasciitis.
Prevention/ Promotion	Avoidance or safe use of tampons
Education	For menstrual TSS instruction about susceptibility to recurrence and avoidance of tampons Education about early signs of TSS

T

Transient Ischemic Attacks (TIAs)

Recurrent, transient, focal neurological disturbances of sudden onset and brief duration characterized by loss of sensory, motor, or visual function

Etiology and Incidence

Most TIAs are caused by cerebral emboli that break off from atherosclerotic plaques in the carotid or vertebral arteries in the neck. The attacks typically last less than 60 minutes but always less than 24 hours followed by full recovery of function. Hypertension (HTN), atherosclerosis, heart disease, diabetes mellitus (DM), and polycythemia serve as predisposing factors. The attacks are most common in adults past middle age, often presage a stroke, and serve as a warning sign of progressing cardiovascular disease. Occasionally TIAs are seen in children with severe cardiovascular disease and an elevated hematocrit. Incidence is 49 cases per 100,000 persons annually in the United States. Males have TIAs more frequently than females and the predominant age is over 60.

Pathophysiology

An atherosclerotic plaque breaks off from an artery in the neck and travels to the brain, where it temporarily impedes the blood flow in the carotid middle or vertebral basilar artery in the circle of Willis.

Clinical Manifestations

TIAs appear suddenly, usually last 2 to 30 minutes, and then subside with no neurological sequelae. They may occur daily or two or three times a year. Manifestations are specific to the artery occluded and the part of the brain affected.

Carotid	Ipsilateral blindness described as a shade being pulled down over the eye; contralateral hemiparesis and homonymous hemianopsia; paresthesia; slurred speech

Vertebrobasilar	Confusion, vertigo, diplopia, or binocular blindness, unilateral or bilateral muscular weakness and paresthesia, drop attacks with buckling of the legs, slurred speech

Complications

TIAs may precede a stroke with 5% to 11% risk within the first year; myocardial infarction (MI) risk if thrombosis is cardiac in origin.

Diagnostic Tests

The diagnosis is made on the clinical history with an ultrasound scan or arteriography, which confirms the presence of stenosis and atherosclerosis of the carotid or vertebral arteries. Head CT scan done to exclude hemorrhage. Echography is done if cardiac source of clot is suspected.

Therapeutic Management

Surgery	Endarterectomy to remove atherosclerotic plaque from the artery is considered if the artery is at least 70% occluded; intracranial anastomosis to revascularize the brain
Medications	Aspirin therapy to interfere with platelet aggregation in carotid involvement; aspirin and/or dipyridamole extended release capsules if aspirin alone not sufficient. Acute and long-term antiplatelet agents and/or anticoagulants are employed in cases with documented cardiogenic emboli, atrial fibrillation, or vertebrobasilar stenosis.
General Prevention/ Promotion	Monitor for bleeding; long-term follow-up Long-term use of low-dose aspirin therapy Smoking cessation Control of HTN, hyperlipidemia, DM Regular exercise and nutritionally sound diet
Education	Educate about TIAs as warning signs of stroke and advancing cerebrovascular disease; instruction in effects and side effects of anticoagulants; emphasize importance of regular follow-up

T

Traumatic Brain Injury (TBI)
(Acquired Brain Injury, Head Injury)

Physical injury occurs to the brain or other structures in the cranium, which may be open with skull fracture and/or penetration or may be closed with impact and rapid jarring. TBI can be classified as mild, moderate, or severe based on level of consciousness or Glasgow coma score.

Etiology and Incidence

Leading causes of head trauma include falls, industrial accidents, vehicular accidents, assaults, sports injuries, intrauterine injury, and birth injury. Alcohol use is a common related factor. More than 1.5 million persons sustain a TBI annually in the United States. It is the most common cause of death and disability in young people, and each year more than 50,000 individuals die and 55,000 more are left with permanent neurological damage.

Pathophysiology

Damage occurs from skull penetration or rapid brain acceleration and deceleration, which injure brain tissue at the point of impact, at its opposite pole (contrecoup), and diffusely in the frontal and temporal lobes. Blood vessels, meninges, and nerves can be ruptured, sheared, and torn. This results in neural disturbances, ischemia, hemorrhage, and cerebral edema. Laceration of meningeal arteries or sinuses can cause subdural or epidural hematomas and leakage of cerebrospinal fluid (CSF).

Risk Factors

Age related: Neonates, adolescents, young adults, elderly (more than 75 years of age)

Male gender

Contact sports involving the head

Extreme sports

Improper use of or lack of use of appropriate headgear in sports

Failure to use seat belts

Failure to use occupational safety gear

Lack of prenatal care

Clinical Manifestations

Clinical manifestations vary by the structures and brain tissue involved, whether the injury was open or closed, and the severity of the injury. Hypoxia, arterial hypotension, and edema of the brain are the most significant secondary effects of TBI. The manifestations listed below are all possible.

Level of Consciousness	Ranges from anxiety and irritability to restlessness, confusion, delirium, stupor, and coma; posttraumatic amnesia
Pain	Mild to severe headache
Cranial Nerve Injuries	Anosmia; diplopia, strabismus, nystagmus, or blindness; deafness; vertigo; trigeminal paresthesia
Motor Function	Weakness, paresis, paralysis; decorticate and decerebrate posturing; areflexia
Meningeal Effects	Nuchal rigidity, positive Kernig's sign, positive Brudzinski's sign
Fractures	*Linear:* No bone displacement, possible epidural hematoma *Depressed:* Focal deficits and cranial nerve injuries *Basilar:* CSF otorrhea or rhinorrhea, periorbital ecchymosis, conjunctival bleeding
Cerebral Edema	Increased intracranial pressure (ICP) with slow respirations, bradycardia, nausea, vomiting, altered or loss of consciousness, seizures, weakness
Hematoma	*Epidural:* Ipsilateral pupil dilation, rapidly increasing ICP *Subdural:* Lethargy, headache, seizures, minimal dilation of pupil on affected side; widening pulse pressure; fixed, dilated pupils; hemiplegia; decorticate rigidity
Vital Signs	Decreased blood pressure (BP); pulse slow (intracranial hypertension [HTV]) or rapid and feeble (hemorrhage); shallow respirations with possible Cheyne-Stokes; hyperthermia with hypothalamic injury

T

Complications

Complications include infection, seizure disorders, hydro-
cephaly, organic brain syndrome, permanent residual neurological deficits (memory loss, loss of impulse control, loss of
initiation skills, decrease in cognition and abstract reasoning,
decrease in judgment and problem solving); physical deficits
(paralysis, weakness, spasticity, loss of fine motor abilities); and
death.

Diagnostic Tests

Clinical Evaluation	Assessment of vital signs, neuro vital signs, reflexes, levels of consciousness/Glasgow coma score (3 to 8 indicative of severe injury; 9 to 12 moderate injury; 13 to 15 mild injury)
Skull and Neck X-rays	To detect fractures and bone fragments, spinal instability
CT Scans/MRI/ Angiography	To detect subdural or intracranial hematoma, shift, or cerebral ventricle distortion
Echoencephalography	To detect midline shifts
Cisternography	To detect dural tear
CSF Sampling	*May be contraindicated with signs of ICP, since it may lead to cerebral herniation;* normal findings with cerebral edema and concussion, increased pressure and blood in CSF with laceration and contusion

Therapeutic Management

Surgery	Débridement of open injuries; ventriculo-stomy or shunting procedures for ICP or hydrocephalus; craniotomy to elevate severe skull depressions, to stop hemorrhage from vessel lacerations, or to evacuate hematoma; trephine to relieve pressure from hematoma; bolt placement to monitor ICP pressure; tracheostomy if necessary for ventilation

Medications   Antiinfective drugs to prevent infection with open injury and leaking CSF; osmotic diuretics to control cerebral edema; polar beta-blockers to control transient hypertension; anticonvulsants for seizures; analgesics for pain *(medullary depressants, such as morphine, are contraindicated since they may interfere with level of consciousness);* muscle relaxants or paralyzing agents for decorticate and decerebrate posturing and restlessness in coma; stool softeners and suppositories to prevent constipation; artificial tears to prevent corneal damage with coma; histamine antagonists and antacids to control gastric reflux with tube feedings and reduce the chance of ulcers developing. *Corticosteroids are contraindicated in TBI.*

General   *Initially:* Secure airway, control bleeding, stabilize body on backboard and transport; mechanical ventilation if necessary with HTN to control intracranial hypertension; maintain brain perfusion; central venous and arterial lines; ICP and cardiac monitoring; blood gases; vital signs and neural vital signs; monitoring of intake and output (I&O); enteral feedings or hyperalimentation; indwelling Foley catheter; seizure precautions; passive range-of-motion (ROM) exercises, turning if comatose; cooling blankets for hyperthermia

Long term: Comprehensive rehabilitation program, including cognitive therapy to address cognitive, memory, and abstract reasoning deficits; speech therapy for communication deficits; physical therapy for residual weakness, paralysis, gait retraining, ataxia; occupational therapy for relearning activities of daily living (ADLs); respiratory therapy to retain vital capacity; vocational therapy for learning vocational skills;

T

counseling of individual and family to aid in adaptation to residual disabilities and amelioration of behavioral sequelae; transitional living placement to return individual to independent or supervised community living; long-term medical follow-up to reduce complications.

Prevention/ Promotion   Wearing seat belt

Use of helmets for bike/motorcycle riding

Use of safety gear in hazardous occupational settings

Use of appropriate headgear in sports (avoidance of "heading" maneuvers for children playing soccer)

Early and consistent prenatal care

Education   Education of individual and/or family about long-term sequelae; instruction in the importance of structure and consistency of environment; detailing of safety issues arising from impaired judgment and lack of impulse control; instruction in the use of memory books and other memory aids; information about community resources

Trichinosis

A roundworm *(Trichinella spiralis)* infection, usually transmitted by eating raw or undercooked pork

Etiology and Incidence

The causal agent is *Trichinella spiralis,* a parasite. Infection occurs when the individual eats contaminated undercooked pork or wild game meat. Because of meat processing and United States Department of Agriculture guidelines in the United States, the disease is uncommon. Approximately 50 to 60 cases are reported each year in the United States. Trichinosis is more prevalent throughout the rest of the world, especially where meats such as undercooked pork, ham, or sausage are eaten. The disease may also be seen in individuals who hunt and prepare their own meat, especially bear, cougar, fox, dog, wolf, horse, seal, walrus, or other wild animals that may be a reservoir for roundworm infection.

Pathophysiology

The muscles of infected animals contain cysts that are ingested. The acid in the human digestive system breaks down the cyst and the larva hatch within the host (human) intestinal tract to produce a roundworm. It takes only 1 or 2 days for the young worm to become an adult roundworm. The adult roundworm then produces numerous larvae that migrate throughout the gastrointestinal (GI) system and bloodstream to muscle tissue. There they produce cysts, and the life cycle repeats.

T

Risk Factors

Eating raw or undercooked pork, ham, or sausage, especially in areas outside of the United States

Eating game meat that has not been properly and fully cooked

Clinical Manifestations

Early:	1 to 2 days after infection, nausea, vomiting, fatigue, fever, and abdominal discomfort

| Late: | About 2 to 8 weeks later, headache, fevers, chills, cough, eye swelling, aching joints and muscle pains, itchy skin, diarrhea, or constipation |
| Serious Late Signs | Difficulty coordinating movements, fatigue, cardiac arrhythmias, respiratory distress |

Complications

Long-term sequelae include headache and myalgias. Untreated serious cases may cause overwhelming infection, respiratory distress, cardiac arrhythmias, and occasional death.

Diagnostic Tests

CBC may indicate increased eosinophils; creatine phosphokinase to identify elevated level of creatine kinase; serology studies to test for *Trichinella;* muscle biopsy to locate evidence of the *T. spiralis* roundworm

Therapeutic Management

Surgery	None
Medications	Antiinfective agents specific to causative organism; analgesics for muscle discomfort; steroids for severe illness
General	Bedrest for myalgias
Prevention/ Promotion	Cook all meat products until the juices run clear or to an internal temperature of 170° F. Cook wild game meat thoroughly. Clean meat grinders thoroughly if you prepare your own ground meats. Curing (salting), drying, smoking, or microwaving meat does not consistently kill infective worms.
Education	Education about preventive food preparation measures

Tuberculosis (TB)

A recurrent, chronic, infectious pulmonary and extrapulmonary disease characterized by formation of granulomas with caseation, fibrosis, and cavitation

Etiology and Incidence

TB is caused by spore-forming mycobacteria *(Mycobacterium tuberculosis, M. bovis, or M. africanum)*. In developed countries the infection is airborne and is spread by inhalation of infected droplets. In underdeveloped countries (Africa, Asia, South America), transmission also occurs by ingestion or by skin invasion, particularly when bovine TB is poorly controlled. The incidence varies widely by country, age, race, gender, and socioeconomic status. The incidence of TB has risen precipitously in the United States with the advent of human immunodeficiency virus (HIV) infection and among certain immigrant populations. Nearly 16,000 new cases of active TB are reported annually in the United States. There are an estimated 10 million to 15 million persons in the United States who are infected but display no symptomatology (latent TB).

Pathophysiology

TB has three stages: (1) primary (initial) infection; (2) latent (dormant) infection; and (3) recrudescent (postprimary) disease. During the first stage, the mycobacteria invade the tissue at the port of entry (usually the lungs) and multiply over a period of approximately 3 weeks. They form a small inflammatory lesion in the lung before traveling to the regional lymph nodes and throughout the body, forming additional lesions. The number of lesions formed depends on the number of invading bacteria and the general resistance of the host. This stage is generally asymptomatic.

Lymphocytes and antibodies mount a fibroblastic response to the invasion, which encases the lesions, forming noncaseating granulomas. This marks the latent stage, and the individual may remain in this stage for weeks to years, depending on the body's ability to maintain specific and nonspecific resistance. Stage three occurs when the body is unable to contain the infection, and a necrotic and cavitation process begins in the lesion at the

T

entry port or in other body lesions. Caseation occurs and the lesions may rupture, spreading necrotic residue and bacilli throughout the surrounding tissue. Disseminated bacteria form new lesions, which in turn become inflamed and form non-caseating granulomas and then caseating necrotic cavities. The lungs are the most common site for recrudescent disease, but it may occur anywhere in the body. Untreated disease has many remissions and exacerbations.

Risk Factors

Age extremes (under age 3 or over age 65)
Smoking
Drug and alcohol abuse
Occupational history as a silicone/asbestos worker (particularly those who smoke)
Malnourished state
Unsanitary, crowded living conditions
Residence in institutional settings
History of chronic illness, general debilitation, immunosuppression, HIV, acquired immunodeficiency syndrome (AIDS)

Clinical Manifestations

Manifestations vary with the systems involved. Symptoms are rarely seen until the recrudescent stage. Individuals are communicable whenever bacilli are present in the sputum.

Pulmonary	Weight loss, fatigue, generalized weakness, anorexia; slight fever with chills and night sweats; nonproductive cough that eventually becomes productive with mucopurulent sputum; tachycardia; dyspnea on exertion; hemoptysis
Cardiovascular	Pericarditis with precordial chest pain, fever, ascites, edema, and distention of neck veins
Gastrointestinal (GI)	Peritonitis with acute abdominal pain, abdominal distention, vomiting, anorexia, weight loss, night sweats, gastrointestinal bleeding, bowel obstruction
Neurological	Meningitis with headache, vomiting, fever, declining consciousness, and neurological deficit

Musculoskeletal	Joint pain, swelling, tenderness, deformities; limitation of motion
Genitourinary	Urgency, frequency, dysuria, hematuria, pyuria; infertility, amenorrhea, vaginal bleeding and discharge; salpingitis with lower abdominal pain
Lymphatics	Enlarged lymph nodes

Complications

Complications include massive destruction of lung tissue, leading to pneumothorax, pleural effusion, pneumonia, and respiratory failure; brain abscess; cardiac tamponade; vertebral collapse and paralysis; liver failure; renal failure; and generalized massive dissemination of disease that usually is fatal. New drug-resistant strains of TB are emerging, leading to more frequent progression to complications.

Diagnostic Tests

Skin Tests	Positive reaction on a Mantoux or purified protein derivative test indicates past infection and presence of antibodies; it is not indicative of active disease
Sputum Culture	Positive for causative agent within 2 to 3 weeks of onset of active disease; it is not positive during latency
Sputum Smear	Acid-fast smear positive for acid-fast bacillus
Biopsy/Culture	Tissue positive for causative agent
Needle Biopsy	Pleural fluid positive for causative agent
Chest X-ray	May reveal cavitation, calcification, parenchymal infiltrate; not diagnostically definitive

Therapeutic Management

| **Surgery** | Drainage of pulmonary abscesses; correction of complications, such as intestinal obstruction or urethral stricture |

T

Medications	Antiinfective drugs in combinations of primary drugs or primary and secondary drugs to combat causative agent (new strains of bacillus are occurring that are resistant to traditional primary drugs)
General	Sputum precautions until no sputum is evident (10 to 14 days after start of drug therapy); management usually on an outpatient basis unless the disease is in an advanced state with complications; skin testing and evaluation of close contacts at the time of initial diagnosis and again in 2 to 3 months; long-term medical follow-up to prevent recurrence
Prevention/ Promotion	Skin testing for screening and early detection Antiinfective drugs (isoniazid) as chemoprophylaxis in individuals who have converted from a negative to a positive skin test, particularly those with HIV or other immunosuppressed conditions, insulin-dependent diabetics, those on prolonged corticosteroid therapy, small children, and health care workers who are regularly exposed Bacille Calmette-Guérin (BCG) vaccine for infants in countries where disease is common Precautions by health care systems to prevent spread (e.g., ultraviolet light, special air filters, special respirators)
Education	Instruction about the importance of uninterrupted drug therapy and the necessity for periodic recultures of sputum throughout drug therapy, which may last a year or longer

Ulcerative Colitis

A chronic inflammatory mucosal disease of the colon and rectum characterized by bloody diarrhea

Etiology and Incidence

The cause of ulcerative colitis is unknown. Immunological factors, infectious agents, toxins, and dietary factors have been studied extensively but with no promising result. The annual incidence of ulcerative colitis in the United States is 7 cases per 100,000 persons. The incidence distribution is bimodal, with peak frequencies between ages 15 and 25, and 50 and 70. It is most prominent in Caucasians, especially American and European Jewish individuals.

Pathophysiology

The disease process usually begins in the rectosigmoid area and spreads proximally. Pathological change starts with degeneration of the reticulin fibers beneath the epithelial mucosa. This causes occlusion of the subepithelial capillaries and infiltration of the lamina propria with lymphocytes, leukocytes, eosinophils, mast cells, and plasma. The result eventually is abscess formation, necrosis, and ulceration of the epithelial mucosa. This in turn reduces the colon's ability to absorb sodium and water.

Clinical Manifestations

The primary sign is the presence of frequent spells of bloody, mucoid diarrhea, accompanied by abdominal cramping. As the ulceration extends proximally, the stools become looser and increase in frequency to as many as 20 times daily. Malaise, fever, anorexia, and weight loss may also be present by this time.

Complications

Complications include perforation, toxic megacolon, massive hemorrhage, and a tenfold increased risk of adenocarcinoma of the colon.

Diagnostic Tests

Clinical Evaluation	Tentative diagnosis made on history and examination of a stool specimen
Sigmoidoscopy	Reveals a granular, friable mucous membrane with crypt abscesses, loss of normal vascular pattern, and scattered areas of hemorrhage
Double Contrast Barium Enemas	Used to visualize and evaluate disease above the reach of a sigmoidoscope
Abdominal X-rays	Assist in gauging the extent and severity of disease
Stool Cultures	To rule out infectious bowel disorders; should be negative in ulcerative colitis
Electrolytes	Serum levels of Na^+, K^+, chloride, bicarbonate, and magnesium may be low
Albumin	Hypoalbuminemia in severe disease
CBC	Anemia with blood loss

Therapeutic Management

Surgery	Colectomy or proctocolectomy with permanent ileostomy for fulminant disease, hemorrhage, perforation, or toxic megacolon
Medications	Sulfasalazine (systemic and/or retention enema) in mild to moderate disease and corticosteroids (retention enema and/or systemic) in active and/or severe disease to help reduce inflammation and maintain remission; antidiarrheal drugs to control diarrhea; folate supplements; analgesics for pain *(avoid aspirin and nonsteroidal antiinflammatory drugs [NSAIDs] because they may be irritating; avoid opiates and anticholinergics if disease is severe and the individual is at risk of toxic megacolon)*; immunosuppressives used to treat severe, nonresponsive disease in individuals who are not surgical candidates

General	Acute attacks treated with bed rest, IV fluids, total parenteral nutrition for severe malnutrition, and blood replacement; perianal skin care, sitz baths to prevent skin breakdown; dietary referral to manage nutritional needs
	Long-term therapy and support groups for coping with disease; counseling to aid adaptation to altered body image with ostomy
Prevention/ Promotion	Drink adequate fluids and avoid irritating foods (e.g., high-fiber foods, raw fruits and vegetables)
	Low-roughage diet at first indication of relapse
	Ongoing colonoscopy and biopsy surveillance because of increased risk for colon cancer starting 8 to 10 years after diagnosis
Education	Dietary education; ostomy care and instructions if necessary; information about available community resources

Ulcers

(See Peptic Ulcer Disease [Gastric or Duodenal Ulcers])

U

Urinary Incontinence

Involuntary leakage of urine classified as instability incontinence (sudden, urgent desire or detrusor contraction with immediate loss of control), stress incontinence (loss of control on sneezing, coughing, laughing, or straining), overflow incontinence (chronic overdistention of the bladder that results in dribbling), and constant incontinence (continual dribbling)

Etiology and Incidence

Causes vary by classification. Instability incontinence is often associated with disease or trauma of the central nervous system (CNS) (e.g., cerebrovascular accident [CVA], parkinsonism, brain tumors, spinal cord injury [SCI]); bladder outlet obstructions (e.g., benign prostatic hypertrophy [BPH]); bladder infection; and bladder irritation (e.g., calculi). Other causes of instability incontinence remain unclear and are labeled idiopathic.

Stress incontinence is caused by pelvic relaxation or sphincter incompetence. Pelvic relaxation leads to cystocele, rectocele, or uterine prolapse. Factors associated with relaxation include multiparity, aging, peripheral neuropathy, diabetes mellitus (DM), and extensive pelvic surgery. Sphincter incompetence is associated with any factor that loosens the sphincter, such as prostate or urinary surgery or repeat urinary procedures, infection, or a reduction in mucus production.

The two causes of overflow incontinence are deficient detrusor function and bladder outlet obstruction. Detrusor function deficiency is associated with cauda equina syndrome, multiple sclerosis (MS), tabes dorsalis, polio, herpes zoster, pelvic trauma, DM, and chronic overdistention. Obstruction is associated with inflammation, BPH, adenocarcinoma of the bladder, urethral stricture in men, and urethral distortion in women.

Constant incontinence results from bypassing of normal sphincter function and failure of the bladder to store urine. Associated factors include urinary fistula, epispadias, urethral ectopia, and surgical conduit.

It is estimated that more than 13 million individuals are affected by incontinence in the United States. It occurs in both men and women and increases with age. As many as 50% of institutionalized elderly individuals experience chronic incontinence, and 20% more experience intermittent incontinence.

Pathophysiology

Stress incontinence occurs when the bladder pressure exceeds the urethral closure pressure. This happens when the urethra is no longer maintained in a normal anatomical position, resulting in inefficient transmission of abdominal pressures along the length of the urethra. Thus sudden increases in abdominal pressure from coughing, sneezing, or straining are not transmitted to the sphincter, and it does not tighten.

Instability incontinence is a result of inappropriate contraction of the detrusor muscle, with loss of coordination between bladder contraction and sphincter release. Overflow incontinence results when the detrusor muscle fails to contract, allowing the bladder to overfill, or when the bladder outlet is blocked and urine backs up and overfills the bladder. Constant incontinence occurs when the sphincter is bypassed and the urine has a new channel or outlet, such as a fistula between the bladder or urethra and the vagina or rectum.

Clinical Manifestations

Involuntary loss of urine is the chief manifestation, and the pattern varies by classification of the incontinence. Abdominal distention and associated urinary tract infection (UTI) are also seen in overflow incontinence.

Complications

Complications include UTI, kidney infection, and skin breakdown.

Diagnostic Tests

Voiding Cystourethrography	*Stress incontinence:* Pelvic descent below the pubis, urethral excursion, and leakage of contrast material with straining
	Instability: Detrusor-sphincter dyssynergia
	Overflow: Large bladder capacity, possible blockage

	Constant: Leakage of contrast material through fistula or ectopic structure
Urodynamic Testing	*Stress:* Normal capacity, sensations, and compliance; stable detrusor; normal electromyographic (EMG) explosive flow with low-pressure detrusor contraction
	Instability: Decreased functional capacity, early sensation, normal compliance, unstable detrusor, normal EMG findings
	Overflow with detrusor dysfunction: Enlarged capacity, delayed sensations, abnormal compliance, poor stream, residuals
	Overflow with obstruction: Normal or enlarged capacity, normal or delayed sensation, normal or impaired compliance, high detrusor contraction with poor flow
	Constant: Impaired urine storage with fistulous tract

Therapeutic Management

Surgery	*Stress:* Vesicourethral suspension to elevate anatomical structures; artificial urinary sphincter, pubovaginal sling to replace or reinforce damaged sphincter
	Instability: Urinary diversions (e.g., suprapubic catheter or ileoconduit)
	Overflow: Transurethral resection of enlarged prostate; urethrotomy to correct urethral stricture; reconstruction of bladder or urethra
	Constant: Repair or removal of ectopic structures or fistulas
Medications	Autonomic drugs, spasmolytics to increase detrusor contractility and tone; autonomic drugs to increase or decrease bladder neck tone; muscle relaxants to diminish external

muscle tone; antispasmodics to decrease detrusor spasms

General   *Stress:* Kegel exercises to strengthen periurethral muscles; electrostimulation therapy to strengthen pelvic muscles; use of pessary to alter anatomical structure

Instability: Use of a timed voiding schedule; manipulation of fluid intake, avoiding large-volume intake periods; intermittent catheterization

Overflow: Double voiding techniques; intermittent catheterization; voiding schedules with manual Credé's maneuvers

All forms: Good skin care with use of barrier cream to protect irritated skin from moisture and urine; use of incontinence aids (e.g., pads, adult diapers, odor elimination substances, external catheters); referral to continence support group; instruction in intermittent catheterization techniques if necessary

Education   Instruction in relevant techniques (e.g., Kegel exercises, double voids, timed voids, Crede's maneuvers, fluid intake schedules); information about available community resources

U

Urinary Tract Infection (UTI), Lower (Cystitis, Urethritis)

An inflammation of the bladder or urethra

Etiology and Incidence

Most UTIs are caused by gram-negative bacteria, with *Escherichia coli* accounting for approximately 80% of cases. *Staphylococcus, Klebsiella, Proteus, Enterobacter,* and mixed infections account for most of the remainder. The infecting bacteria are commonly normal intestinal and fecal flora. Interference in urine flow dynamics puts an individual at greater risk. Women are 10 times more likely than men to have a UTI because of anatomical construction of the female urinary system. Approximately 20% of women have at least one UTI in their lifetime.

Pathophysiology

Bacteria invade the urethra and bladder when the body defense mechanisms (regular emptying and cleansing of the lower urinary tract by urine flow) are diminished or absent. When urine flow is impeded or interrupted, or when the bladder is retaining residual and static urine, bacteria can ascend the urethra, move into the bladder mucosa, colonize, and multiply; this sets up the inflammatory process.

Risk Factors

Obstructions (e.g., strictures, calculi, tumors, prostatic hypertrophy)

Retention (e.g., neurogenic bladder, low bladder wall compliance, infrequent voiding)

Underlying disease/conditions (e.g., neurological, diabetes mellitus [DM], renal disease, human immunodeficiency virus [HIV], pregnancy)

Anatomical abnormalities (e.g., bladder outlet obstruction, ectopia, vesicourethral reflux)

Personal practices (e.g., frequent sexual activity, poor hygiene, douching, tampon use, diaphragm use)

Medical or surgical procedures, such as catheterization, cystoscopy, ureteral stents

Clinical Manifestations

Common signs and symptoms include pain; burning on urination; frequency; urgency; nocturia; cloudy, foul-smelling urine; hematuria.

Complications

The major complications include damage and scarring to the lining of the urinary tract with recurrent infection and ascension of the infection to the kidneys, causing pyelonephritis.

Diagnostic Tests

The diagnosis is based on the history and on urine culture and sensitivity to identify the causative agent and its response to a given antiinfective drug. A complete urodynamic work-up may be done in those with recurrent infection or to identify factors contributing to infection, such as obstruction, stricture, and detrusor abnormality.

Therapeutic Management

Surgery	Revision of abnormalities in urinary tract
Medications	Antiinfective drugs to kill pathogen and render urine sterile; urinary analgesics for pain
General	Warm soaking baths, increased fluid intake (avoid caffeinated beverages, alcohol, and citrus juices as they irritate bladder); repeat of culture after drug therapy
Prevention/ Promotion	Empty bladder regularly and completely and evacuate bowel regularly
	Good hygiene practices (e.g., front to back perianal wiping, thorough wiping, regular bathing/showering, prompt changing of tampons)
	Careful sexual practices (urinating and cleaning after sexual intercourse, avoidance of vaginal penetration after anal penetration during intercourse, proper use and removal of diaphragm)
	Adequate daily fluids

U

	Daily intake of cranberry juice and/or tablets for high-risk individuals
	Avoidance of unnecessary catheterization, early removal of indwelling catheters
Education	Education about importance of completing medication cycle; evaluation and instruction about voiding patterns, sexual practices, and hygiene practices for prevention of future UTIs

Urticaria (Hives, Angioedema)

An allergic reaction that produces wheals and erythema in the dermis (urticaria) or the dermis and subcutaneous structures (angioedema)

Etiology and Incidence

Urticaria and angioedema are caused by an allergen that provokes a histamine-mediated response. Common allergens include drugs, insect bites or stings, miscellaneous environmental factors, desensitization injections, and foods (eggs, shellfish, nuts, fruits). About 20% of the general population have had an episode of urticaria or angioedema at some time. The peak incidence occurs in adults in their 30s.

Pathophysiology

A histamine response to the allergen induces vascular changes that result in vasodilation and itching. The histamine-mediated response also causes endothelial cells to contract, which allows vascular cells to leak between the cells via the vessel wall to form a wheal on the skin. A more diffuse swelling of subcutaneous tissue accompanies angioedema and is typically seen in the hands, feet, face, and upper airways.

Clinical Manifestations

Pruritus is followed by the appearance of wheals 1 to 5 cm in diameter. These may enlarge and develop a clear center and erythematous border. The wheals may occur singly or in crops. They may appear in one site, remain for several hours, disappear, and then appear in a new site. Angioedema involves edema of subcutaneous tissue, and the wheals are typically larger. Respiratory distress and stridor may be seen if the upper airways are affected.

U

Complications

Skin abrasion and secondary infection may occur as a result of scratching, and laryngeal edema may occur in angioedema.

Diagnostic Tests

The diagnosis is made by history and clinical evaluation. Other tests are unnecessary unless the urticaria is chronic and has no apparent allergic cause. In such cases underlying disease (e.g., lymphoma, polycythemia, systemic lupus erythematosus [SLE]) should be ruled out.

Therapeutic Management

Surgery	None
Medications	Antihistamines to control histamine response; H_1 receptor agonists for chronic cases; addition of H_2 agonists in refractory cases; corticosteroids if H_1 and H_2 receptor agonists fail
General	Identification and elimination of allergens; avoidance of scratching; specialized baths (e.g., Starch, Aveeno) effective in some individuals
Prevention/ Promotion	Avoidance of allergen triggers in susceptible individuals
Education	Instruction in allergen avoidance and prompt treatment

Uterine Bleeding, Dysfunctional

Abnormal uterine bleeding not associated with recognizable organic lesion, inflammation, ovulation, or pregnancy

Etiology and Incidence

Dysfunctional uterine bleeding (DUB) is usually caused by anovulation (90%), which creates an imbalance in the hormone-endometrium relationship when unopposed estrogen stimulates the endometrium. The remaining cases are caused by a dysfunction in the corpus luteum. Variation in uterine bleeding is the most frequently encountered health problem in women, and DUB is the most common cause of abnormal bleeding. It is typically seen at the extremes of reproductive life, with 50% of cases occurring after 45 years of age and another 20% in adolescence.

Pathophysiology

Unopposed estrogen stimulation resulting from anovulation often causes an endometrial hyperplasia. The endometrium becomes thickened by the estrogen, and when it can no longer be maintained, the endometrial lining sloughs in an incomplete and irregular pattern, leading to irregular, prolonged bleeding.

Risk Factors

History of anovulation from factors such as polycystic ovaries, follicle depletion
Obesity
Nulliparity
Use of exogenous estrogen

U

Clinical Manifestations

The main sign is painless, irregular, heavy vaginal bleeding. Midcycle spotting, oligomenorrhea, or amenorrhea may also be present.

Complications

Anemia is the chief complication.

Diagnostic Tests

The diagnosis is made on the basis of the history, a pelvic examination, and laparoscopy to rule out other bleeding disorders or underlying disorders. Endometrial biopsy can rule out cancer.

Therapeutic Management

Surgery	Laser ablation or fulguration of endometriosis; presacral neurectomy when bleeding is severe and does not respond to other treatment
Medications	Combination contraceptives to control bleeding
General	Iron replacement or packed cells for associated anemia; adequate nutritional intake; cessation of extreme exercise schedules

Uterine Cancer (Endometrial Cancer)

Adenocarcinomas account for most endometrial cancer; other tumor types include adenoacanthoma and clear cell and squamous cell tumors.

Etiology and Incidence

The cause of endometrial cancer has not yet been firmly established although a long-established link exists to hormone-related disorders. However, approximately 40% of endometrial tumors appear to be autonomous with no known cause.

Endometrial cancer is the most common of the gynecological malignancies, with more than 40,000 new cases a year in the United States. There are 6800 reported deaths annually. This cancer is found primarily in postmenopausal women between ages 55 and 60. The women tend to be from highly industrialized countries, and the prevalence has increased sharply.

Pathophysiology

Cells begin as endometrial hyperplasia and change to cancer cells, beginning in the fundus of the uterus and spreading to the entire endometrium. The tumor may then extend down the endocervical canal and involve the cervix and vagina. It also spreads through the uterine wall to the abdominal cavity and adjacent structures and metastasizes to the pelvic and paraaortic lymph nodes, lungs, bone, and brain.

Risk Factors

Infertility

Early onset of menarche (before age 12), late onset of menopause (after age 52)

Nulliparity

Use of unopposed estrogen

Extended periods of anovulation

Morbid obesity

History of hyperplasia of the endometrium, diabetes mellitus (DM), hypertension (HTN), or gallbladder disease

History of breast or ovarian cancer

History of pelvic radiation

Familial history of the disease

U

Clinical Manifestations

The only significant clinical sign of endometrial cancer is inappropriate uterine bleeding. Approximately one third of postmenopausal women who experience such bleeding have endometrial cancer.

Complications

Advanced disease leads to complications such as bowel obstruction, ascites, and respiratory distress, and the prognosis is poor. Prognosis with early detection is excellent, with a greater than 96%, 5-year survival rate.

Diagnostic Tests

A Pap smear is helpful but undependable, because 30% to 40% of smears yield false-negative results. Malignant cells on endometrial biopsy and fractional curettage yield a definitive diagnosis.

Therapeutic Management

Surgery	Hysterectomy
Medications	Chemotherapy for recurrent lesions and metastasis; hormones (e.g., progestin) to treat metastasis or precancerous lesions
General	Radiation as an adjunct to surgery and palliation; counseling for alterations in body image and sexual functioning
Prevention/ Promotion	Annual screening with endometrial biopsy starting at age 35 for women at increased risk for hereditary nonpolyposis colon cancer
	Prompt medical follow-up for any unexplained and/or unexpected vaginal bleeding or spotting

Uterine Fibroids (Leiomyomas, Myomas)

Well-circumscribed, nonencapsulated, benign tumors of the uterus

Etiology and Incidence

The cause is unclear, but the tumors tend to grow in response to excess estrogen levels and shrink after menopause. Steroid hormones including estrogen and progestin, and several growth factors have been implicated as causal factors. Fibroids are the most common benign uterine tumor and occur in more than 40% of women over age 40. In the United States, the incidence is higher in African-American women.

Pathophysiology

Fibroids arise from the smooth muscle within the myometrium of the uterus. They may be seen on the intramural, submucosal, or subserous surface of the uterus or in the musculature of the cervix or broad ligaments. Tumor growth often outstrips blood supply, causing the tumor to hyalinize. The hyaline tissue may then liquefy and calcify.

Clinical Manifestations

Most fibroids are asymptomatic. Symptoms, when present, include prolonged or excessive menstrual bleeding with no change in the cycle interval. Pain, heaviness, or tenderness in the lower abdomen may also be present.

Complications

Complications include hemorrhage, torsion, infection, adhesions, and infertility.

Diagnostic Tests

The diagnosis is made on abdominal and bimanual palpation of the uterus. Ultrasound scanning may be used to distinguish endometriosis from leiomyomas. Cytological tests and cervical biopsy may be done to rule out cancer.

U

Therapeutic Management

Surgery	Hysteroscopic or laparoscopic myomectomy to preserve uterus for childbearing; hysterectomy to control heavy bleeding
Medications	Gonadotropin-releasing hormone (GnRH) agonists can be used to reduce uterine volume as surgical alternative or before surgery or to preserve fertility in women attempting to become pregnant
General	Ongoing gynecological examinations to monitor fibroids

Vaginitis (Vulvovaginitis)

Infection and inflammation of the vaginal mucosa, often extending secondarily to the vulva

Etiology and Incidence

Most vaginitis is caused by bacteria *(Gardnerella vaginalis)*, protozoa *(Trichomonas vaginalis)*, fungi (*Candida* sp.), and viruses (human papilloma virus). Other causes include mechanical forces (foreign objects, vigorous wiping, or cleansing); irritating chemicals found in douches, deodorant sprays, laundry soaps, and bath water additives; and sensitivity to spermicides, latex condoms, or latex diaphragms. Tight, nonporous, nonabsorbent underclothing or poor hygiene may foster growth of pathogens. Women exposed to diethylstilbestrol have vaginal adenosis, which can produce a vaginal discharge. Older, postmenopausal women have vaginal and mucosal atrophy, which predisposes them to infection. Vaginitis is a common disorder, and most women can expect to have at least one vaginal infection in their lifetime. All age groups are at risk. In the reproductive years, vaginitis is usually caused by infection. Premenopausal and postmenopausal causes are more often mechanical or chemical.

Pathophysiology

The causative agent sets up an infective or inflammatory process. Infective agents invade and grow in the warm, moist environment of the vagina, often aided by a decrease in acidity and an increase in the sugar level in the vaginal environment. Infective agents are often introduced by sexual activity (*Trichomonas* and *Gardnerella* sp., papilloma virus) or are part of the normal vaginal flora *(Candida albicans)* that overgrow when vaginal conditions are ripe, such as before menstruation and during pregnancy. Inflammation occurs with mechanical, chemical, or other sensitivity, often with an inadequately lubricated or a thinning vaginal mucosa.

V

Clinical Manifestations

The most common presenting sign is vaginal discharge with or without itching, odor, or pain.

Mechanical/Chemical	Increase in clear, viscous discharge; burning; redness; itching
Bacterial (*Gardnerella*)	Malodorous (fishy) white or grayish yellow discharge; itching, burning
Protozoan (*Trichomonas*)	Copious frothy, bubbly, greenish gray, malodorous discharge; itching, dyspareunia, vulvar edema, hyperemia
Viral (papilloma virus)	Vaginal or vulvar warts, discharge, odor, spotty bleeding
Fungal (*C. albicans*)	Thick, cheesy white or yellow discharge; intense itching, redness
Atrophic	Itching, dryness, redness, irritation, burning, spotty bleeding

Complications

Chronic vulvitis and vulvar dystrophies can occur and are most often seen after menopause.

Diagnostic Tests

The diagnosis is made through a history, a pelvic examination, and a wet smear or culture to identify the causative organisms. Pap smears and biopsies may be done to rule out cancer.

Therapeutic Management

Surgery	Laser therapy, cautery, or cryotherapy to remove warts
Medications	Topical or systemic antiinfective drugs to treat specific causative pathogen; treatment of sex partner for *Trichomonas* infections; topical estrogen applications for atrophic vaginitis
General	Removal of chemical, mechanical, or other sources of irritation; refrain from scratching

Prevention/ Promotion	Good vaginal hygiene/cleanliness to prevent environment for pathogen growth
	Avoid mechanical irritants (e.g., vigorous perianal cleansing, scratching, insertion of foreign objects)
	If sensitive, avoid chemical irritants (e.g., vaginal deodorants, bath water additives, spermicides)
	If sensitive to latex, avoid latex condoms and diaphragms
	Avoid douching as it destroys protective vaginal environment
	Avoid tight, nonporous, nonabsorbent underclothing
	Use vaginal lubricants if necessary
	Safe sex to prevent sexually transmitted disease (STD) transmission (condoms, spermicides)
Education	Instruction in application of vaginal medications; education about precautions to prevent repeat infection

V

Varicose Veins

Elongated, dilated, and tortuous superficial and/or subcutaneous veins usually seen in the lower extremities

Etiology and Incidence

Varicose veins occur because of incompetency in the valves of the vein, which permits a backflow of blood in the dependent position. The cause of valvular incompetence is unclear but may be associated with an inherent weakness in the vein walls. Approximately 30% of the adult population in the United States have varicose veins. Varicosities increase with age and are more common in women than in men.

Pathophysiology

The prevailing hypothesis for pathogenesis is that valve failure occurs at the perforator veins in the lower leg, resulting in high-pressure flow and increased volume in the superficial veins during muscular contraction. Over time the superficial veins become dilated, separating the valve cusps and reversing blood flow in the affected veins.

Risk Factors

Familial tendency
Underlying conditions such as congenital arteriovenous fistulas, ascites
Vein trauma or occlusion
Pregnancy
Occupations necessitating prolonged standing
Obesity
Aging
Oral contraceptive use

Clinical Manifestations

Initially the vein may be palpated but invisible, and the individual may have a feeling of heaviness in the legs that gets worse at night and in hot weather. Aching also occurs after prolonged standing or walking, during menses, when fatigued, and at night. Over time, the veins can be seen as dilated, purplish, and ropelike.

Complications

Venous insufficiency and venous stasis ulcers are the two most common complications.

Diagnostic Tests

The initial diagnosis is made on inspection and palpation and is checked by a manual compression test that reveals a palpable impulse. A Trendelenburg's test can help pinpoint the location of incompetent valves. Plethysmography and duplex ultrasound scans can be used to detect venous backflow.

Therapeutic Management

Surgery	Stripping and ligation of severely affected veins that have not responded to conservative therapy
Medications	Sclerotherapy (injection of chemicals designed to sclerose the affected veins)
General	Leg elevation and rest; lightweight compression hosiery and avoidance of prolonged standing for mild varicosities; custom-fitted, surgical-weight antiembolism stockings with graduated pressure (high at ankle, lower at top) with prescribed exercise program to promote circulation and prevent stasis with moderate varicosities; weight loss in obesity cases
Prevention/ Promotion	Weight loss if obese. Avoidance of restrictive and/or occlusive clothing. Regular aerobic exercise (e.g., walking). Avoidance of prolonged sitting or standing or frequent position changes with prolonged sitting or standing
Education	Instruction in correct application of compression/antiembolism stockings

V

West Nile Virus Infection (West Nile Fever)

A viral infection that affects the central nervous system (CNS)

Etiology and Incidence

The West Nile virus is a mosquito-borne virus belonging to the Flaviviridae family. This viral infection is endemic in Africa, West Asia, and the Middle East. The first cases were reported in the United States in 1999. It has since spread to 44 states, and the number of cases is increasing. There were 4156 laboratory positive cases with 284 deaths in the United States in 2002. It occurs primarily in midsummer to midfall and is most severe in individuals over the age of 50.

Pathophysiology

West Nile virus is transmitted to humans primarily through a bite from infected mosquitoes that have acquired the virus from feeding on infected birds. *Culex* mosquitoes most commonly carry the virus. During an incubation period of 3 to 15 days, the virus replicates, causing a brief viremia. If body defenses fail to clear the virus, it enters the CNS via the bloodstream. Once in the brain, virions spread from cell to cell, causing meningeal congestion, inflammation, brain edema, and widespread encephalitis. Other forms of transmission are very rare but have been documented through blood transfusion, breast milk, organ transplant, and lab samples.

Risk Factors

Exposure to infected mosquitoes
Transfusion with contaminated blood products
Transplant with infected organs
Lab workers who handle West Nile viral samples or cultures
Breastfeeding from infected milk

Clinical Manifestations

The majority of cases are asymptomatic or produce flulike symptoms, including sudden fever, chills, cough, headache, eye pain, myalgia, malaise, anorexia, and lymphadenopathy. Occasionally a pale maculopapular rash develops on the trunk and arms. In severe cases, high fever, headache, nuchal rigidity, enlarged spleen and liver, stupor, disorientation, coma, tremors, convulsions, muscle weakness, and paralysis occur. Severe disease symptoms last for weeks and are accompanied by profound fatigue.

Complications

Severe disease may produce myocarditis, pancreatitis, hepatitis, and permanent neurological sequelae, such as residual paralysis. Death occurs in 3% to 15% of diagnosed patients, and the elderly and those who are immunocompromised are at highest risk.

Diagnostic Tests

Clinical Evaluation	Symptom pattern of febrile illness (greater than 100° F) and/or neurological involvement, including altered mental status, nuchal rigidity, cranial nerve palsies, paresis and/or paralysis, and convulsion
Lumbar Puncture	Abnormal cerebrospinal fluid (CSF) profile with pleocytosis and/or elevated protein; WNV-IgM antibodies detected in CSF and/or serum samples

Therapeutic Management

Surgery	Tracheotomy if indicated for mechanical ventilation
Medications	Analgesics for pain; effectiveness of both ribavirin and interferon are in testing phase
General	Supportive at home for mild cases Hospitalization with severe cases: IV hydration; airway management, mechanical ventilation as indicated; prevention of secondary infection; rehabilitation for neurological impairment; report all suspected cases to local health authorities

W

Prevention/ Promotion	Mosquito control programs in community (surveillance, spraying, clean-up of breeding grounds)
	Report dead bird activity to local health authorities
	Prevent mosquito bites (apply DEET repellents and wear long sleeves, long pants, and socks when outdoors particularly at dawn, dusk, and early evening)
	Drain standing water and install screens at home
	Blood bank screening by all blood banks effective in 2003
Education	Individual, neighborhood, and community education on prevention tactics

Wilms' Tumor

A complex mixed embryonal cancer of the kidneys usually seen in children; cell types include blastema, epithelial, and stroma

Etiology and Incidence

The cause is unclear, but it involves hereditary or sporadic forms of gene mutation. The WT-1, WT-2, and WT-3 genes have been associated with the development of both the inherited and sporadic forms.

Incidence has been estimated at 8 cases per million in children less than 15 years of age in the United States. It occurs most frequently in children from age 2 to 5 and is the second most common abdominal malignancy in childhood.

Pathophysiology

The tumor probably arises from an undifferentiated cluster of primordial cells in the kidney that grow into a large solitary well-circumscribed mass composed of variable stromal, epithelial, and blastemic cells. The percentage of the cell types seems to be linked to tumor aggressiveness. Those that are predominantly epithelial are less aggressive, and tumors with a high percentage of blastemic cells are highly aggressive. Metastasis occurs via venous or lymphatic routes, and the most common sites are the abdomen and peritoneum, lungs, liver, bone, and opposite kidney.

Risk Factors

Genetic abnormalities
Familial tendencies
Presence of syndromes (WAGR, Denys-Drash, Beckwith-Wiedemann, Klippel-Trenaunay)
Paternal occupation (e.g., machinist, welder, auto mechanic)

Clinical Manifestations

Generally asymptomatic; usually present with a palpable nontender abdominal mass on one side; abdominal pain, fever, fatigue, weight loss, and hematuria may also be present.

W

Complications

Complications include metabolic alterations and respiratory distress from metastasis; development of secondary malignancies (e.g., leukemia, lymphoma, and soft tissue sarcoma). Prognosis varies with aggressiveness and histology of tumor and is 90% with stage I or II tumors and 60% overall.

Diagnostic Tests

Clinical evaluation, ultrasound, and CT scans to detect masses; biopsy for definitive diagnosis, identification of cell types and staging

Therapeutic Management

Surgery	Radical nephroureterectomy with inspection of contralateral kidney and regional lymph nodes; resection of involved abdominal structures (e.g., colon, diaphragm, vena cava); kidney transplant for bilateral renal involvement
Medications	IV combination chemotherapy regimens as an adjunct to surgery or for inoperable tumors; analgesics for pain
General	Radiotherapy for postoperative residual disease; preoperatively to decrease tumor size; for palliation; routine postoperative care for abdominal surgery; family support
Education	Education about disease, effects of chemotherapy and radiation; preoperative and postoperative instruction (e.g., *no preoperative palpation of abdomen*; turn, cough, deep breathing)
	Education about long-range precautions of living with one kidney (e.g., avoiding contact sports, prompt treatment of any genitourinary symptoms); information on community resources

Zollinger-Ellison Syndrome (ZES)

A syndrome marked by hypergastrinemia, gastric acid hypersecretion, and recurrent peptic ulcerations

Etiology and Incidence

The cause of ZES is excessive gastrin secretion produced by a non beta islet cell tumor in the pancreas. Most individuals have several tumors, and about 50% of the tumors are malignant. ZES often occurs in conjunction with other endocrine abnormalities, particularly of the parathyroids. About 60% of cases are seen in men. The peak incidence occurs between 30 and 50 years of age.

Pathophysiology

The high serum gastrin levels continuously stimulate hydrochloric acid (HCl) hypersecretion from parietal cells. This constant production of HCl overcomes the duodenum's ability to neutralize the acid, and peptic ulcers result. The gastrin stimulates intestinal motility and increases secretion of water and electrolytes, and the HCl increases peristalsis. Intestinal pH and fat breakdown are diminished, which inactivates pancreatic lipase and interferes with absorption of a variety of substances in the intestine. Gastrin also stimulates intrinsic factor secretion and interferes with vitamin B_{12} absorption.

Clinical Manifestations

The major manifestations stem from peptic ulcer formation and include burning epigastric pain (relieved by food) and coffee grounds or bloody emesis. Diarrhea, steatorrhea, foul-smelling stools, anorexia, and weight loss may also be present.

Complications

The mortality rate is high because of malignant metastasis to the liver, spleen, bone, skin, and peritoneum, and perforation and hemorrhage of the peptic ulcers.

Z

Diagnostic Tests

Serum Gastrin	Elevated to 500 pg/ml or higher
Endoscopy/ X-ray	To detect ulcers
Provocative Tests	Serum gastrin rises within 30 minutes of injection of secretin and calcium
Arteriography	To locate pancreatic tumors

Therapeutic Management

Surgery	Resection of tumor possible in 20% of cases; total gastrectomy or vagotomy when ulcers are not responding to medication
Medications	Proton pump inhibitors (omeprazole, lansoprazole) to reduce gastric acid; cytoprotectives (Sucralfate) to form a protective coating in the base of the ulcer; chemotherapy to treat malignant tumors; vitamin B_{12} injections, iron and calcium supplements
General	Fluid replacement with diarrhea; monitoring for dehydration and electrolyte imbalance; support to aid in adaptation; hospice care for terminal malignancy

Bibliography

Adenoviral-based SARS vaccine shows promise in macaques, Lancet 362:1895-1896, 2003.

Adkinson NF, et al: Middleton's Allergy: Principles and Practice, ed 6, St Louis, 2003, Mosby.

American Cancer Society: Cancer facts and figures, Atlanta, 2003, The Society (www.cancer.org).

American Psychological Association: Diagnostic and statistical manual of mental disorders, text revision (DSM-IV-TR), Washington, DC, 2000, The Association.

American Society of Internal Medicine, Guidelines for thyroid disease screening, Ann Int Med 129(2):141-158, 1998.

Armstrong D: Infectious diseases, St Louis, 1999, Mosby.

Beck AT, Weissman A, Lester D, Trexler L: The measurement of pessimism: the hopelessness scale, J Consult Clin Psych 42:861-865, 1974.

Beers MH, Berkow R: The Merck manual of diagnosis and therapy, ed 17-Internet, Rahway, NJ, 1999-2003, Merck.

Behrman RE: Nelson textbook of pediatrics, ed 17, Philadelphia, 2004, WB Saunders.

Bender K, Thompson FE: West Nile Virus: a growing challenge, Am J Nurs 103(6):32-39, 2003.

Bolduc C, Lui H: *Alopecia areata,* eMedicine.com, Inc. Sept 11, 2002.

Bonner LT: Pharmacologic treatments of dementia, Med Clin North Am 86(3):657-674, 2002.

Braunwald E, Zipes DP, Libby P: Heart disease: a textbook of cardiovascular medicine, ed 6, Philadelphia, 2001, WB Saunders.

Centers for Disease Control and Prevention, National Center for Health Statistics: Fast Stats A to Z, 2003 (www.cdc.gov/nchs/fastats.htm).

Centers for Disease Control and Prevention: Health Topics A-Z, 2003 (www.cdc.gov/nccdphp/index.htm).

Centers for Disease Control and Prevention: Severe Acute Respiratory Syndrome, 2003 (www.cdc.gov/ncidod/sars/).

Centers for Disease Control: West Nile Virus, 2003 (www.cdc.gov/ncidod/dvbid/westnile/index.htm).

Chatfield J: AAP guideline on treatment of children with ADHD, Am Fam Physician 65(4):726, 728, 2002.

Clinical Topic Tours: Primary Hyperparathyroidism, Apr 10, 2002 (http://home.mdconsult.com/das/news/body).

Clinical Topic Tours: Carpal Tunnel Syndrome, Sep 17, 2002 (http://home.mdconsult.com/das/news/body).

Clinical Topic Tours: Tuberculosis, Oct 9, 2002 (http://home.mdconsult.com/das/news/body).

Clinical Topic Tours: Carpal Tunnel Syndrome, Nov 6, 2002 (http://home.mdconsult.com/das/news/body).

Clinical Topic Tours: Anthrax, Dec 31, 2002 (http://home.mdconsult.com/das/news/body).

Clinical Topic Tours: Sudden Infant Death Syndrome, Mar 4, 2003 (http://home.mdconsult.com/das/news/body).

Clinical Topic Tours: Age-related Macular Degeneration, Apr 23, 2003 (http://home.mdconsult.com/das/ news/body).

Clinical Topic Tours: Lead Poisoning, April 30, 2003 (http://home.mdconsult.com/das/news/body).

Clinical Topic Tours: Multiple Sclerosis, Jul 17, 2003 (http://home.mdconsult.com/das/news/body).

Clinical Topic Tours: Severe Acute Respiratory Syndrome, July 24, 2003 (http://home.mdconsult.com/das/news/body).

Clinical Topic Tours: Intracranial Aneurysm, Aug 1, 2003 (http://home.mdconsult.com/das/news/body).

Clinical Topic Tours: Meningitis, Aug 7, 2003 (http://home.mdconsult.com/das/news/body).

Clinical Topic Tours: Traumatic Brain Injury, Aug 14, 2003 (http://home.mdconsult.com/das/news/body).

Clinical Topic Tours: West Nile Virus, Aug 28, 2003 (http://home.mdconsult.com/das/news/body).

Clinical Topic Tours: Peptic Ulcer Disease, Oct 24, 2003 (http://home.mdconsult.com/das/news/body).

Clinical Topic Tours: Tourette's Syndrome, Oct 30, 2003 (http://home.mdconsult.com/das/news/body).

Cotran RS: Robbins pathologic basis of disease, ed 6, Philadelphia, 1999, WB Saunders.

Dambro MR: Griffith's 5-minute consult, ed 11, Philadelphia, 2003, Lippincott, Williams and Wilkins.

DeLisa JA: Rehabilitation medicine: principles and practice, ed 3, Philadelphia, 1998, JB Lippincott.

DeVita VT, Hellman S, Rosenberg SA: Cancer: principles and practice of oncology, ed 6, Philadelphia, 2001, Lippincott, Williams and Wilkins.

Duthie EH, Katz PR: Practice of geriatrics, ed 3, Philadelphia, 1998, WB Saunders.

Fanaroff AA, Martin RJ: Neonatal-perinatal medicine: diseases of the fetus and infant, ed 7, St Louis, 2002, Mosby.

Feldman M, Friedman LS, Sleisenger MH: Sleisenger & Fordtran's gastrointestinal and liver disease, ed 7, Philadelphia, 2002, WB Saunders.

Ferri F: 2004 Ferri's clinical advisor instant diagnosis and treatment, 2004 ed, St Louis, 2004, Mosby.

Finelli L, Levine WC, Valentine J: Syphilis outbreak assessment, Sex Transm Dis 28(3):131-135, 2001.

FluMist, Med Immune Vaccines, Sept 2003
(www.flumist.com/con about.asp).

Fortinash KM, Holoday-Worret PA: Psychiatric mental health nursing, ed 3, St Louis, 2004, Mosby.

Gabbard GO: Treatments of psychiatric disorders, ed 3, Washington DC, 2001, American Psychiatric Press.

Gabbe SG, Niebyl JR, Simpson JL: Obstetrics—normal and problem pregnancies, ed 4, New York, 2002, Churchill Livingstone.

Garrison LE, Bausch DG: Hantavirus pulmonary syndrome: The essentials of an emerging disease, Clinical Insights: Mar 27, 2003.
(http://home.mdconsult.com/das/news/body).

Gershenson DM: Operative gynecology, ed 2, Philadelphia, 2003, WB Saunders.

Goetz CG: Textbook of clinical neurology, ed 2, Philadelphia, 2003, WB Saunders.

Goldman L, Bennett JC: Cecil textbook of medicine, ed 22, Philadelphia, 2004, WB Saunders.

Heart attack and angina statistics, American Heart Association, 2002
www.americanheart.org/presenter.jhtml/identifier=4591.

Hodgson BB, Kizior RJ: Saunders nursing drug handbook 2003, Philadelphia, 2003, WB Saunders.

Hordirisky M: Alopecia areata
http://npntserver.mcg.edu/html/alopecia/documents/AAconcept.html.

Jacobson JL: Psychiatric secrets, ed 2, St Louis, 2001, Hanley and Belfus.

Jenson HB: Pediatric infectious diseases: principles and practice, ed 2, Philadelphia, 2003, WB Saunders.

Kaufman D: Adult ADD and ADHD problems can be addressed by primary care physicians, This Week in Medicine, July 11, 2003, MD Consult.

Kaufman D: Ten year study finds first genes involved in psoriasis susceptibility, This Week in Medicine, Nov 13, 2003, MD Consult.

Kelley KJ, Walsh-Kelly CM: Latex allergy: A patient and health care system emergency. J Emer Nursing, Vol 24, No 6, December 1998, pp 539-545.

Kryger MH, Roth T, Dement WC: Principles and practice of sleep medicine, ed 3, Philadelphia, 2000, WB Saunders.

Latex allergy: a prevention guide, US Department of Health and Human Services, NIOSH Publication No. 98-113, February 25, 1999.

Lewis SM, Heitkemper MM, Dirksen SR: Medical surgical nursing, ed 6, St Louis, 2004, Mosby.

Lowdermilk DL, Perry SE: Maternity and women's health care, ed 8, St Louis, 2004, Mosby.

Mandell GL, Bennett JE, Dolin R: Mendell's principles and practice of infectious diseases, ed 5, Philadelphia, 2000, Churchill Livingstone.

Marx JA: Rosen's emergency medicine: concepts and clinical practice, ed 5, St Louis, 2002, Mosby.

Murphy-Lavoie H, Preston C: Cardiomyopathy, dilated, 2003, eMedicine.com, Inc (www.emedicine.com/emerg/topic80.htm).

National Center on Elder Abuse, US Department of Health and Human Services, Administration on Aging, Washington, DC, 1999.

National Clearinghouse on Child Abuse and Neglect Information, Washington, DC, 1999.

National Institutes of Health, National Cancer Institute, Cancer Statistics Branch, Bethesda, MD, 2003 (www.ninds.nih.gov).

National Institutes of Health, Spinal cord injury: emerging concepts, July 1, 2001 (www.ninds.nih.gov/health-and-medicine/pubs/sci-report.htm).

Noble J: Textbook of primary care medicine, ed 3, St Louis, 2001, Mosby.

Poutanan SM, Low DE: The diagnosis and clinical management of SARS, Clinical Insights: Oct 17, 2003 (http://home.mdconsult.com/das/news/body).

Rakel RE, Bope ET: Conn's current therapy 2003, ed 55, St Louis, 2003, Elsevier.

Raskind MA, Peskind ER: Alzheimer's disease and related disorders, Med Clin North Am 85(3):803-817, 2001.

Rosenthal M, Pentland B, Kreutzer JS: Rehabilitation of the adult and child with traumatic brain injury, ed 3, Philadelphia, 1999, FA Davis.

Rubin P: Clinical oncology, ed 8, Philadelphia, 2001, WB Saunders.

Rudolf AM, Rudolf CD: Rudolph's pediatrics, ed 21, New York, 2002, McGraw-Hill.

SARS deaths double with pollution; Environ Health, Nov 21, 2003 (www.ehjournal.net/content/2/1/15).

Schlossberg D: Current therapy of infectious disease, ed 2, St Louis. 2001, Mosby.

Schroeder BM: Obstructive sleep apnea syndrome in children, Am Fam Physician 66(7):1342-1345, 2002.

Soeken K, et al: The abuse assessment screen: a clinical instrument to measure frequency, severity, and perpetrator of abuse against women. In Campbell JC, editor: Empowering survivors of abuse: health care for battered women and their children, Newbury Park, California, 1998, Sage.

Stenchever MA: Comprehensive gynecology, ed 4, St Louis, 2001, Mosby.

Strickland GT: Hunter's tropical medicine and emerging infectious diseases, ed 8, Philadelphia, 2000, WB Saunders.

Stuart GW, Laraia MT: Principles and practice of psychiatric nursing, ed 7, St Louis, 2001, Mosby.

Technical Information Bulletin: Potential for allergy to natural rubber latex gloves and other latex products. US House Subcommittee on Oversight and Investigation Hearing of the Education and Workforce Committee, US Newswire release, March 25, 1999.

Tjaden P, Thoennes N: Full report of prevalence, incident, and consequences of violence against women, Washington DC, 2000, National Institute of Justice (NCJ-183781).

Vega C, Kwoon JV, Lavine SD: Intracranial aneurysms: current evidence and clinical practice, Am Fam Physician 66(4):601-608, 2002.

Volkmar FR, Cohen DJ: Autism: current concepts, Child and Adolescent Psychiatric Clinics of North America 3(1):43-52, 1994.

Weiss M: Advances in the treatment of adult ADHD—landmark findings in nonstimulant therapy, Therapeutic Focus, New York, 2003, Rogers Medical Intelligence Solutions.

Weiss M, Murray C: Assessment and management of attention-deficit hyperactivity disorder in adults, Canad Med Assoc J 168(6):715-722, 2003.

Wilcock GK: Mematine for the treatment of dementia, Lancet Neurol 2(8):503-505, 2003.

Wong DL, Hockenberry-Eaton M: Wong's essentials of pediatric nursing, ed 6, St Louis, 2001, Mosby.

Workowski KA, Levine WC: Sexually transmitted diseases treatment guidelines 2002, Morbidity and Mortality Weekly Report 51 (RR-6):1-128, 2002.

Index